CHILD PSYCHOPATHOLOGY:
Diagnostic Criteria and Clinical Assessment

CHILD PSYCHOPATHOLOGY:
Diagnostic Criteria and Clinical Assessment

Edited by

Stephen R. Hooper
University of North Carolina at Chapel Hill

George W. Hynd
University of Georgia
Medical College of Georgia

Richard E. Mattison
Washington University

LAWRENCE ERLBAUM ASSOCIATES, PUBLISHERS
1992 Hillsdale, New Jersey Hove and London

Lawrence Erlbaum Associates, Inc., Publishers
365 Broadway
Hillsale, New Jersey 07642

Library of Congress Cataloging-in-Publication Data

Child psychopathology : diagnostic criteria and clinical assessment / edited by Stephen R. Hooper, George W. Hynd, Richard E. Mattison.
p. cm.
Companion v. to: Developmental disorders.
Includes bibliographical references and indexes.
ISBN 0-8058-0328-9 (c)
1. Mental illness—Diagnosis. 2. Child psychopathology.
I. Hooper, Stephen R. II. Hynd, George W. III. Mattison, Richard E.
[DNLM: 1. Mental Disorders—diagnosis. 2. Mental Disorders—in adolescence. 3. Mental Disorders—in infancy & childhood. WS 350 C53785]
RJ503.5.C48 1992
618.92′89075—dc20
DNLM/DLC
for Library of Congress 91-6502
CIP

Printed in the United States of America
10 9 8 7 6 5 4 3 2 1

To my wonderful families—old and new. *S.R.H.*

To Ben, above all a good friend and valuable colleague who sensitized me to the many divergent issues related to childhood and adolescent psychopathology. *G.W.H.*

To my parents, my wife Christine, and my children Lara and Brian. *R.E.M.*

Contents

Foreword

It is indeed a pleasure to write the foreword to this text and its companion volume. One text focuses on child and adolescent psychopathology, and the other focuses on developmental disorders. Both volumes deal directly with evaluating the diagnostic criteria for these disorders, with a particular eye toward improving these criteria based on contemporary literature. Both volumes also focus on the clinical assessment of these disorders and related issues. Taken together, these two volumes should contribute to advancing the scientific study of child psychopathology and developmental disorders.

The scientific study of child and adolescent psychopathology does not have a very long history. Child psychiatry and the delivery of child mental health services grew up in the child guidance clinic movement of the 1920s. These clinics were designed for service delivery and operated on what became known as the "Holy Trinity Approach" to service delivery. That is, the child psychiatrist, who had no officially approved training in child and adolescent psychopathology, generally saw the child for play therapy; the psychologist saw the child for testing; and the social worker generally saw the family. These service delivery clinics did not promote research into the nature of the disorders that they were evaluating and treating and, as a result, there does not exist a serious body of scientific literature emanating from the large number of patients who were seen in those early years.

It wasn't until 1959 that the American Board of Psychiatry and Neurology accepted child and adolescent psychiatry as a legitimate board certifiable specialty. Concurrent with this, an increased number of research reports began to appear in the areas of childhood psychopathology and developmental disorders. But a perusal of the content of child psychology and child psychiatry journals of even the late 1950s and 1960s, as well as the content of programs of the annual meetings of the American Academy of Child and Adolescent Psychiatry of those years, also reveals that most of the publications and presentations were of the clinical and case report variety. Although these works were noteworthy, the scientific study of childhood psychopathology and developmental disorders was clearly in its infancy.

In addition to the few number of scientific endeavors in the field at that time, at least part of the difficulty with the early literature on child and adolescent psychopathology was the lack of a modern classification system. Relatedly, contemporary assessment approaches to the delineation of the clinical picture and possible subtypes of child and adolescent psychiatric disorders were not well developed or refined. Although the field has addressed these areas of concern over the past several decades, it is clear that many of these issues continue into the present. Some of these issues, along with a variety of classification approaches, are reviewed by Drs. Mattison and Hooper in chapter 1 of *Child Psychopathology* and by Dr. Hooper in chapter 1 of *Developmental Disorders*. Contemporary assessment approaches and related issues also are discussed more generally in each of these introductory chapters and in more detail in the subsequent chapters in each volume.

With respect to classification issues, Kraeplin's psychiatric taxonomy, published in 1883, ignored disorders of children. Nearly 70 years later, the Diagnostic and Statistical Manual of Mental Disorders,[1] the first version of the American Psychiatric Association's classification system, contained only three psychiatric diagnoses for children and adolescents: childhood schizophrenia, adjustment reaction of childhood, and childhood special symptom reactions. Subsequently, Anna Freud's Developmental Profile[2] was considered by many to be the first diagnostic classification system that dealt extensively with child psychiatric disorders. This system was based on psychoanalytic constructs and presented a variety of diagnostic categories. For example, these categories included variations of normality, transitory by-products of developmental strain, infantile neurosis, character disorders,

[1]American Psychiatric Association (1952). *Diagnostic and statistical manual of mental disorders*. Washington, DC: author.

[2]Freud, A. (1965). *Normality and pathology in childhood*. New York: International Universities Press.

retarded defective or nontypical personality, and disruptions of mental growth. Not surprisingly, the categories in Anna Freud's Developmental Profile or, for that matter, any of these early classification attempts, were not subjected to the type of empirical validity and reliability studies that one would demand today.

In 1966, the Group for the Advancement of Psychiatry (GAP) produced a detailed classification of child and adolescent psychiatric disorders.[3] This was revised in 1974 to reflect a system of categorical diagnoses that were primarily descriptive as opposed to the psychodynamic, etiological focus of Freud's Developmental Profile. Ten major categories comprised the GAP Classification System, but this system did not enjoy wide usage among researchers in child and adolescent psychopathology.

Two of the more widely used classification systems have been the International Classification of Diseases (ICD) and the Diagnostic and Statistical Manual of Mental Disorders (DSM). The various editions of the ICD, including the currently used ICD-9, have had greater or lesser numbers of categories dealing with child and adolescent psychopathology as the years have progressed. While the ICD-9 has a greater number of diagnoses than its predecessors, the draft of ICD-10 suggests that the section on child and adolescent psychopathology will be quite detailed and come somewhat closer to the DSM-III, DSM-III-R, and the proposed DSM-IV than its predecessors. Although it appears that the latest editions of the DSM and ICD correspond more closely to each other than in the past, there remains a number of differences between the two systems.

As noted earlier, the first version of the DSM was published in 1952 and contained only three diagnoses for children and adolescents. The second edition, DSM-II, was published by the American Psychiatric Association in 1968 and did include a section titled "Behavior Disorders of Childhood and Adolescence."[4] This section specifies six disorders: hyperkinetic reaction, overanxious reaction, withdrawing reaction, runaway reaction, unsocialized aggressive reaction, and group delinquent reaction. It was not until DSM-III was published in 1980, however, that a truly comprehensive classification of child and adolescent psychopathology was attempted in the DSM system.[5] The revised

[3]Group for the Advancement of Psychiatry. (1966). *Psychopathological disorders in childhood: Theoretical considerations and a proposed classification*. New York: Author.

[4]American Psychiatric Association (1968). *Diagnostic and statistical manual of mental disorders*. (2nd ed.). Washington, DC: Author.

[5]American Psychiatric Association (1980). *Diagnostic and statistical manual of mental disorders*. (3rd ed.). Washington, DC: Author.

version of this attempt, DSM-III-R, was published in 1987 and included some substantial changes.[6] Many of these specific changes have been reviewed elsewhere (e.g., Cantwell & Baker, 1988)[7] and are reflected in nearly all of the chapters contained within these two volumes. Some of these changes were considered positive, but some of them were not. Furthermore, many of the changes were made with a lack of empirical support. A major strength of these two volumes is that all of the contributors were encouraged to suggest specific changes in diagnostic criteria for a selected disorder, but they were encouraged to do this based on the available scientific literature for that disorder. Perhaps these efforts will contribute to improving the scientific basis for many of the childhood disorders and their associated diagnostic criteria.

It is highly likely that the DSM and ICD, and their future versions (i.e., DSM-IV and ICD-10), will be the two major systems that will set the tone for the future with regard to official classification attempts; however, both systems consist of categories of psychiatric disorders that were initially derived from clinical experience. Other approaches to the classification of child and adolescent disorders, such as the dimensional classification approach, have been developed in an attempt to address this issue. The dimensional classification approach is based on numerical scores obtained with specific behavioral assessment tools. Statistical procedures, such as factor analysis, are used to determine the tendency of specific items of behavior to co-occur. As dimensions of behavior, or factors, are identified by these statistical procedures, individuals can be classified into mutually exclusive groups using statistical clustering techniques. Systematic comparative studies have suggested that the clinical syndromes that arise from dimensional classification correspond somewhat to the clinically derived syndromes, but there is less than a perfect correspondence. More specifically, there are ICD and DSM syndromes that are not exactly reproduced in these dimensional systems, and, conversely, the reverse also is true.

Proponents of the dimensional approach suggest that because dimensional classification is empirically derived, the groups that result from this approach are more reliable, valid, and clinically homogeneous. Further, they assert that the diagnoses tend to be tied to the assessment process more directly than those produced in the DSM and ICD systems. However, there are criticisms of the dimensional approach as well. In particular, the dimensions of behavior created by the

---

[6]American Psychiatric Association (1987). *Diagnostic and statistical manual of mental disorders.* (3rd ed., rev.). Washington, DC: Author.

statistical procedures may not turn out to be either clinically or theoretically meaningful. In the future, it is likely that the dimensional and categorical approaches may be combined and, consequently, result in a more useful classification system than is currently in existence. In fact, some of the categorically defined disorders in the DSM and ICD systems already may have dimensional aspects to them. For example, the developmental learning disorders and mental retardation do have dimensional components to their classification (e.g., slow and/or disrupted learning), but the exact nature of this relationship requires further investigation.

The chapters in these two volumes reflect the major DSM types of childhood and adolescent psychopathology that are currently the focus of intense study. These include the disruptive behavior disorders (i.e., conduct disorder, attention deficit-hyperactivity disorder), schizophrenia, major depression, some of the anxiety disorders, some of the eating disorders, gender disorders, tic disorders, elimination disorders, elective mutism, mental retardation, autism, developmental learning disorders, developmental language and speech disorders, and motor skill disorders. Each chapter presents a thorough review of the ontogeny of each diagnosis and its scientific status (i.e., reliability and validity) according to contemporary literature. Suggestions are proposed for possible changes in diagnostic criteria based on this literature. It is hoped that such a detailed review of each of these disorders will contribute to the processes of revising and generating future versions of the ICD and DSM and, ultimately, result in improved classifications systems (e.g., ICD-10 and DSM-IV).

The issues for each of the disorders discussed in these two volumes differ slightly with regard to their place in the nosological system. For the disruptive behavior disorders, there is the question of whether this overall rubric should be retained for attention deficit-hyperactivity disorder, conduct disorder, and oppositional defiant disorder. For example, the role and place of attention deficit disorder without hyperactivity need to be explicated further, and its association with other disorders should receive more intense study as well. The relationship of oppositional defiant disorder to conduct disorder also needs to be delineated, particularly from a developmental perspective. Subtyping and severity ratings of all of the disruptive disorders need to be extensively studied and more fully described.

Related questions can be asserted for other disorders as well. For example, with schizophrenia there is the problem of defining a disorder based primarily on its manifestations in adulthood and late adolescence and then extending it downward to prepubertal children. Russell challenges this notion in his chapter in *Child Psychopathology* and indicates that the literature on such children is sparse. Whether these children present with the same phenomonologic picture as adults or whether there is a "pre-schizophrenic" picture in children which is phenomonologically different that eventually melds into the adult picture needs to be explored further.

Similar questions exist with regard to the mood disorders. The nosologic status of mood disorders in childhood and adolescence versus their adult counterparts needs further exploration. Systematic studies have suggested that children and adolescents do present with clinical pictures very similar to those seen in adults with mood disorders. But whether there are meaningful modifications of the diagnostic criteria that should be made in preschool children, grade school children, and adolescents remains a subject for scientific inquiry.

The relationship between childhood and adult onset anxiety disorders also needs to be explored further. For example, some of the anxiety disorders regularly begin in childhood and are listed under the category of anxiety disorders of childhood and adolescence. Others, such as obsessive-compulsive disorder, which often do occur for the first time in childhood and adolescence are listed with other anxiety disorders. Again, the question of whether there are meaningful modifications of the clinical picture that occur as a function of age and developmental stage remains to be studied.

For the eating disorders, some of the issues include whether anorexia nervosa should be subtyped according to the presence or absence of bulimic symptoms, and whether there should be a separate category of binge eating disorder that might be somewhat different from the current definition of bulimia. The relationship of the eating disorders of infancy and early childhood to the later developing eating disorders also remains an area for future research efforts. With the gender identity disorders, one of the major questions revolves around whether these disorders are on a continuum. Some investigators might suggest that the clinical separations, such as those found in the DSM-III and DSM-III-R, are rather arbitrary in nature and lack a scientific base. The clinical literature also suggests that there may be gender identity disorders that are secondary to documented Axis III conditions. Many of these issues are addressed in the chapters contained in *Child Psychopathology*.

A wide array of similar concerns can be raised with respect to the developmental disorders. For example, mental retardation could be primary in nature, or it could be secondary to a known Axis III condition. One of the classification systems currently in use (e.g., DSM-III-R) specifies severity to be based largely on IQ measures, although the diagnosis and its severity should be made on the basis of the presence of both intellectual and adaptive behavior deficiencies. Only the American Association of Mental Retardation (AAMR) classification system takes into account the level of adaptive behavior impairment with regard to severity. The AAMR classification also is much more detailed than the DSM-III-R system, although the correspondence between the two is closer than ever before. Reschly addresses many of these issues in his chapter on this topic in *Developmental Disorders*.

The pervasive developmental disorder category was created for DSM-III-R. At that time, two major subtypes were proposed: classical infantile autism and a residual category of pervasive developmental disorder childhood onset. However, recent literature suggests that conditions such as Aspergers Syndrome, Retts' Syndrome, and disintegrative disorder of childhood all may be possible inclusions under the rubric of pervasive developmental disorder. Further confusion was created in this general category of disorders with revision of the DSM-III. Specifically, the differences between the diagnostic criteria for the more classical infantile autism in the DSM-III and DSM-III-R have contributed to the likelihood of clinicians and researchers obtaining significantly different groups of children for examination and study. This undoubtedly has hindered the comparison of the research findings on this population. Future classification systems need to specify criteria that will correctly include and exclude those children who represent the more classical autistic picture. The similarities and differences of all of the pervasive developmental disorders also will require intensive study.

The developmental learning, language and speech, and motor skill disorders are treated rather simply in the DSM classification schemes, and it is not coincidence that most of the chapters in *Developmental Disorders* advocate for significant changes in diagnostic criteria for these disorders. The chapters in *Developmental Disorders* discuss in much more detail this available literature. Possible underlying etiologic factors that may affect some of these disorders also are presented. Whether these hypothesized underlying problems should be part of the core criteria is an issue for further discussion, but it is clear that the criteria associated with these disorders in the DSM system should be expanded and/or totally revised.

For any classification system of child and adolescent phenomenon to be useful, it must meet minimal standards of reliability and validity, show adequate coverage, observability, and age sensitivity, and maintain clinical feasibility (Cantwell & Baker, 1988).[7] None of the current

---

[7]Cantwell, D. P., & Baker, L. (1988). Issues in the classification of child and adolescent psychopathology. *Journal of the American Academy of Child and Adolescent Psychiatry*, *27*, 521–533.

systems is perfect in any of these areas. Future classification systems, if they are going to advance the field, must reflect increasingly sophisticated knowledge about the disorders of childhood and adolescence. For this to occur, much more research is needed in a variety of areas. For example, one area that should receive intense attention is in the external validation of the various categories and possible subtypes of childhood and adolescent psychopathology. Research on the assessment process itself also is sorely needed, especially in the very sticky aspect of combining data from a variety of sources (e.g., parents, teachers, significant others, and the children themselves) into a diagnostic statement. In this regard, sophisticated techniques of assessment are emerging almost on a yearly basis, and this should contribute to refining diagnostic criteria and associated characteristics of these disorders. Although these efforts in assessment and external validation should contribute to increasing the reliability, validity, and clinical utility of the classification systems, there is a danger that these clinical assessment procedures and techniques (e.g., structured interviews, behavioral rating scales) will be so tightly bound to specific classification systems that they will result in a reification of those systems and the disorders that they delineate.

Although the study of child psychopathology and developmental disorders has shown considerable growth over the past several decades, it is clear that there are a large number of issues that remain to be addressed and/or resolved. These issues not withstanding, these two volumes contribute to advancing our understanding of child psychopathology and developmental disorders, and they produce an empirical basis upon which one can build for the future.

—Dennis P. Cantwell, MD.
—Joseph Campbell Professor of Child Psychiatry
University of California, Los Angeles

Preface

In what some would perhaps consider an historical piece of writing, Smoller (1985) wrote a satirical article about the etiology and treatment of childhood. In his treatise, Smoller noted that "Childhood is a syndrome which has only recently begun to receive serious attention from clinicians" (p. 3). With this conjecture, Smoller acknowledged the "growing acceptance of childhood as a distinct phenomenon" and its pending inclusion in the upcoming DSM-IV. Although the focus of this work was on the origins and treatments of this "syndrome," there was significant discussion regarding its evolution, core clinical components, associated features, and issues surrounding its assessment and diagnosis.

Although tongue-in-cheek, Smoller's work certainly highlighted several of the most important aspects of any childhood diagnosis (e.g., core components, associated features). Furthermore, although the diagnosis of "childhood" has not really captured the clinical spotlight, the study and classification of childhood developmental and psychiatric disorders truly has progressed in the past two decades. This is particularly illustrated by the fact that the DSM-I and DSM-II devoted precious little space and attention to the conceptualization of psychiatric disorders in children and adolescents, whereas more recent versions of the DSM (DSM-III and DSM-III–R) have devoted a significant amount of energy and space to these diagnostic considerations. A similar pattern can be seen in the evolution of the International Classification of Diseases (ICD) system.

Despite this increased interest in developmental and psychiatric disorders, with the evolution of how one conceives of childhood and adolescent disorders comes the potential for confusion among practicing clinicians and researchers. This confusion is created by issues related to: (a) how to diagnose psychopathology, (b) what correspondence exists between currently employed criteria and research findings with children and adolescents, (c) how the criteria were developed, with particular concerns directed toward how decisions were made to retain or eliminate specific criteria for inclusion, and (d) what particular assessment strategies or models would be most useful in arriving at a specific diagnosis. To address these issues, there have been a number of texts published on the general topic of childhood and adolescent psychopathology (e.g., Quay & Werry, 1986; Rutter & Hersov, 1985; Rutter, Tuma, & Lann, 1988; Solnit, Cohen, & Schowalter, 1986), and there have been single volumes devoted to selected child psychiatric and developmental disorders such as Attention Deficit Disorder (Barkley, 1981), affective disorders (Cantwell & Carlson, 1983), anxiety disorders (Gittelman, 1986), eating disorders (Garner, 1988), autism and pervasive developmental disorders (Cohen, Donnellan, & Paul, 1987), dyslexia (Hynd & Cohen, 1983), and speech and language disorders (Cantwell & Baker, 1987). Although the current volume was designed to complement these works, it also was designed to address the diagnostic criteria and clinical assessment of childhood and adolescent psychiatric disorders from a more critical perspective. In particular, this text was designed to review and critique the diagnostic criteria for most of the major psychiatric disorders that are used to describe children and adolescents in the DSM-III-R. As such, it is hoped that the data-based nature of these chapters will provide some guidance for the continued evolution of classification for children and adolescents (i.e., DSM-IV), particularly those with psychiatric disorders.

This text and its companion volume, *Developmental Disorders*, were designed to provide a critical evaluation of literature with respect to the diagnostic criteria set forth for selected child and adolescent diagnoses. The major goal of these volumes is to provide contemporary diagnostic criteria and assessment guidelines for the clinician and researcher that are based on the scientific literature in each clinical domain. Consequently, this volume and its companion were written for professionals and graduate students in the fields of clinical child psychology, child psychiatry, pediatrics, pediatric psychology, school psychology, social work, special education, and other child mental health specialties. Each chapter contains a discussion of the historical background of the diagnosis; definitional issues; a critical, selective review of the literature addressing the diagnosis in question; proposed changes in the diagnostic criteria based on the available literature; and proposed assessment models and methods based on the designated criteria. Given the scientific basis for much of this discussion of diagnostic criteria, many of these chapters also should serve to provide researchers in a wide variety of fields with practical guidelines.

This volume contains 13 chapters and, although several other key diagnoses are presented, it is organized largely around the Disorders Usually First Evident in Infancy, Childhood, or Adolescence identified in the current DSM-III-R classification system. Chapter 1 (Mattison & Hooper) reviews the modern classification of these disorders. This introductory chapter also discusses contemporary efforts in the classification of these disorders and related diagnostic assessment technology. Chapters 2 (Russell) and 3 (Newman & Garfinkel) deal with disorders that have recently been applied to children and adolescents. Chapters 4 (Routh & Daugherty) and 5 (Guevremont & Barkley) discuss the primary disruptive behavior disorders that occur in childhood and adolescence. Chapter 6 (Mattison) addresses the diagnostic criteria and assessment of anxiety disorders in children, and chapters 7 (Mayes) and 8 (Garner, Shafer, & Rosen) deal with specific eating disorders seen in this population. Gender Disorders (Zucker), Tic Disorders (Towbin, Riddle, Leckman, & Cohen), Elimination Disorders (MacLean & Brayden), and Elective Mutism (Hooper & Linz) are presented in chapters 9, 10, 11, and 12, respectively. The volume concludes with an Epilogue highlighting the major changes suggested by the authors. Although it is not a comprehensive listing of topics, this volume attempts to provide specific suggestions for clinicians and researchers for the major psychiatric diagnoses typically used with children and adolescents. As such, it is hoped that these chapters will contribute to the ongoing evolution and refinement of an accurate and clinically useful classification system for children and adolescents with psychiatric disorders.

ACKNOWLEDGMENTS

In addition to the large number of expert contributors, without whom this project would never have been possible, we would like to extend our sincere gratitude to several important individuals. We would like to thank Teresa Buckner and Cheryl Hunter at the Clinical Center for the Study of Development and Learning for their expert and timely assistance on a number of endeavors related to this project. Our sincere appreciation also goes out to Carolyn Anderson, Barb Kaylor, and Ann Moore at the Hershey Medical Center, and to Dora Ervin at the University of Georgia for their assistance in selected aspects of manuscript preparation. Finally, although we could not have completed this project without considerable assistance and support, any shortcomings of this volume remain our own doing.

Stephen R. Hooper
George W. Hynd
Richard E. Mattison

REFERENCES

Barkley, R. A. (1981). *Hyperactive children. A handbook for diagnosis and treatment.* New York: Guilford Press.

Cantwell, D., & Baker, L. (1987). *Developmental speech and language disorders.* New York: Guilford Press.

Cantwell, D., & Carlson, G. (1983). *Affective disorders in childhood and adolescence: An update.* New York: Spectrum.

Cohen, D. J., Donnellan, A. M., & Paul, R. (Eds.). (1987). *Handbook of autism and pervasive developmental disorders.* New York: Wiley.

Garner, D. M. (1988). *Diagnostic issues in anorexia nervosa and bulimia nervosa.* New York: Brunner/Mazel.

Gittleman, R. (Ed.). (1986). *Anxiety disorders of childhood.* New York: Guilford.

Hynd, G. W., & Cohen, M. (1983). *Dyslexia: Neuropsychological theory, research, and clinical differentiation.* New York: Grune and Stratton.

Quay, H. C., & Werry, J. S. (Eds.) (1986). *Psychopathological disorders of childhood* (3rd ed.). Somerset, NJ: Wiley.

Rutter, M., & Hersov, L. (Eds.). (1985). *Child and adolescent psychiatry. Modern approaches* (2nd ed.). Boston: Blackwell Scientific Publication.

Rutter, M., Tuma, A. H., & Lann, I. S. (Eds.). (1988) *Assessment and diagnosis in child psychopathology* New York: Guilford Press.

Smoller, J. W. (1985). The etiology and treatment of childhood. *Journal of Polymorphous Perversity, 2,* 3–7.

Solnit, A. J., Cohen, D. J., & Schowalter, J. E. (Eds.). (1986). *Psychiatry, Volume 6: Child psychiatry.* New York: Basic Books.

CHAPTER 1

The History of Modern Classification of Child and Adolescent Psychiatric Disorders: An Overview

Richard E. Mattison
Washington University School of Medicine

Stephen R. Hooper
University of North Carolina School of Medicine

Over the past two decades, the classification of childhood and adolescent psychopathology has evolved as a result of increasing attention devoted to issues surrounding the diagnostic criteria pertinent to specific disorders. In particular, the scientific parameters of classification systems have been emphasized, and the development of objective instrumentation has improved the diagnostic capabilities of clinicians and researchers. This volume and its companion (*Developmental Disorders*) are devoted to presenting expert appraisals of the scientific merits of the child and adolescent diagnostic categories described in the DSM-III (American Psychiatric Association, 1980) and in the DSM-III-R (American Psychiatric Association, 1987), with a particular eye toward proposing refinements in the current diagnostic criteria based on the available empirical literature.

This chapter serves as a brief introduction to the history of modern classification of childhood and adolescent psychopathology, with primary emphasis devoted to efforts in the United States. In addition, several of the major scientific parameters crucial to developing a psychiatric nosology are reviewed. Finally, an overview of the current empirical assessment methodology that is available for diagnostic evaluations is provided.

HISTORY OF MODERN CLASSIFICATION

DSM-II

The more recent history for classification of child and adolescent psychopathology in the United States began with the *Diagnostic and Statistical Manual of Mental Disorders* (DSM-II; American Psychiatric Association, 1968). The earlier DSM-I (American Psychiatric Association, 1952) contained no specific section for childhood or adolescent diagnostic categories, although it did have a variety of diagnoses that likely were used for child and adolescent populations (e.g., adjustment reaction of childhood, mental deficiency, special symptom reaction: learning disturbance). Following the development of the DSM-I, classification schemes for childhood disorders were proposed nationally by the Group for the Advancement of Psychiatry (1966) and internationally through the work of Rutter and his colleagues for the World Health Organization (WHO, 1965). These events culminated in the development of the DSM-II in 1968.

Unlike the DSM-I, the DSM-II contained a section entitled Behavior Disorders of Childhood and Adolescence, which enumerated six specific categories: hyperkinetic reaction, withdrawing reaction, overanxious reaction, runaway reaction, unsocialized aggressive reaction, and group delinquent reaction. This section also included a diagnosis termed "other reaction of childhood," which was designed to include children showing serious behavioral disorders not listed in the previous categories. Each diagnosis was described in one paragraph listing typical symptoms and, for selective categories (e.g., unsocialized aggressive reaction), included information to guide differential diagnosis. In addition, adjustment reactions of infancy, childhood, or adolescence were specific diagnoses that could be coded, along with childhood schizophrenia, with each of these diagnoses having a brief description of distinguishing symptoms. A section of special symptoms included potential child and adolescent diagnoses such as enuresis, feeding disturbance, and specific learning disturbance, but none of these diagnoses had accompanying definitions or related information. Lastly, digits could be added to the diagnostic codes to indicate severity of the dysfunction (i.e., mild, moderate, and severe).

Although the inclusion of these diagnoses was a noteworthy improvement over DSM-I, these child and adolescent diagnostic categories received limited scientific scrutiny, because their brief descriptions and lack of operational criteria did not lend the diagnoses to proper investigation. Indeed, the reliability of the childhood diagnoses of

DSM-II were not investigated until after the DSM-III appeared (Mattison, Cantwell, Russell, & Will, 1979). Furthermore, the state-of-the-art with respect to diagnostic assessment tools and methodology was not well interrelated to DSM-II classification—nor to any classification, for that matter.

DSM-III

The childhood section of DSM-II evolved into the DSM-III section entitled Disorders Usually Evident in Infancy, Childhood, or Adolescence. Based on the limited coverage of child and adolescent psychiatric disorders provided by the DSM-II, the number of possible diagnoses for children and adolescents expanded to 32 categories (excluding atypical diagnoses). Furthermore, the DSM-III featured a multiaxial format, including five specific developmental disorders that could be coded on Axis II.

In addition to the increased number of diagnoses available to child practitioners, the meager information provided to guide diagnosis in DSM-II was enhanced in DSM-III by the inclusion of considerable descriptive information for each diagnosis. For example, specific diagnostic criteria were provided for each category. In addition, standard information was provided for each diagnosis. This included information related to associated features, age at onset, course, impairment, complications, predisposing factors, prevalence, sex ratio, and familial pattern. A discussion of differential diagnosis was included for each diagnostic category. Finally, an appendix of decision trees was proposed, and a glossary of technical terms was also included.

As a consequence of the more objective and descriptive nature of the DSM-III, the number of scientific investigations of this psychiatric classification system increased. For example, the DSM-III itself included an appendix of the results for two field trials testing the interrater reliability for 126 cases selected by pairs of raters. Subsequently, other research teams also focused on general reliability studies of the childhood and adolescent categories contained in DSM-III (Mattison et al., 1979; Mezzich, Mezzich, & Coffman, 1985; Strober, Green, & Carlson, 1981; Werry, Methven, Fitzpatrick, & Dixon, 1983). A host of reliability and validity studies also surfaced with respect to specific diagnoses, and these are presented in the individual chapters in this volume.

Simultaneously, instrumentation also was developed to take advantage of the improved objectivity of the DSM-III. In particular, structured interviews were created that utilized the operational criteria of the child diagnostic categories in providing a scope and sequence for interviewers. Measurement technology for specific categories also was improved, thus lending greater clarity to the operational criteria listed in the DSM-III.

Although many criticisms were levied against the DSM-III diagnoses and its multiaxial system on its introduction to the field (e.g., Rutter & Shaffer, 1980), including its basis in the medical model (Achenbach, 1980) and the high number of unvalidated diagnostic categories (Achenbach, 1980; Rutter & Shaffer, 1980; Werry, 1985), the attempt at providing an empirical foundation for many of the diagnoses in the DSM-III set the stage for further development of a useful nosology for child psychiatry. Mezzich and Mezzich (1987) listed 10 reasons for the general acceptance of the DSM-III system in the field. These included:

1. its multiaxial framework for conceptualizing problem behaviors;
2. an increased number of child and adolescent diagnoses;
3. greater specification of criteria for each diagnosis;
4. its inclusion of additional descriptive information along with specific criteria;
5. its phenomenological approach;
6. its recognition of developmental parameters in conceptualizing childhood disorders;
7. its attempt to recognize the impact of stress (i.e., Axis IV) and adaptive functioning (i.e., Axis V);
8. the coding of psychosocial stressors;
9. its recognition of continuity of selected disorders into adulthood; and
10. its ability to define a problem without employing a specific psychiatric label.

DSM-III-R

Published 7 years after the third edition, the DSM-III-R (American Psychiatric Association, 1987) sought to refine the improvements noted in the preceding edition to a greater degree by incorporating the interim advancements in the field. Within the section on child and adolescent disorders, some diagnostic criteria and standard clinical information were updated. Perhaps the most important revisions included the combining of the DSM-III attention deficit disorders and conduct disorders under the major DSM-III-R section of Disruptive Behavior Disorders, and the inclusion of mental retardation and pervasive developmental diagnoses on Axis II.

Efforts also were made to increase the objectivity of the DSM-III-R. For example, field trials were conducted for certain child diagnoses (e.g., autism) to determine the optimal number of items required to satisfy specific diagnostic criteria and thereby improve sensitivity and specificity. Severity ratings for Axis IV (Psychosocial Stressors) and Axis V (Global Assessment of Functioning) were also improved and more distinctly defined.

The scientific investigations of the DSM-III-R child and adolescent diagnostic categories should prove more numerous and rigorous than the study of DSM-III. As the DSM classification system has evolved in its empirical underpinnings, so has the clarity of specific diagnostic entities. A chronology and evolution of selected child and adolescent psychiatric diagnoses pertinent to this volume are presented in Table 1.1, which shows the ebb and flow of diagnostic trends with respect to specific terminology up through the current DSM-III-R. These changes are important to note, particularly given the relatively short history of the DSM classification system, in that the system is dynamic and amenable to change in accordance with current research and clinical practice. Along with the evolution of the diagnoses and the dynamic nature of the DSM nosology, the sophistication of diagnostic methodology and instrumentation has improved and become more integrated with DSM-III-R criteria, thus making it somewhat easier to research proposed psychiatric taxonomies. Despite its multitude of problems, the DSM-III system and the more recent version of this classification system (i.e., DSM-III-R) represent "a landmark in the development of a psychiatric classification system" (Mezzich & Mezzich, 1987, p. 49).

ICD-9

The International Classification of Diseases, 9th revision (ICD-9; WHO, 1978) and its comparison to the DSM-III have been extensively reviewed (Gould, Rutter, Shaffer, & Sturge, 1988; Quay, 1986; Werry, 1985). Overall, this more conservative international taxonomy has fewer axes, and the selection of a proper diagnostic category is assisted by a glossary rather than specific diagnostic criteria. Whereas the ICD-9 shares some childhood diagnoses in common with the DSM-III, there are some important differences between these two classification systems. For example, the DSM-III-R contains attention deficit-hyperactivity disorder while the comparable major diagnosis in ICD-9 is hyperkinetic syndrome of childhood, with more specific diagnostic categories being listed (e.g., simple disturbance of activity and attention, hyperkinesis with developmental delay, and hyperkinetic con-

TABLE 1.1
A Chronology and Evolution of Selected Child and Adolescent Psychiatric Disorders

DSM-I (1952)	*DSM-II (1968)*
Schizophrenia	
Hebephrenic →	Hebephrenic →
Catatonic →	Catatonic →
Paranoid →	Paranoid →
Chronic undifferentiated →	Chronic undifferentiated →
Mood disorders	
Depressive reaction →	Depressive neurosis →
Depressive reaction →	Depressive neurosis →
—— →	—— →
Manic-depressive reaction, manic type →	Manic-depressive illness, manic type →
Manic-depressive reaction, depressed type →	Manic-depressive illness, depressed type →
Manic-depressive reaction, other →	Manic-depressive illness, circular type →
—— →	—— →
Disruptive-behavior disorders	
—— →	Unsocialized aggressive reaction of childhood (or adolescence) →
—— →	Runaway reaction of childhood (or adolescence) →
—— →	Group delinquent reaction of childhood (or adolescence) →
—— →	Hyperkinetic reaction of childhood (or adolescence) →
Anxiety disorders of childhood or adolescence	
Phobic reaction →	[Phobic neurosis → Withdrawing reaction of childhood (or adolescence) → Overanxious reaction of childhood →]

DSM-III (1980)	DSM-III-R (1987)
Disorganized →	Disorganized
Catatonic →	Catatonic
Paranoid →	Paranoid
Undifferentiated →	Undifferentiated
Major depression →	Major depression
Dysthymic disorder →	Dysthymia
Atypical depression →	Depressive disorder NOS
Bipolar disorder, manic →	Bipolar disorder, manic
Bipolar disorder, depressed →	Bipolar disorder, depressed
Bipolar disorder, mixed →	Bipolar disorder, mixed
Atypical bipolar disorder →	Bipolar disorder NOS
Conduct-disorder-undersocialized, aggressive →	Conduct-disorder-isolated, aggressive type
Conduct-disorder-undersocialized, nonagressive →	———
Conduct-disorder-socialized, aggressive →	———
Conduct-disorder-socialized, nonagressive →	Conduct-disorder, group type
Conduct-disorder-atypical →	Conduct-disorder-undifferentiated
ADD with hyperactivity →	Attention-deficit-hyperactivity
ADD without hyperactivity →	Undifferentiated ADD
ADD residual type	ADHD (residual state)
Separation anxiety →	Separation anxiety
Avoidant disorder of childhood or adolescence →	Avoidant disorder of childhood or adolescence
Overanxious disorder →	Overanxious disorder

(Continued)

TABLE 1.1
(Continued)

DSM-I (1952)		*DSM-II (1968)*	
Eating disorders			
Other special symptom reaction	→	Feeding disturbance	→
Gender identity disorders			
Sexual deviation	→	Unspecified sexual deviation	→
Tic disorders			
Other special symptom reaction	→	Tic	→
Elimination disorders			
Enuresis	→	Enuresis	→
Other special symptom reaction	→	Encopresis	
Other disorders of infancy, childhood or adolescence			
———	→	Other reaction of childhood (or adolescence)	→

Note. This information was abstracted from *DSM-II* (APA, 1968), *DSM-III* (APA, 1980), and *DSM-III-R* (APA, 1987).

duct disorder). Despite these differences, however, reliability studies of the two systems have yielded similar results (Quay, 1986). Although Rutter (1988) noted the increasing comparability between these two systems, largely due to their empirical evolution, the upcoming ICD-10 will likely continue to manifest major differences in diagnostic categories from the DSM-III-R and the DSM-IV (Cantwell & Baker, 1988).

Dimensional Classification

In contrast to the categorical approach of the DSM classification systems, this alternative approach to psychiatric classification utilizes

DSM-III (1980)	DSM-III-R (1987)
Anorexia nervosa →	Anorexia nervosa
Bulimia →	Bulimia nervosa
Pica →	Pica
Rumination disorder of infancy →	Rumination disorder of infancy
Atypical eating disorder →	Eating disorder NOS
Gender identity disorder of childhood →	Gender identity disorder AANT Gender identity disorder of childhood
Atypical gender identity disorder →	Gender identity disorder NOS
Transient tic disorder →	Transient tic disorder
Chronic motor tic disorder →	Chronic motor or vocal tic disorder
Tourette's disorder →	Tourette's disorder
Atypical tic disorder →	Tic disorders NOS
Atypical stereotyped movement disorder →	Stereotypy/habit disorders
Functional enuresis →	Functional enuresis
Functional encopresis →	Functional encopresis
Elective mutism →	Elective mutism

empirically derived dimensions of childhood and adolescent psychopathology (i.e., homogeneous groups of behaviors that are statistically intercorrelated). A diagnostic profile can then be determined by plotting the child's score for each dimension in relation to normative data. Although this conceptualization of psychopathology has been present for over four decades (Hewitt & Jenkins, 1946), the predominant taxonomies representing this approach have been developed by Achenbach and Edelbrock (1983, 1986) and by Quay and Peterson (1983). Millon (1981) also presented an empirically based dimensional approach for the classification of personality disorders.

One major characteristic of dimensional classification systems is strong reliability, which tends to be a by-product of the statistical derivation of the dimensions. Furthermore, similar dimensions are proving constant among different raters, with different populations of children and adolescents, and with different instruments (Achenbach & Edelbrock, 1978). Quay (1986) recently summarized these major dimensions to include: undersocialized aggressive conduct disorder, socialized aggressive conduct disorder, attention deficit disorder, and anxiety-withdrawal-dysphoria. Quay also considered other dimensions as promising, but in need of additional confirmation. These included schizoid-unresponsive, social ineptness, psychotic disorder, and motor overactivity. Achenbach (Achenbach, Conners, & Quay, 1985) already proposed more narrow dimensions.

Both Achenbach (1980) and Quay (1986) already noted similarities between established dimensions and some DSM-III childhood categories. At the same time, both researchers noted that several DSM-III child diagnoses are not confirmed by dimensional studies. Studies of the convergence of DSM-III categories and comparable dimensions have been few thus far. One notable report (Edelbrock & Costello, 1988), however, investigated relationships between scales of the parent Child Behavior Checklist (CBCL; Achenbach & Edelbrock, 1983) and the DSM-III diagnoses determined by diagnostic algorithms from parent interviews with the Diagnostic Interview Schedule for Children–Parent Version (DISC-P; Edelbrock & Costello, 1987). The strongest linear relationships were obtained between the hyperactive, delinquent, and depressed scales of the CBCL and the DSM-III diagnoses of attention deficit disorder, conduct disorder, and depression/dysthymia, respectively. Specifically, the higher the obtained score on the specific scale of the CBCL, the more probable the comparable diagnosis would be applied. Also, the more diagnostic criteria a child fulfilled for a specific DSM-III diagnosis, the more likely that a high *T* score would be generated on the comparable scale. Such studies will prove invaluable for the development of both types of classification approaches.

Similar to the DSM-III and the DSM-III-R, however, dimensional classification has its own unique set of problems that must be addressed (Achenbach, 1985). For example, the relevance of established dimensions to important criteria (e.g., etiology, course, treatment response, etc.) requires much additional study. Also, the meaningful integration of dimensional information from different sources must be developed, as it appears that agreement among different observers is not good (Achenbach, McConaughy, & Howell, 1987). Finally, the actual clinical use of information from multisource checklists is still at a fledgling stage (Achenbach & McConaughy, 1987), and its eventual role in traditional diagnosis and treatment will need to be explored further.

Other Classification Systems

In addition to the DSM, ICD, and the dimensional nosological systems, a variety of other classification systems for child and adolescent psychiatric disorders have been proposed. From a psychodynamic perspective, Freud (1965) and Anthony (1970) proposed comprehensive classification models based on developmental parameters. In addition, a variety of multiaxial systems have been proposed. For example, the Rutter system (Rutter et al., 1969) was designed as a triaxial system that included axes for clinical psychiatric syndromes, intellectual level, and medical conditions. This system was further developed by Rutter, Shaffer, and Sturge (1975) to include two additional axes: one for specific delays in development and another for abnormal psychosocial situations. This system was noteworthy in that it inspired the development of the Multiaxial system (MAS 81; Isager, 1982), a five axes system designed to obtain additional information for the development of the ICD-10.

Another triaxial system has been proposed by Spiel (1981), who classified symptoms according to somatic, psychic, and social functioning. Sadoun, Casadebaig, and Hatton (1976), Kreisler, (1977), and Rocha (1977) proposed classification systems for psychiatric disturbance that include four axes, with the Sadoun and colleagues' and Kreisler systems being proposed primarily for infants. Multiaxial systems for family pathology also have been proposed (Tseng & McDermott, 1979). In general, although these classification systems have not achieved the notoriety of the ICD and DSM systems, the importance of obtaining clear descriptions of psychiatric disorders for children and adolescence continues to be challenged and evolve.

SCIENTIFIC PARAMETERS OF A CLASSIFICATION SYSTEM

As each of the contributors to the two volumes review individual DSM-III-R diagnostic categories, they focus on specific scientific parameters that any specific diagnosis should demonstrate. For example, Remschmidt (1988) noted that the basic aim of any classification system should be to classify disorders, not children, and that the system must be defined in operational terms covering a broad range of symptom manifestations. Although the parameters that should be addressed in any classification system can be debated, nearly all researchers in the classification of childhood and adolescent psychopathology basically agree that these parameters should encompass issues of reliability, validity, and clinical utility (Achenbach, 1985; Cantwell, 1975; Cantwell & Baker, 1988; Quay, 1983; Rutter, 1965; Rutter & Gould, 1985).

Reliability

Issues pertaining to reliability pervade psychiatric diagnosis in general. One of the primary mechanisms for determining the reliability of a diagnosis is *interrater reliability* (i.e., the degree of agreement that different raters show in assigning specific cases to the same diagnostic categories). The primary statistic now utilized in such investigations is the kappa statistic, with a recommended minimum value of ≥ .6 (Achenbach, 1985). Earlier investigations utilized percentage of interrater agreement, but that calculation did not take into account the likelihood of chance agreements.

Although the determination of interrater reliability may seem at first to be a straightforward matter, several issues involving methodological variance may have a potential impact on the findings. Foremost is the clarity and specificity of the diagnostic criteria, which some researchers believe should be empirically derived. Closely related to the quality of the diagnostic criteria is the format of the clinical interview and assessment strategies that are utilized to elicit information for diagnosis. In general, it will be important for the clinical interview and accompanying assessment strategies to include sufficient structure and breadth in order to obtain a comprehensive history and mental state symptoms for final diagnostic conclusions to be asserted.

At a more macroscopic level, studies of interrater reliability can also be affected by different approaches to judging cases, such as joint interview, joint diagnosis by videotape, consecutive interviews by the same clinician, or diagnosis of the same written case material by different clinicians. Also, raters of the same research team may tend to show higher rates of agreement than raters from different research teams.

Achenbach (1985) offered further discussion of cognitive factors that can influence clinical assessment. Such sources of bias include illusory correlation, inability to assess covariation, the representativeness heuristic, the availability heuristic, and the confirmatory bias. Thus, diagnosis also can be affected by several aspects of clinical information processing which may require consideration in future interrater reliability (e.g., circumvention via computer algorithms).

Although contributors to both volumes cite interrater reliability studies more specific to their individual diagnoses, general findings should be mentioned for the interrater reliability of DSM-III child and adolescent categories (such studies are just beginning for DSM-III-R).

Cantwell and Baker (1988) succinctly summarized these results and noted that, across studies, overall reliability has ranged from .37 to .70, and the reliability of DSM-III has generally fared as well as, if not better than, direct comparisons with DSM-II. The reliability of individual diagnostic categories have varied greatly, however, demonstrating the ongoing need for reliability studies of DSM-III-R diagnoses, particularly for diagnoses that have been newly refined.

Validity

Initially, face validity, based on the general agreement between clinicians, was important to the architects of DSM-III. Now, logically, other types of validity have become the foci of investigations (e.g., the uniqueness and mutual exclusivity of individual diagnostic categories). Kazdin and Petti (1982) emphasized the importance of convergent and discriminant validity in psychiatric diagnosis. A specific diagnostic category should correlate or converge with measures where agreement is anticipated. On the other hand, the same category should be discriminated by measures with which it would not be expected to correlate. Ideally, convergent and discriminant validity should be demonstrated at the same time by the proper selection of measures for the study of a specific child or adolescent diagnosis.

Clinically, predictive validity has primary importance for psychiatric classifications. A diagnosis with predictive value should be associated with specific natural history, biological correlates, familial pattern, response to treatment, and prognosis. Operationally, Cantwell (1975) proposed a six-stage model to validate child and adolescent psychiatric diagnoses. These stages include: (a) essential and associated features of the disorder as well as exclusionary criteria; (b) physical and neurological studies; (c) laboratory studies; (d) family psychopathology and interaction studies; (e) follow-up studies; and (f) treatment studies. Although predictive validity studies have been conducted for several DSM-III categories (and consequently the comparable DSM-III-R categories), such studies have not been conducted for other categories, and it will be important for the number of these investigations to increase with respect to planning for DSM-IV.

Clinical Utility

Terms such as feasibility, coverage, and utility describe different practical facets of a classification system that are integral to the actual usage of a taxonomy by clinicians and researchers. In today's computer terminology, a system of diagnoses must be "user friendly." The taxonomy should provide consistent communication among clinicians who employ the system. Diagnostic criteria should be clear, and accompanying information relevant and up-to-date. Similarly, the coding process should be unambiguous and easy to use. The range of diagnoses should adequately cover disorders encountered in actual clinical practice, but at the same time not be too over- or underinclusive.

DSM-III was the first classification system investigated for its practical value to clinicians. Cantwell and his colleagues (Cantwell, Mattison, Russell, & Will, 1979; Russell, Mattison, & Cantwell, 1983) surveyed clinicians for their reactions to initial usage of DSM-III. The clinicians felt the diagnostic coverage was adequate and showed an easy transition from DSM-II to comparable DSM-III categories. Axis II was well utilized, and a wide range of DSM-III diagnoses was used as opposed to a few general "wastebasket" diagnoses. The participants rated few difficulties in using DSM-III and, in general, preferred the new system over the DSM-II. Thus, qualities that should be important to practicing clinicians were found to be satisfied, although given the changes in DSM-III-R ongoing studies of this nature should be pursued.

DIAGNOSTIC ASSESSMENT TECHNOLOGY

As DSM-III and DSM-III-R have become empirical in their underpinnings, instruments for use with these classification systems have increased both in terms of number and objectivity. Furthermore, this emphasis on empiricism has led to more rigorous requirements to be satisfied with respect to instrument usage and development. This section provides an overview of the current status and issues with respect to the diagnostic assessment technology available for clinical and research investigations in child and adolescent psychopathology.

Diagnostic Interviews

Historically, the diagnostic interview (e.g., the mental status examination) has been one of the major cornerstones of the standard psychiatric evaluation. However, given the lack of objectivity, standardization, and normative base for the unstructured diagnostic interview, attention shifted to the importance of structured and semistructured interviews with children and their parents as pioneered by Rutter and colleagues during the Isle of Wight research (Rutter & Cox, 1981). Generally, semistructured interviews have been developed for use by experienced clinicians in the identification of specific diagnoses, while structured interviews have been developed for use by trained lay interviewers for diagnosis in epidemiological studies.

The value and importance of these types of interviews for children received support from the adult literature as these techniques were gaining credibility among researchers in adult psychiatric disorders, particularly as these interviews were being developed simultaneously with diagnostic criteria for individual DSM-III categories. Thus, these events gave impetus to researchers in child and adolescent psychopathology to develop specific interviews for use with youth and their parents.

Currently, several structured (e.g., Diagnostic Interview for Children and Adolescents, Diagnostic Interview Schedule for Children) and semistructured (e.g., Kiddie-Schedule for Affective Disorders and Schizophrenia, Child Assessment Schedule) interviews are in various stages of development, and their strengths and weaknesses have been extensively reviewed (Edelbrock & Costello, 1988; Gutterman, O'Brien, & Young, 1987). In general, the primary critique holds that much more work will be required to establish the reliability and validity of these techniques, particularly with respect to their psychometric integrity for individual diagnostic categories. In addition, the need for such work has been complicated further by the need to revise the instruments to coincide with DSM-III-R, thus necessitating more current reliability and validity studies relating the instruments to DSM-III-R diagnostic categories—especially categories with changed criteria. The methodology required for proper reliability and validity studies also has increased in complexity and sophistication, thus making such research all the more difficult to perform.

As noted earlier, structured and semistructured psychiatric interviews are becoming more bound to the existing DSM-III child and adolescent diagnostic categories. Although these linkages are necessary and without argument, at the same time these linkages make the search for potential new categories difficult. One possible remedy, as exemplified by the dimensional classification approach, might be a greater dependence on factor analytic studies of these instruments in divergent, but sufficiently large populations of children and adolescents. Another a priori remedy might be the expansion of instrument items beyond the criteria of DSM-III-R so as to encourage and explore new avenues of diagnosis. This latter suggestion is currently being pursued by Achenbach and McConaughy (1987) in their development of a new semistructured clinical interview.

While the aforementioned issues continue to be debated and investigated, the ongoing development of structured and semistructured interviews for use with children and adolescents has produced important benefits. Noteworthy among these benefits has been that the importance of comprehensive inquiry during initial interviewing has gained acceptance as opposed to a narrow-focused inquiry based on clinical judgment. Moreover, the emphasis on the use of these types of interviews has led to a healthy re-examination of what information is gathered from children and their parents during the initial evaluation period. Relatedly, the extent of clinical information and the number of sources necessary for the most optimal diagnostic decision making are being reconsidered. This concern has been addressed, in part, by the development of child and parent versions of structured and semistructured diagnostic interviews. Also, the "gold standard" diagnostic thinking of clinicians is undergoing closer scrutiny through simultaneous diagnosis by computer algorithms. Thus, the quality of the diagnostic interview and the diagnostic process continues to experience healthy evolution influenced by research results with these types of diagnostic techniques.

Rating Instruments

The development of several types of clinical rating instruments, both general and specific, has flourished in the past 10 to 15 years. This flurry of activity has seen the development of parent and teacher behavior checklists, clinician rating forms, self-reports for children and adolescents, and direct observational measures. In general, parent and teacher checklists tend to be used most frequently. From an evolutionary perspective, the initial focus of rating instruments was on the development of parent checklists because parental information was deemed the most valid. However, teacher checklists have now gained equal status, largely because teachers continually observe children of similar ages on a daily basis under relatively consistent environmental circumstances. Needless to say, the rating instruments that have begun to dominate the field (e.g., the Child Behavior Checklist) tend to be those that have been most carefully researched for their scientific parameters and clinical utility (Barkley, 1988).

In addition to their relatively low cost, rating techniques take advantage of observers in the child's natural surroundings, thus minimizing possible changes in the child's behavior due to the presence of a stranger. Furthermore, the use of raters other than the clinician (e.g., parents, teachers) capitalizes on the fact that these raters often have observed the child over extended periods of time that, in turn, will tend to increase the reliability and validity of the findings (Martin, Hooper, & Snow,

1986). Not surprisingly, because of their format, scientific parameters also have been more readily obtained for these instruments and these findings, in general, have been relatively superior to those obtained for semistructured and structured diagnostic interviews.

Although rating scales have become some of the most widely used measurement devices in clinical and research endeavors in child psychopathology (Martin et al., 1986), these instruments are prone to purposeful distortions and inadvertent biases that need to be considered. Eliminating purposeful distortions for the moment, a number of specific reasons makes rating instruments prone to inadvertent biases. Generally, these ratings are a function of the complexity of the mental (e.g., motivation to perform the ratings, prior expectations) and emotional (e.g., affective involvement such as parental stress) processes that occur when a rating is conducted (Cooper, 1981). Furthermore, although it has become clear that observers of the same child in different situations show poor agreement on behavior ratings (Achenbach et al., 1987; Pfeffer & Martin, 1983), these differences in ratings are distinctly important and must be synthesized for the best overview of the child. Indeed, this integration problem, referred to as the aggregation principle, is now receiving considerable attention (Achenbach & McConaughy, 1987; Ghiselli, Campbell, & Zedeck, 1981; Martin et al., 1986).

Although most of the attention regarding rating scales and checklists has been focused on their empirical qualities, particularly with respect to their utility in establishing taxonomies of psychopathology, other clinical advantages should be mentioned. For example, rating instruments can assist a clinician to understand or review which symptoms have been observed by parents and teachers, thus enhancing communication in the clinical arena. The results of rating instruments also can improve or confirm the focus of clinical inquiry. Relatedly, after the initial interview, a clinician can examine rating instruments to be certain that major symptoms and concerns presented by parents have been addressed. Finally, the rating instrument technology provides an economical and efficient baseline of behavior from which to judge ongoing treatment results, thus extending observations of the clinical impact of treatment beyond the clinician's office.

In addition to the more general rating instruments, more specific measures have been developed for use with individual diagnostic categories, many of which are integral to the discussions in the ensuing chapters. Such instruments have been tailored for use with a variety of specific disorders such as attention deficit disorder, conduct disorder, depression, and anxiety. Specificity has been extended to include target areas of symptoms within selected disorders, such as hopelessness and suicidal behavior within the category of depressive disorders, and different raters often can be utilized (e.g., parent, teacher, self) so as to reinforce and/or differentiate observations across settings. Although many of these more specific measures continue to require the establishment of basic scientific parameters (e.g., reliability, validity, normative data), they do have the potential to become useful components of clinical and research protocols.

SUMMARY

The modern evolution toward more objective classification of childhood and adolescent psychopathology has led to improved communication between clinicians and researchers with respect to psychiatric taxonomies and specific diagnoses within these taxonomies. This communication has been promoted by the widespread use of DSM-III and DSM-III-R, despite continued debate and varying degrees of approval. In addition to professionals utilizing the same diagnoses provided by the DSM taxonomies, these same professionals have begun to employ the same technology, if not the same instrumentation, in their investigations of various aspects of these diagnoses. Interestingly, many of these instruments have been developed in accordance with the DSM criteria. Thus, the common ground for professionals has been extended to include not only a specific taxonomy, but vehicles for exploring the diagnoses in the taxonomy. This common ground now serves as a substantial base to determine the "true" clinical validity of the diagnostic categories. Furthermore, the evolution of the DSM taxonomy is being driven through healthy competition from other evolving classification systems such as ICD-9/ICD-10 and the noncategorical approach to classification represented by dimensional taxonomies.

In the following chapters contributors provide selected critical reviews of individual diagnostic categories within the DSM system, and hopefully build on the legacy that has been evolving with respect to classification of child and adolescent psychiatric disorders. The modern history of the specific diagnosis is traced and concludes with the most recent diagnostic criteria listed in the DSM-III-R. The concordance of the present criteria with research findings is discussed, with recommendations for future criteria offered for specific diagnoses. Finally, clinical instruments that have proven useful for identifying a particular diagnosis are presented. Thus, it is hoped that the current status of many of the child and adolescent DSM categories will be thoroughly assessed, with practical suggestions being offered for future work with these disorders, particularly with respect to their contributions to the continual evolution of child and adolescent psychiatric diagnosis.

REFERENCES

Achenbach, T. M. (1980). DSM-III in light of empirical research on the classification of child psychopathology. *Journal of the American Academy of Child Psychiatry, 19,* 395–412.

Achenbach, T. M. (1985). *Assessment and taxonomy of child and adolescent psychopathology.* Beverly Hills, CA: Sage Publications.

Achenbach, T. M., Conners, C. K., & Quay, H. C. (1985). *The ACQ Behavior Checklist.* Burlington, VT: University of Vermont (unpublished).

Achenbach, T. M., & Edelbrock, C. (1978). The classification of child psychopathology: A review and analysis of empirical efforts. *Psychological Bulletin, 85,* 1275–1301.

Achenbach, T. M., & Edelbrock, C. (1983). *Manual for the Child Behavior Checklist and Revised Child Behavior Profile.* Burlington, VT: University of Vermont, Department of Psychiatry.

Achenbach, T. M., & Edelbrock, C. (1986). *Manual for the Teacher's Report Form and Teacher Version of the Child Behavior Profile.* Burlington, VT: University of Vermont, Department of Psychiatry.

Achenbach, T. M., & McConaughy, S. H. (1987). *Empirically based assessment of child and adolescent psychopathology: Practical applications.* Beverly Hills, CA: Sage Publications.

Achenbach, T. M., McConaughy, S. H., & Howell, C. T. (1987). Child/adolescent behavioral and emotional problems: Implications of cross-informant correlations for situational specificity. *Psychological Bulletin, 101,* 213–232.

American Psychiatric Association (1952). *Diagnostic and statistical manual of mental disorders.* Washington, DC: Author.

American Psychiatric Association (1968). *Diagnostic and statistical manual of mental disorders* (2nd ed.). Washington, DC: Author.

American Psychiatric Association (1980). *Diagnostic and statistical manual of mental disorders* (3rd ed.). Washington, DC: Author.

American Psychiatric Association (1987). *Diagnostic and statistical manual of mental disorders* (3rd ed., rev.). Washington, DC: Author.

Anthony, E. J. (1970). The behavior disorders of childhood. In P. H. Mussen (Ed.), *Charmichal's manual of child psychology* (Vol. 1, pp. 667–764). New York: Wiley.

Barkley, R. A. (1988). Child behavior ratings scales and checklists. In M. Rutter, A. H. Tuma, & I. S. Lann (Eds.), *Assessment and diagnosis in child and adolescent psychopathology* (pp. 113–155). New York: Guilford Press.

Cantwell, D. P. (1975). A model for the investigation of psychiatric disorders: Its application in genetic studies of the hyperkinetic syndrome. In E. J. Anthony (Ed.), *Explorations in child psychiatry* (pp. 57–59). New York: Plenum.

Cantwell, D. P., & Baker, L. (1988). Issues in the classification of child and adolescent psychopathology. *Journal of the American Academy of Child and Adolescent Psychiatry, 27,* 521–533.

Cantwell, D. P., Mattison, R., Russell, A. T., & Will, M. A. (1979). A comparison of DSM-II and DSM-III in the diagnosis of childhood psychiatric disorders: IV. Difficulties in use, global comparison, and conclusions. *Archives of General Psychiatry, 36,* 1227–1228.

Cooper, W. H. (1981). Ubiquitous halo. *Psychological Bulletin, 90,* 218–244.

Edelbrock, C., & Costello, A. J. (1987). A review of structured diagnostic interview schedules for children. In M. Rutter, H. Tuma, & I. Lann (Eds.), *Assessment and diagnosis child and adolescent psychopathology* (pp. 87–112). New York: Guilford Press.

Edelbrock, C., & Costello, A. J. (1988). Convergence between statistically derived behavior problem syndromes and child psychiatric diagnoses. *Journal of Abnormal Child Psychology, 16,* 219–231.

Freud, A. (1965). *Normality and pathology in childhood.* New York: International Universities Press.

Ghiselli, E. E., Campbell, J. P., & Zedeck, S. (1981). *Measurement theory for the behavioral sciences.* San Francisco, CA: W. H. Freeman.

Gould, M. S., Rutter, M., Shaffer, D., & Sturge, C. (1988). UK/WHO study of ICD-9. In M. Rutter, A. H. Tuma, & I. S. Lann (Eds.), *Assessment and diagnosis in child psychopathology* (pp. 37–65). New York: Guilford Press.

Group for the Advancement of Psychiatry. (1966). *Psychopathological disorders in childhood: Theoretical considerations and a proposed classification.* New York: Author.

Gutterman, E. M., O'Brien, J. D., & Young, J. G. (1987). Structured diagnostic interviews for children and adolescents: Current status and future directions. *Journal of the American Academy of Child and Adolescent Psychiatry, 26,* 621–630.

Hewitt, L. E., & Jenkins, R. L. (1946). *Fundamental patterns of maladjustment: The dynamics of their origin.* Springfield, IL: State of Illinois.

Isager, T. (1982). Multiaxial diagnostic system in a department of child psychiatry. Preliminary experience as an introduction to revision. *Ugeskr-Laeger, 144,* 400–403.

Kazdin, A. E., & Petti, T. A. (1982). Self-report and interview measures of child and adolescent depression. *Journal of Child Psychology and Psychiatry, 23,* 437–457.

Kreisler, L. (1977). Psychopathology of infancy: A nosological regrouping. *Psychiatrie de L'enfant (Paris), 20,* 521–532.

Martin, R. P., Hooper, S., & Snow, J. (1986). Behavior rating scale approaches to personality assessment in children and adolescents. In H. M. Knoff (Ed.), *The psychological assessment of children and adolescents* (pp. 309–351). New York: Guilford Press.

Mattison, R. E., Cantwell, D. P., Russell, A. T., & Will, M. A. (1979). A comparison of DSM-II and DSM-III in the diagnosis of child psychiatric disorders: II. Interrater agreement. *Archives of General Psychiatry, 36,* 1217–1222.

McConaughy, S. H., & Achenbach, T. M. (1990). *Guide for the Semistructured Clinical Interview for Children.* Burlington, VT: University of Vermont.

Mezzich, J. E., & Mezzich, A. C. (1987). Diagnostic classification systems in child psychopathology. In C. L. Frame & J. L. Matson (Eds.), *Handbook of assessment in childhood psychopathology. Applied issues in differential diagnosis and treatment evaluation* (pp. 33–60). New York: Plenum.

Mezzich, A. C., Mezzich, J. E., & Coffman, G. A. (1985). Reliability of DSM-III vs. DSM-II in child psychopathology. *Journal of the American Academy of Child Psychiatry, 24,* 273–281.

Millon, T. (1981). *Disorders of personality.* DSM-III: *Axis II.* New York: Wiley.

Pfeffer, J., & Martin, R. P. (1983). Comparisons of mothers' and fathers' temperament ratings of referred and non-referred preschool children. *Journal of Clinical Psychology, 39,* 1013–1020.

Quay, H. C. (1983). A critical analysis of DSM-III as a taxonomy of psychopathology in childhood and adolescence. In T. Millon & G. Klerman (Eds.) *Contemporary issues in psychopathology* (pp. 151–165). New York: Guilford Press.

Quay, H. C. (1986). Classification. In H. C. Quay & J. S. Werry (Eds.), *Psychopathological disorders of childhood* (3rd ed., pp. 1–34). New York: Wiley.

Quay, H. C., & Peterson, D. R. (1983). *Interim manual for the Revised Behavior Problem Checklist*. Miami, FL: Authors.

Remschmidt, H. (1988). German study of ICD-9. In M. Rutter, A. H. Tuma, & I. S. Lann (Eds.), *Assessment and diagnosis in child psychopathology* (pp. 66–83). New York: Guilford Press.

Rocha, Z. (1977). Child behavior disorders in daily practice (a multidimensional diagnostic approach). *Neurobiologia, 40*, 269–296.

Russell, A. T., Mattison, R., & Cantwell, D. P. (1983). DSM-III in the clinical practice of child psychiatry. *Journal of Clinical Psychiatry, 44*, 86–90.

Rutter, M. (1988). DSM-III-R: A postscript. In M. Rutter, A. H. Tuma, & I. S. Lann (Eds.), *Assessment and diagnosis in child psychopathology* (pp. 453–464). New York: Guilford Press.

Rutter, M. (1965). Classification and categorization in child psychiatry. *Journal of Child Psychology and Psychiatry, 6*, 71–83.

Rutter, M., & Cox, A. (1981). Psychiatric interviewing techniques: I. Methods and measures. *British Journal of Psychiatry, 138*, 273–282.

Rutter, M., & Gould, M. (1985). Classification. In M. Rutter & L. Hersov (Eds.), *Child and adolescent psychiatry: Modern approaches* (2nd ed., pp. 304–324). Boston: Blackwell Scientific Publications.

Rutter, M., Lebovici, S., Eisenberg, L., Sneznevskij, A. V., Sadoun, R., Brooke, E., & Lin, T. Y. (1969). A triaxial classification of mental disorders in childhood. *Journal of Child Psychology and Psychiatry, 10*, 41–61.

Rutter, M., & Shaffer, D. (1980). DSM-III: A step forward or back in terms of the classification of child psychiatric disorders? *Journal of the American Academy of Child Psychiatry, 19*, 371–394.

Rutter, M., Shaffer, D., & Sturge, C. (1975). *A guide to a multiaxial classification scheme for psychiatric disorders in childhood and adolescence*. London: Institute of Psychiatry.

Sadoun, R., Casadebaig, R., & Hatton, F. (1976). Studies of the infant population placed in charge of the A. Binet Mental Health Center in 1970 and 1971. *Social Psychiatry (Berlin), 11*, 179–205.

Spiel, W. (1981). Some critical comments on a systematic approach to diagnosis: Contribution to a documentation and classification system in child neuropsychiatry. *Acta Paedopsychiatrica, 47*, 269–278.

Strober, M., Green, J., & Carlson, G. (1981). Reliability of psychiatric diagnosis in hospitalized adolescents—interrater agreement using DSM-III. *Archives of General Psychiatry, 38*, 141–145.

Tseng, W., & McDermott, J., Jr. (1979). Tri-axial family classification. *Journal of the American Academy of Child Psychiatry, 18*, 22–43.

Werry, J. S. (1985). ICD-9 and DSM-III classification for the clinician. *Journal of Child Psychology and Psychiatry, 26*, 1–6.

Werry, J. S., Methven, R. J., Fitzpatrick, J., & Dixon, H. (1983). The interrater reliability of DSM-III in children. *Journal of Abnormal Child Psychology, 11*, 341–354.

World Health Organization (1965). *International classification of diseases* (8th ed.). Geneva: Author.

World Health Organization (1978). *International classification of diseases* (9th rev.). Geneva: Author.

CHAPTER 2

Schizophrenia

Andrew T. Russell
UCLA Neuropsychiatric Institute

What is schizophrenia? Since the term *dementia praecox* was coined by Kraepelin at the turn of the century, the precise answer to this question has remained stubbornly elusive (Meltzer & Liberman, 1982). In 1983 the World Psychiatric Association (WPA) published a compilation of 15 different sets of diagnostic criteria for schizophrenia (WPA, 1983). The criteria ranged from the work of Kraepelin and Bleuler to the Research Diagnostic Criteria (Spitzer, Endicott, & Robins, 1978) and DSM-III (American Psychiatric Association, 1980). The differences between the criteria demonstrated that for a complex disorder such as schizophrenia there is no single, universally accepted diagnostic schema. The clinical and research implications of this lack of agreement are considerable. For example, one study applied six different sets of diagnostic criteria for schizophrenia to the same 168 adult patients (Endicott et al., 1982). The rate of diagnosing schizophrenia varied as much as sevenfold, depending on which diagnostic criteria were used.

If controversy exists concerning the diagnosis of schizophrenia in adults, it is not surprising that this controversy is even greater in regard to schizophrenia occurring in childhood. The problem begins with terminology. Seriously ill children have been described with a multitude of terms that mean different things to different people. Some have used *psychosis* as a term denoting severity of illness (i.e., more severe than neurosis), and others to indicate the presence of such symptoms as hallucinations or delusions. Similarly, the term *childhood psychosis* has been used in a variety of different ways, generally as a broad generic term covering what some would argue are a variety of different disorders, (e.g., autism, pervasive developmental disorders, schizophrenia, atypical variants). As a generic term childhood psychosis has also encompassed such categories as symbiotic psychosis, the atypical child, and so forth. Finally, *childhood schizophrenia* has been used by some in the narrow sense—referring to a classical schizophrenic syndrome occurring in childhood, and by others as a more generic term virtually synonymous with childhood psychosis. As is discussed later, this lack of agreement on basic terminology has had a serious detrimental impact on the field to the point that many older studies are simply uninterpretable.

There is confusing terminology in this area, thus the use of terms in this review need to be made explicit. The terms *childhood psychosis* and *childhood schizophrenia* are avoided whenever possible, but when used they serve as "umbrella" terms referring to a poorly differentiated group of children encompassing the wide range of categories listed earlier (e.g., autism, etc.). *Schizophrenia* and *schizophrenia occurring in childhood* are used synonymously, and in accordance with the DSM-III definition of the adult syndrome. Reflecting the organization of DSM-III, *autism* is used to refer to a separate disorder, although the controversy concerning the overlap between autism and schizophrenia is discussed. The ages covered by schizophrenia occurring in childhood will generally range from age 5 through early adolescence (roughly age 14) although, where appropriate, distinctions are made between prepubertal and postpubertal onset. Finally, *schizotypal* is used in the DSM-III-R sense of schizotypal personality disorder. As is discussed, this term probably covers most children described by Wolff as "schizoid" (Wolff & Barlow, 1979) and by others as exhibiting "borderline schizophrenia" (not Borderline Personality Disorder).

If clinicians and researchers cannot agree on what basic term to use for a disorder, or on the subsequent diagnostic criteria, the usual underlying reason is a lack of adequate research. As is described, this is the case with schizophrenia occurring in childhood. As clinical researchers have attempted to distinguish between very different children previously lumped together under the rubric of childhood schizophrenia, one group of children (i.e., children with autism) have been the subject of intensive study. Ironically, as pointed out by Beitchman (1983), this focus on children with autism has led to the "benign neglect" of those children who may be comparable to autistic children in the severity of their disorder, but who tend to be older at the time of diagnosis and present with symptoms characteristic of adult onset schizophrenia (i.e., hallucinations, delusions, thought disorder). We are belatedly realizing that we may know less about these children than we once thought (Beitchman, 1983; Tanguay, & Asarnow, 1985; Volkmar, Cohen, Hoshino, Rende, & Paul, 1988). This chapter reviews some of what we do know about the phenomenology, diagnostic classification, and assessment of this fascinating group of children.

Several themes recur throughout this review and should be highlighted now. The first, already alluded to, has been the attempt to divide a rather heterogeneous group of children described as psychotic or having childhood schizophrenia into more diagnostically homogeneous and valid subgroups. A second related theme concerns the degree of overlap, if any, between autism and schizophrenia. A third theme stems from the growing recognition (as with adults) that positive symptoms such as hallucinations, delusions, and thought disorder are not pathognomonic of schizophrenia but are seen in a variety of disorders, particularly the affective disorders. To what extent do our current diagnostic schemes and assessment tools for children take this into account? A fourth theme concerns the effects of development on phenomenology and diagnostic reliability. A final theme that has been the subject of only limited research, is the downward extension of "Schizophrenic Spectrum Disorder" to children and adolescents. This search suggests that there are a group of children, roughly comparable to adults with DSM-III-R Schizotypal Personality Disorder, that do not exhibit the full syndrome of schizophrenia. Are they at risk for developing schizophrenia later in life?

These five themes recur throughout this chapter. They are evident during a historical review of the concept of schizophrenia occurring in childhood. They are especially important as certain definitional problems are examined, and they help to organize a review of pertinent research literature. This review leads to some suggestions for the revision of current DSM-III-R criteria and categories for children and adolescents. Available methods and tools for the diagnostic assessment of schizophrenia occurring in childhood are described. Finally, the need for new phenomenological, epidemiological, and treatment research is emphasized.

HISTORY

The classification of schizophrenia occurring in childhood has undergone dramatic revisions since the turn of the century. The swings of the nosological pendulum, particularly in this country, have tended to follow theoretical stances and only occasionally have been based on careful empirical observations. The empirically based studies are emphasized in this brief historical review. For a more comprehensive review the reader is referred to Cantor (1988).

It is difficult to discuss the history of the diagnosis of schizophrenia without first considering the work of the great European psychiatrists, Kraepelin and Bleuler. They developed different diagnostic criteria, with Kraelpelin establishing a narrower concept of schizophrenia (dementia praecox) emphasizing chronicity, and Bleuler a somewhat broader view emphasizing more difficult to define symptoms (the four "As"—association, affect, ambivalence, autism) (Goodwin & Guze, 1989). This distinction between narrow and broader conceptualizations unknowingly anticipated the controversy concerning childhood schizophrenia in the 1960s. Both Kraepelin and Bleuler recognized that schizophrenia could arise before adolescence in a small number of cases, with Kraepelin pointing out that 3.5% of his series of 1,054 cases had an onset before age 10 and 6.2% prior to age 15. He also felt that this was an underestimate reflecting the nonreferral of less severe young cases (Green et al., 1984; Kraepelin, 1919).

One of the first descriptions of a schizophrenic child was reported by De Sanctis in 1906. Building on Kraepelin's term, he labeled schizophrenia occurring in childhood as *dementia praecocissima* and distinguished it from mental retardation and neurological disorders. He also stated "the prognosis of which is perhaps not always as grave as that of dementia praecox in adolescents and in adults, but which . . . is sometimes cured" (De Sanctis, 1906, p. 599). In the United States, Potter (1933) was among the first to carefully describe schizophrenic children and drafted the first set of diagnostic criteria for the disorder in this age group. Potter presented case descriptions of six hospitalized prepubertal children, all of whom were severely disturbed, and several exhibited features of catatonia. Perhaps because of the nature of his sample, Potter's criteria tended to emphasize profound disturbances in affect, relatedness, form of thought, and motor activity. Although mentioned in the case histories, hallucinations and delusions were not part of these diagnostic criteria. These criteria can be seen in Table 2.1. Potter's work is notable for its rich clinical descriptions, the attempt to develop diagnostic criteria, the careful search for "organic" etiologies, and the emphasis on the importance of developmental factors in modifying symptom presentation. According to Potter (1933):

> It is necessary to bear in mind that children cannot be expected to exhibit psychopathology with all the elaborations of the adult. . . . Children, therefore, do not possess the facility to fully verbalize their feelings, nor are they capable of complicated abstractions. Consequently, delusional formations seen in childhood are relatively simple and the symbolization is particularly naive. (p. 1253)

This observation anticipated much of the criticism of the DSM-III-R

TABLE 2.1
Diagnostic Criteria for Childhood Psychosis 1933–1961

Potter, 1933	*Bradley & Bowen 1941*	*British Working Party Creak et al., 1961*
1. Generalized retraction of interests from environment	1. Seclusiveness	1. Gross and sustained impairment of emotional relationships with people
2. Dereistic thinking, feeling, and acting	2. Irritability	2. Apparent unawareness of their own personal identity to a degree inappropriate to their age
3. Disturbances of thought through blocking, symbolization, condensation, perseveration, incoherence, diminution, and mutism	3. Day-dreaming	3. Pathological preoccupation with particular objects or certain characteristics of them, without regard to their accepted functions
4. Defect in emotional rapport	4. Bizarre behavior	4. Sustained resistance to change in the environment and a striving to maintain or restore sameness
5. Diminution, rigidity, and distortion of affect	5. Diminuition of interests	5. Abnormal perceptual experience (in the absence of discernible organic abnormality)
6. Alterations of behavior with either increase of motility leading to complete immobility or bizarre behavior with a tendency to perseveration or stereotypy	6. Regressive interests	6. Acute, excessive, and seemingly illogical anxiety as a frequent phenomenon
	7. Sensitivity	7. Speech either lost, or never acquired, or showing failure to develop beyond a level appropriate to an earlier age
	8. Physical inactivity	8. Distortion in motility patterns
		9. A background of serious retardation in which islets of normal, near normal, or exceptional intellectual function or skill may appear

Note: Adapted from Werry, 1979, by permission.

criteria, which, in essence, apply adult criteria to children without much consideration of developmental issues.

The next important contribution to the field also came from an institution specializing in the long-term care of severely disturbed children, the Bradley Hospital. In 1941, Bradley and Bowen published a study that is often overlooked but has been described by Werry (1979) as "one of the classics in the nosology of child psychiatry" (p. 47). Bradley identified 14 children felt to be schizoid or schizophrenic and contrasted their symptomatology with the other hospitalized children. From this careful comparison they developed a list of eight diagnostic criteria with definitions (Table 2.1). Their criteria emphasized observable behavior (e.g., irritability, bizarre behavior) but did not mention hallucinations, delusions, or disturbances in form of thought. Bradley was among the first to make phenomenological distinctions between schizoid and schizophrenic disorders in children. Indeed, the majority of the sample was less profoundly regressed than Potter's cases, and 10 of the 14 were given the diagnosis of schizoid rather than schizophrenia. Furthermore, some of the Bradley and Bowen criteria (e.g., seclusiveness, day-dreaming) appeared to be precursors to criteria for schizotypal personality disorder in DSM-III-R.

The period from 1940 to 1970 encompassed a rather dramatic swing in the nosological pendulum. The "unitary view" of the childhood psychoses emerged from the work and influence of Loretta Bender at New York University. Endorsing a similar perspective was the British Working Group who, led by Creak (Creak et al., 1961), presented nine diagnostic criteria for childhood psychoses (Table 2.1). In fact, such was the influence of the unitary view, that 20 years ago this book probably would have had a different organization and this chapter would have had a different title, probably "Childhood Schizophrenia." Included here would have been an amalgam of psychiatric disorders linked as much by severity as by phenomenological distinctiveness. Over Leo Kanner's protests, infantile autism would have been found here, and there certainly would not have been a separate chapter on autism in a separate volume entitled *Developmental Disorders*. Moreover, the careful reader would have found "symbiotic psychosis," "atypical child," and other diagnostic terms applied to a severely disturbed but symptomatically heterogeneous group of children.

How did this shift from the narrow view of schizophrenia, espoused by Kraepelin, to a broader conceptualization of this disorder take place? Many factors were involved. The first factor undoubtedly was the lack of careful descriptive and epidemiological research into schizophrenia occurring in childhood. Second was the fact that psychodynamic theory, the predominate viewpoint in American psychiatry during this time period, tended to deemphasize empirical classification systems. Third, as already noted, was the influential work of Loretta Bender and her colleagues at New York University. At Bellevue hospital, Bender had the opportunity to study a large number of seriously disturbed hospitalized children. In her most quoted paper Bender (1947) defined childhood schizophrenia as

> a clinical entity, occurring in childhood before the age of eleven years, which . . . reveals pathology in behavior at every level and in every area of integration or patterning within the functioning of the central nervous system, be it vegetative, motor, perceptual, intellectual, emotional or social. (p. 40)

This definition has been criticized as overly broad and cutting across many different forms of psychopathology (Rutter, 1972; Tanguay & Asarnow, 1985; Werry, 1979). Although it was subsequently narrowed and more completely operationalized by Fish (Fish & Shapiro, 1965), this definition remains an extremely broad view of prepubertal schizophrenia, which has largely been set aside by a return to Kraepelinian concepts as manifested in DSM-III-R. What has not been set aside has been Bender and her colleagues' emphasis on developmental, neurological, and cognitive deficits in schizophrenic children. The work of Bender and Fish also had a great influence on the development of research that emphasizes vulnerabilities or risk factors, noted in the offspring of schizophrenic mothers (Asarnow, 1988; Fish, 1986).

Along with Bender, a unitary view of the childhood psychoses was supported by the British Working Group who developed a set of "9 diagnostic points" (Table 2.1) meant to cover all forms of childhood psychosis (Howells & Guirguis, 1984). From a contemporary perspective, these criteria most closely resemble various criteria developed to describe infantile autism. They make no specific mention of hallucinations or delusions, or to other Schneiderian criteria incorporated into DSM-III-R. Also notable is criterion number 9, which is described as "an indispensable condition for diagnosing childhood psychosis, a sine qua non" (Howells & Guirguis, 1984, p. 124). Criterion number 9 adds the element of a background of "serious retardation" and therefore raises the whole issue of the relationship between mental retardation, autism, and schizophrenia. The British Working Group criteria, therefore, do not seem to account adequately for descriptions of children and young adults with classical autism and average or above-average intellectual functioning (e.g., Rumsey, Rapoport, & Sceery, 1985) and the fact that the majority of studies of children with DSM-III schizophrenia report IQ's in the normal range (Asarnow, Tanguay, Bott, & Freeman, 1987; Green et al., 1984; Russell, Bott, & Sammons, 1989). Other problems with the "9 points" criteria set are illustrated by a follow-up study of 20 children originally diagnosed using the criteria and rediagnosed 20 years later (Howells & Guirguis, 1984). One of the questions posed by the study was whether the childhood schizophrenics would meet diagnostic criteria for schizophrenia when followed-up as adults. It was found that none of the adults were diagnosed as having schizophrenia using Schneider's first rank symptoms (similar to DSM-III criteria). However, using a broad interpretation of Feighner's criteria set (Feighner et al., 1972), they found that all of the adult subjects met criteria for schizophrenia. As pointed out by Tanguay and Cantor (1986), this latter conclusion required counting "suspected" delusions or hallucinations in 55% of the subjects, and such a broad application of Feighner's criteria would be "unacceptable to many." Howells and Guirguis (1984) concluded that "whether or not our patients have become adult schizophrenics remains mostly unanswered" (p. 127). Perhaps it is also reasonable to conclude that the question was not answered because the diagnostic criteria employed both originally and at follow-up were too imprecise or interpreted too broadly to be able to prove or disprove the hypothesis.

The 1970s brought with them another swing of the nosological pendulum. In essence, the pendulum swung away from a unitary view of the childhood psychoses and returned to a Kraepelinian viewpoint. This viewpoint saw schizophrenia occurring in childhood as essentially similar to schizophrenia seen in adults, and it carefully established autism as a phenomenologically and developmentally distinct disorder. This return swing of the pendulum began almost 30 years earlier with the work of Leo Kanner. In 1943, Kanner described 11 children with a disorder he termed *infantile autism* in a classic paper of the child psychiatry literature. Interestingly, Kanner (1943) originally felt autism to be related to "the schizophrenias," but subsequently felt it to be a separate entity (Kanner, 1971). Kanner's description of autism had a major impact on the conceptualization and nosology of schizophrenia occurring in childhood. It led directly to the work of Rutter (1972) and Kolvin (1971), who empirically demonstrated the distinctions between autism and schizophrenia. As noted previously, it also led to a tremendous clinical and research interest in autism, and ironically, to a relative neglect of other forms of childhood psychosis.

Rutter (1972) clearly presented the position that schizophrenia and autism were distinct entities. After reviewing a variety of research, including his own (Rutter & Lockyer, 1967a, 1967b), Rutter bluntly concluded: "The inescapable conclusion is that, so far as one can judge from the available evidence, autism has nothing to do with schizophrenia" (Rutter, 1972, p. 329). This conclusion was based to an important degree on the classic study of Kolvin and colleagues conducted in

England in the late 1960s (Kolvin, 1971; Kolvin, Garside, & Kidd, 1971a; Kolvin, Humphrey, & McNay, 1971b; Kolvin, Ounsted, Humphrey, & McNay, 1971c; Kolvin, Ounsted, Richardson, & Garside, 1971d; Kolvin, Ounsted, & Roth, 1971e). Over a period of years Kolvin identified 80 hospitalized children who met one of two sets of diagnostic criteria. The first set of criteria specified onset before the age of 3 years, "a self isolating pattern of social behavior," and either catastrophic reactions to environmental changes or gross stereotypies. The second set of criteria specified onset between 5 and 15, Schneiderian first rank symptoms, and "other adult schizophrenic symptoms in the field of affect, motility and volition" (Kolvin, 1971, p. 384). At some risk of circularity, Kolvin then carefully studied the phenomenology of both groups and found that the late onset group differed from the early onset (infantile psychosis) in significant ways. The most frequent and highly discriminant symptoms for the late onset group were hallucinations, disorder of thought content, and blunting and incongruity of affect. Similarly, for the infantile psychosis group the most frequent and discriminating symptoms were gaze avoidance, abnormal preoccupations, stereotypy, poor supervised play, disinterest in people, echolalia, and overactivity (Kolvin et al., 1971c). In summary, the early onset and late onset groups looked very differently phenomenologically. In this landmark study Kolvin also demonstrated differences between the groups on the basis of family, genetic, social class, maternal personality, and cerebral dysfunction variables.

The work of Kolvin and Rutter has been extremely influential. According to Beitchman (1983), it has provided evidence "sufficiently convincing to end this debate" (p. 26) (i.e., whether autism and schizophrenia are similar or different illnesses). It directly led to the classification system now employed in DSM-III and DSM-III-R in which autism is established as a separate category, and unmodified adult criteria are used to diagnose schizophrenia occurring in the childhood years. It is only recently that some intriguing new evidence has been presented suggesting that in a small number of children the phenomenological picture and longitudinal course may indeed show considerable overlap between classical autism and schizophrenia. This "minority view" is discussed later in this review. Suffice it to say, the preponderance of current evidence establishes autism and schizophrenia in childhood as distinct entities.

From a historical standpoint, before reviewing recent research, one more set of criteria for the diagnosis of schizophrenia must be considered. This was the criteria developed by the Group for Advancement of Psychiatry (GAP, 1966). This classification scheme is notable for its developmental viewpoint, dividing the psychoses seen in childhood into three major categories: psychoses of infancy and early childhood, psychoses of later childhood, and psychoses of adolescence. The first category includes autism and "interactional psychotic disorder" (e.g., symbiotic psychosis). The second category is the most interesting for this review in that it deals with the question of adult-type schizophrenia occurring before adolescence, and describes a typical course for the onset of psychosis in childhood. The text points out that the course may be insidious, beginning with "neurotic symptoms," progressing to "looseness of association," and later to "marked withdrawal, intense involvement with fantasy, . . . true disorders in thinking and a breakdown in reality testing." It is mentioned that true hallucinations may not be noted until the late school-age period. The text for this section concludes: "The term schizophreniform is preferred by the Committee, to indicate the parallels between this disorder and the adult form of schizophrenia, but to emphasize as well the developmental differences and the clinical impression that children with this disorder do not necessarily develop the later form" (GAP, 1966, pp. 254–256).

The descriptions included in the GAP classification can be criticized as vague and not operationalized, but the classification system is notable for its emphasis on development, the longitudinal progression of the disorder(s), the identification of less severe forms with a better prognosis, and the realization that there may be personality disturbances that may reflect the basic disorder (e.g., Is schizotypal personality disorder of DSM-III-R an attenuated form of schizophrenia?) Unfortunately, the GAP classification was virtually ignored between Kolvin's work and the return to Kraelpelinian concepts codified in DSM-III.

In summary, the history of the concept of childhood schizophrenia has been tortuous. In the last two decades, some clarity has emerged, and virtually all recent research uses criteria (e.g., DSM-III, ICD-9) that clearly differentiate between autism and schizophrenia occurring in childhood. In addition, schizophrenia occurring in childhood is generally diagnosed in a narrow sense and requires the presence of typical adult symptoms such as auditory hallucinations, delusions, or severe disturbances of thought. This approach presents numerous definitional issues, particularly in young children, and tends to de-emphasize developmental patterns of the disorder. In addition, the narrowing of the criteria for schizophrenia occurring in childhood has led to new problems of differential diagnosis. As newer research has demonstrated, there are clearly a significant number of severely disturbed children who do not meet either the criteria for autism or schizophrenia occurring in childhood (Volkmar et al., 1988). These children, using DSM-III-R, have been categorized as pervasive developmental disorder—NOS, atypical psychosis, schizotypal personality disorder and other diagnostic variants. To what extent recent research validates these distinctions in children, as well as issues of diagnostic reliability, is discussed later in the chapter.

DEFINITIONAL ISSUES

The DSM-III and DSM-III-R criteria for schizophrenia are outlined in Table 2.2. These criteria have been developed from the Feighner criteria (Feighner et al., 1972) and the Research Diagnostic Criteria (RDC; Spitzer et al., 1978), which both pioneered the use of specific inclusionary and exclusionary criteria. There are four basic elements to the DSM-III-R criteria that can be described as phenomenological (the presence of certain "psychotic" symptoms during an active phase of illness with or without prodromal or residual symptoms), chronological (duration 6 months), exclusionary (not due to affective disorder, organic factors, autism), and an element of severity (deterioration in level of functioning).

There were several changes to the schizophrenia criteria in DSM-III-R (Fenton, McGlashan, & Heinssen, 1988; Kendler, Spitzer, & Williams, 1989). Interestingly, two of the revisions were related to diagnostic issues with children and adolescents. The first came from difficulties encountered when applying DSM-III to schizophrenia occurring in childhood and involved the issue of deterioration. Cantor, Evans, Pearce, and Pezzot-Pearce (1982) argued that the deterioration in previous level of functioning criteria could not be applied to certain schizophrenic children who had demonstrated abnormalities from birth and had been seriously impaired in numerous domains in a continuous manner. Although Cantor's sample of children raises certain diagnostic controversies (Prior & Werry, 1986), the basic point that certain children who develop schizophrenia are impaired over long periods of time and insidiously develop the full syndrome is well taken (Asarnow & Ben-Meir, 1988; Russell, Bott, & Sammons, 1989). As a result, the DSM-III-R criterion B includes the qualifying phrase "when the onset is in childhood or adolescence, [there is] failure to achieve expected level of social development" (p. 194). The effect of this change has not been empirically studied, but probably allows for more chronically and developmentally impaired children to meet the diagnostic criteria. The second revision related to childhood disorders involved the differential diagnosis of autism and schizophrenia. It was felt that it was possible for an adolescent or adult who had met full criteria for autism as a child to receive a diagnosis of schizophrenia based on the DSM-III thought

TABLE 2.2a
Comparison of DSM-III and DSM-III-R Criteria for Schizophrenia
Criterion A

DSM-III	*DSM-III-R*
A. At least one of the following during a phase of the illness: (1) bizarre delusions (content is patently absurd and has *no* possible basis in fact), such as delusions of being controlled, thought broadcasting, thought insertion, or thought withdrawal (2) somatic, grandiose, religious, nihilistic, or other delusions without presecutory or jealous content (3) delusions with persecutory or jealous content if accompanied by hallucinations of any type (4) auditory hallucinations in which either a voice keeps up a running commentary on the individual's behavior or thoughts, or two or more voices converse with each other (5) auditory hallucinations on several occasions with content of more than one or two words, having no apparent relation to depression or elation (6) incoherence, marked loosening of associations, markedly illogical thinking, or marked poverty of content of speech if associated with at least one of the following: (*a*) blunted, flat, or inappropriate effect (*b*) delusions or hallucinations (*c*) catatonic or other grossly disorganized behavior	A. Presence of characteristic psychotic symptoms in the active phase: either (1), (2), or (3) for at least one week (unless the symptoms are successfully treated); (1) two of the following: (*a*) delusions (*b*) prominent hallucinations (throughout the day for several days or several times a week for several weeks, each hallucinatory experience not being limited to a few brief moments) (*c*) incoherence or marked loosening of associations (*d*) catatonic behavior (*e*) flat or grossly inappropriate affect (2) bizarre delusions (i.e., involving a phenomenon that the person's culture would regard as totally implausible, e.g., thought broadcasting, being controlled by a dead person) (3) prominent hallucinations [as defined in (1) (*b*) above] of a voice with content having no apparent relation to depression or elation, or a voice keeping up a running commentary on the person's behavior or thoughts, or two or more voices conversing with each other

disorder criteria (A6) coupled with abnormalities of affect (A6a) and that this was "undesirable" (Kendler et al., 1989). Therefore, Criterion F was added to DSM-III-R, which only allows the diagnosis of schizophrenia in a person who previously met criteria for autism if hallucinations and delusions are present. Interestingly, and perhaps uninten-

TABLE 2.2b
Comparison of DSM-III and DSM-III-R Criteria for Schizophrenia
Other Criteria

DSM-III	*DSM-III-R*
B. Deterioration from a previous level of functioning in such areas as work, social relations, and self-care. C. Duration: Continuous signs of illness for at least six months at some time during the person's life, with some signs of illness at present. The six-month period must include an active phase during which there were symptoms from A, with or without a prodromal or residual phase, as defined [in Table 2.2c]. *Prodromal phase*: A clear deterioration in functioning before the active phase of the illness not due to a disturbance in mood or to a Substance Use Disorder and involving at least *two* of the symptoms noted [in Table 2.2c] *Residual phase*: Persistence, following the active phase of the illness, of at least *two* of the symptoms noted [in Table 2.2c], not due to a disturbance in mood or to a Substance Use Disorder. D. The full depressive or manic syndrome (criteria A and B of major depressive or manic episode), if present, developed after any psychotic symptoms, or was brief in duration relative to the duration of the psychotic symptoms in A. E. Onset of prodromal or active phase of the illness before age 45. F. Not due to any Organic Mental Disorder or Mental Retardation	B. During the course of the disturbance, functioning in such areas as work, social relations, and self-care is markedly below the highest level achieved before onset of the disturbance (or, when the onset is in childhood or adolescence, failure to achieve expected level of social development). C. Schizoaffective Disorder and Mood Disorder with Psychotic Features have been ruled out, i.e., if a Major Depressive or Manic Syndrome has ever been present during an active phase of the disturbance, the total duration of all episodes of a mood syndrome has been brief relative to the total duration of the active and residual phases of the disturbance. D. Continuous signs of the disturbance for at least six months. The six-month period must include an active phase (of at least one week, or less if symptoms have been successfully treated) during which there were psychotic symptoms characteristic of Schizophrenia (symptoms in A), with or without a prodromal or residual phase, as defined [in Table 2.2c] *Prodromal phase*: A clear deterioration in functioning before the active phase of the disturbance that is not due to a disturbance in mood or to a Psychoactive Substance Use Disorder and that involves at least two of the symptoms listed below. *Residual phase*: Following the active phase of the disturbance, persistence of at least two of the symptoms noted [in Table 2.2c], these not being due to a disturbance in mood or to a Psychoactive Substance Use Disorder. E. It cannot be established that an organic factor initiated and maintained the disturbance. F. If there is a history of Autistic Disorder, the additional diagnosis of Schizophrenia is made only if prominent delusions or hallucinations are also present.

tionally, DSM-III-R now allows what was prohibited in DSM-III; that is receiving a diagnosis of both autism and schizophrenia. Although the prevalent view holds that autism and schizophrenia are different disorders, there are several reports in the literature describing a small number of children who met full criteria for autism in childhood and

TABLE 2.2c
Comparison of DMS-III and DMS-III-R Criteria for Schizophrenia Prodromal or Residual Symptoms

DSM-III	*DSM-III-R*
(1) social isolation or withdrawal (2) marked impairment in role functioning as wage-earner, student, or homemaker (3) markedly peculiar behavior (e.g., collecting garbage, talking to self in public, or hoarding food) (4) marked impairment in personal hygiene and grooming (5) blunted, flat, or inappropriate affect (6) digressive, vague, overelaborate, circumstantial, or metaphorical speech (7) odd or bizarre ideation, or magical thinking, e.g., superstitiousness, clairvoyance, telepathy, "sixth sense," "others can feel my feelings," overvalued ideas, ideas of reference (8) unusual perceptual experiences, e.g., recurrent illusions, sensing the presence of a force or person not actually present *Examples*: Six months of prodromal symptoms with one week of symptoms from A; no prodromal symptoms with six months of symptoms from A; no prodromal symptoms with two weeks of symptoms from A and six months of residual symptoms; six months of symptoms from A, apparently followed by several years of complete remission, with one week of symptoms in A in current episode.	(1) marked social isolation or withdrawal (2) marked impairment in role functioning as wage-earner, student, or home-maker (3) markedly peculiar behavior (e.g., collecting garbage, talking to self in public, hoarding food) (4) marked impairment in personal hygiene and grooming (5) blunted or inappropriate affect (6) digressive, vague, overelaborate, or circumstantial speech, or poverty of speech, or poverty of content of speech (7) odd beliefs or magical thinking, influencing behavior and inconsistent with cultural norms e.g., superstitiousness, belief in clairvoyance, telepathy, "six sense," "others can feel my feelings," overvalued ideas, ideas of reference. (8) unusual perceptual experiences, e.g., recurrent illusions, sensing the presence of a force or person not actually present (9) marked lack of initiative, interests, or energy *Examples*: Six months of prodromal symptoms from A; no prodromal symptoms with six months of symptoms from A; no prodromal symptoms with one week of symptoms from A and six months of residual symptoms.

Note: DSM-III criteria are from *Diagnostic and Statistical Manual of Mental Disorders* by the American Psychiatric Association, 1980, Washington, DC: Author. DSM-III-R criteria are from *Diagnostic and Statistical Manual of Mental Disorders* (3rd. ed., rev.), by the American Psychiatric Association, 1987, Washington, DC: Author.

subsequently developed the full DSM-III schizophrenic syndrome (Petty, Ornitz, Michelman, & Zimmerman, 1984; Watkins, Asarnow, & Tanguay, 1988). DSM-III-R now allows for these children and adults to be categorized, which hopefully will lead to further studies of this rare combination of disorders.

The other changes in the criteria apply equally to children and adults. Although criterion A was "simplified" (Kendler et al., 1989), this investigator finds the new DSM-III-R criterion A1 to be somewhat less than intuitive, and it allows certain combinations of symptoms that would not have met criteria in DSM-III (e.g., the presence of delusions and hallucinations without qualification as to type or content). In addition, frequency criteria have been included for hallucinations. Auditory hallucination must now be "prominent," which means that "throughout the day for several days or several times a week for several weeks, each hallucinatory experience [is] not . . . limited to a few brief moments" (194). Fenton and colleagues (1988) studied the consequences of these changes in an adult sample. They reported that for a sample of 532 patients, 182 met DSM-III criteria for schizophrenia and only 164 met DSM-III-R criteria. Thus, the revised criteria narrowed the concept of schizophrenia by 10%. Twelve patients did not receive the DSM-III-R diagnosis because they exhibited nonbizarre delusions (criterion A2) without hallucinations. An additional five patients had hallucinations of insufficient frequency and duration to meet the stricter DSM-III-R criteria. Only one patient was excluded because of the addition of the autism criteria. These investigators argued that the further narrowing of the DSM-III-R criteria did not improve diagnostic validity and cautioned against frequent changes in criteria (DSM-IV and ICD-10 take note!). It is unknown to what extent the DSM-III-R changes affected diagnostic patterns in schizophrenia occurring in childhood.

A more basic problem than criterion differences is whether hallucinations, delusions, and thought disorder have the same phenomenological significance in children as in adults. For example, when a child "hears a voice," does this imply the presence of serious psychopathology, much less schizophrenia? To attempt to answer this question, some of what is known about the significance and differential diagnosis of hallucinations, delusions, and thought disorder in children is considered here. The issue of whether such symptoms can be reliably elicited in younger children is covered in the section on assessment.

Hallucinations

Of the major psychotic symptoms occurring in children, hallucinations have received the most study (for a review see Simonds, 1986). Egdell and Kolvin (1972) emphasized issues of differential diagnosis. They pointed out that it is generally insufficient to assume the presence of hallucinations by behavioral observation and "at some time the child should describe the hallucinatory experience" (p. 281). They remarked that true auditory hallucinations must be distinguished from other, nonpathological phenomena occurring in children. These include imaginary companions, eidetic imagery (the production of vivid visual images that are not confused with reality), pseudo-hallucinations (frightening but vague experiences similar to illusions), night terrors, and hypnogogic experiences (hallucinations when falling asleep). Egdell and Kolvin also mentioned the need to rule-out organic brain syndromes and the fact that hallucinations may occur in children subjected to extreme stress. The DSM-III-R has indirectly taken some of this into account by including, for the first time, frequency and severity criteria to be applied to hallucinatory phenomenon. As many of the non-diagnostic hallucinatory phenomena tend to be fragmentary, of brief duration, and periodic rather than prominent and frequent, the new criteria should help reduce the number of false positive diagnoses of schizophrenia in children, especially when those diagnoses are based primarily on the presence of hallucinations.

In addition to distinguishing true hallucinations from other phenomena, the clinician must also be aware to what extent hallucinations are found in disorders other than schizophrenia. Garralda (1984a) carried out a retrospective and a follow-up (1984b) study of hallucinations in children with conduct and emotional disorders (i.e., not schizophrenic). Reviewing the records of 4,767 children seen at the Maudsley hospital, she found hallucinations noted in only 1.1% of the records. Hallucinations were common in children with "late-onset psychosis" (i.e., schizophrenia occurring in childhood), but were noted in only 0.5% of the rest of the sample, after excluding organic and sleep disorders. She followed-up 20 of the children with conduct and emotional disturbance and hallucinations into adulthood and found that while 16 continued to hallucinate, only one developed schizophrenia. In summary, Garralda established, more carefully than had been done previously, that hallucinations may occur in children who are not schizophrenic, and the presence of such symptomatology does not imply that these children are at risk for psychoses later in life.

Hallucinations may also occur in children with major affective disorder. Chambers, Puig-Antich, Tabrizi, and Davies (1982) studied 58 prepubertal children who met RDC Criteria (Spitzer et al., 1978) for major depressive disorder based on structured interview with the Schedule for Affective Disorders and Schizophrenia for School-Age Children—Present Episode (K-SADS-P). About one third (36%) of the sample reported "diagnostic auditory hallucinations" (i.e., "one or more voices saying at least one word other than one's own name"). About a quarter of the children who hallucinated were convinced the voice was real and reported that it significantly affected their behavior. Chambers and associates concluded that the hallucinations were similar to those reported in adult samples of individuals with major depressive disorder although they occurred more frequently. In a rather similar study, (Freeman, Poznanski, Grossman, Buchsbaum, & Banegas, 1985) reported an 18% rate of psychotic symptoms in a sample of 33 children with major depressive disorder. Four of the six children received a DSM-III diagnosis of schizoaffective disorder.

Among other disorders associated with hallucinations, special mention must be made of multiple personality disorder (MPD). MPD often originates in childhood and is particularly notable in children with histories of severe abuse, especially sexual abuse and neglect (Kluft, 1985). In frank multiple personality disorder, or in its early forms, auditory hallucinations (i.e., one alter conversing with another) may be reported. This may result in an incorrect diagnosis of schizophrenia (Bliss, Larson, & Nabashima, 1983; Malenbaum & Russell, 1987). Clinically, it would seem essential that MPD is carefully ruled out in a child who reports auditory hallucinations in the presence of relatively normal affect and thought processes.

Thus, auditory hallucinations in children (and in adults) should never be considered pathognomonic of schizophrenia. They need to be carefully distinguished from normal phenomena in childhood (i.e., imaginary companions) and may be found associated with several important psychiatric disorders in childhood. In short, they require a careful, systematic, and comprehensive assessment. The new frequency criteria developed for DSM-III-R should reduce the number of false positive diagnoses of schizophrenia occurring in childhood, although this has not been empirically demonstrated.

Delusions

In contrast to hallucinations, little is found in the literature regarding delusional symptomatology in childhood. Kolvin and colleagues (1971c) reported delusional thinking in 57% of his 33 cases of late-onset psychosis. The most common types of delusions were persecutory and "fantastic." In a study of 57 children with a diagnosis of schizophrenia (exact diagnostic criteria were not reported), Eggers (1978) contrasted types of delusions seen in children under 10 with delusional thinking in children ages 10 to 14. In the younger group delusions of identity and "coenesthetic" delusions were characteristic. In the older children diffuse fears had coalesced into paranoid thinking, ideas of reference, and hypochondriacal delusions. These conclusions supported the historical observations of Despert (1948), who noted, based on her experience with 50 schizophrenic children, that in children over 10 years of age delusions are similar to those seen in adults with the exception that they are simpler and less organized and systematic. In particular, she notes somatic delusions in older children and delusions of identification (often with animals) in younger children. Russell and associates (1989) reached a similar conclusion. Delusions were noted in 63% of 35 children who received a DSM-III diagnosis of schizophrenia. These investigators reported a wide variety of delusional thinking with verbatim examples and observed that, in general, the delusions reported were less complex and less likely to be rigidly sustained than those reported by adult patients.

The major differential diagnostic problem, as noted by several authors, is distinguishing elaborate childhood fantasies from firmly held delusional ideation. Developmentally, we tend to encourage active and vivid fantasy in our children as this is regarded as cognitively healthy. But at what point does this become pathological? The extent to which this distinction can be made with reliability and validity awaits empirical study. Once again, DSM-III-R is of little specific help in dealing with young children, stating that delusions must be ideas that involve "a phenomenon that the person's culture would regard as totally implausible." What is totally implausible to an 8-year-old child?

Thought Disorder

Even more problematic is thought disorder, the third major category of positive symptoms leading to a diagnosis of schizophrenia. There were some subtle changes in the definitions and criteria for formal thought disorder between DSM-III and DSM-III-R. In DSM-III thought disorder is described as "incoherence, marked loosening of associations, markedly illogical thinking, or marked poverty of content of speech when associated with other symptoms" (see Table 2.2). "Marked(ly)" is not defined or operationalized. In DSM-III-R, illogical thinking is not mentioned and poverty of content of speech is moved to the Prodromal or Residual Symptom category. The rationale for these changes is not clear, is not mentioned in the manual, and is not discussed in Kendler and associates (1989). One empirical paper suggests that illogical thinking may be an important component of thought disorder in schizophrenia occurring in childhood, and that it can be reliably assessed, which argues against the DSM-III-R changes (Caplan, Guthrie, Fish, Tanguay, & David-Lando, 1989).

Two modern studies have been conducted examining thought disorder in schizophrenic children (Arboleda & Holzman, 1985; Caplan et al., 1989). The methodology of these two studies are discussed in more detail in the section on assessment. However, several clinical findings are important as we consider issues of differential diagnosis of thought disorder in children. Using the Thought Disorder Index, Arboleda and Holzman were able to identify significantly higher rates of formal thought disorder in a sample of hospitalized psychotic children and a high-risk sample of children born to psychotic mothers when compared to a group of normal children and a group of nonpsychotic hospitalized children. Importantly, they also demonstrated that mild forms of thought disorder are present in young normal children and decrease with age, suggesting that one must control for cognitive development in children under 10 years of age. Caplan and colleagues (1989) studied thought disorder using the Kiddie Formal Thought Disorder Scale, which was based on the DSM-III categories of content of speech. They used carefully diagnosed children with schizophrenia and schizotypal disorder as subjects and compared them with normal controls. They found significantly higher rates of illogical thinking and loose associations in subjects compared with the controls. Like Arboleda and Holzman, they also found a developmental trend, with younger (particularly under age 7) target and control children exhibiting more thought disorder than older children. The results from both of these studies suggest that DSM-III-R's criteria for formal thought disorder in the acute phase is perhaps unrealistically limited to only incoherence and loosening of associations when other aspects of thought disorder may also be characteristic of the acute schizophrenic picture (Andreasen, 1979). The results also suggest that the DSM should include some cautions about the reliability of rating thought disorder, especially in younger children, without employing special assessment techniques.

The preceding selective review of pertinent features of the DSM-III-R criteria for schizophrenia in childhood has focused on recent changes in the criteria, and has included a review of pertinent literature regarding hallucinations, delusions, and thought disorder in children. The prodromal or residual symptoms have not been discussed, primarily because they seldom have been the subject of systematic study in children (Asarnow & Ben-Meir, 1988). What is striking about these so-called residual symptoms, however, is how closely they approximate the criteria for schizotypal personality disorder. This raises the whole issue of schizotypy in childhood, which is considered in the next section.

SELECTIVE LITERATURE REVIEW

There are relatively few studies, using modern diagnostic criteria, of schizophrenia occurring in childhood. There are several reasons for this lack of useful research (Russell et al., 1989). As noted previously, early studies tended to use broad or unspecified diagnostic criteria that led to serious problems of diagnostic heterogeneity. Another inherent difficulty is the rarity of the disorder. The prevalence rate for autism is around 4 to 5 per 10,000, and schizophrenia occurring in childhood is probably even less common (Tanguay & Asarnow, 1985; Volkmar et al., 1988). Thus, large referral centers and considerable amounts of time are required to accumulate a useful sample, especially prospectively. Finally, there has been a lack of standardized diagnostic interviews and other instruments available to the researcher interested in this area.

Despite these difficulties, three major modern studies have appeared and are reviewed here (Green et al., 1984; Kolvin, 1971; Russell et al., 1989). All meet the basic criteria of using modern diagnostic criteria (DSM-III or equivalent), carefully distinguishing between autism and schizophrenia, and employing a sample of useful size. A carefully done retrospective chart review by Volkmar and associates (1988) is also described. To reduce the scope of this section, the few other studies that have appeared in the last 10 years are not reviewed in-depth for a variety of reasons: Kydd and Werry (1982) used a small sample size; Cantor (1982, 1988) had problematic diagnostic criteria; Eggers (1978) had unspecified diagnostic criteria.

Kolvin's series of studies has been mentioned earlier in this chapter. From a sample of 80 hospitalized children, Kolvin and colleagues identified 33 children who were characterized by an onset of psychosis after age 5 and another group of children with an onset of significant symptoms prior to 30 months. The entire sample was rated for the presence or absence of symptoms typically associated with autism as well as adult schizophrenia. The early onset group was characterized by autistic symptomatology and the late onset psychosis group exhibited a high frequency of symptoms characteristic of schizophrenia. The features of the late-onset group are presented in Table 2.3 (from Russell et al., 1989). Of note is the male-to-female ratio and the relative rates of major psychotic symptoms, with auditory hallucinations noted in over 80% of the sample.

The Bellevue group (Green et al., 1984) conducted a retrospective chart review of 5 years of admissions to an acute inpatient unit and discovered 24 children who met DSM-III criteria for schizophrenia based on the consensus of two child psychiatrists. Based on the stated average number of admissions per year to the unit, this represented approximately 7% of the admissions to the service. Contrast groups of 25 autistic children and 25 conduct disordered children were also described. The demographic and basic clinical presentations are presented in Table 2.3. The authors noted that only one of the children reported visual hallucinations without also describing auditory hallucinations.

The third major phenomenological study was conducted by the author and colleagues as part of the UCLA Child Psychiatry Clinical Research Center (CPCRC) (Russell et al., 1989). This prospective study differed from the others in that it utilized a structured diagnostic interview and protocol. For inclusion in the UCLA study subjects had to have a full scale IQ greater than 75 and no diagnosable neurological disorder. This was in contrast to the Kolvin studies in which five children had IQs less than 69 and five had "unequivocal evidence of brain dysfunction" (Kolvin et al., 1971e, p. 409). Among those children were three with temporal lobe epilepsy with onset prior to the appearance of schizophrenic symptoms. In the Bellevue study three schizophrenic children had IQs in the mildly retarded range (65 to 70). Despite these differences in sample composition, the three groups did not show significant differences in mean IQ which was in the normal range. The demographic and clinical characteristics of the 35 children in the UCLA sample are presented in Table 2.3.

These three studies provide the major sources of phenomenological data concerning schizophrenia occurring in childhood using modern diagnostic criteria. All represent samples of adequate size requiring several years for recruitment in major metropolitan centers. Comparisons between the three samples, collected using different methods and with somewhat different criteria, are illuminating. All show a positive male-to-female ratio, although this is smaller than the ratio reported for autism. This is in contrast to schizophrenia diagnosed in adulthood, which shows a roughly equal ratio. The racial and socioeconomic differences between the samples probably reflect different catchment areas and referral biases. Large-scale epidemiological studies are required to demonstrate whether childhood-onset schizophrenia is more common in lower socioeconomic groups (as may be true in adult schizophrenia) (APA, 1987, p. 191). Despite the differences between the samples, the phenomenological similarities are striking. Auditory hallucinations were the most common positive symptom, reported in approximately 80% of the subjects. Delusions of various types were found in over half the subjects. The major symptom category that differed significantly in frequency between the three samples was thought disorder. It is unclear, however, whether these differences reflect true differences or simply reflect rating distinctions and definitional issues.

What do these three studies say about the adequacy of the current DSM-III-R criteria? First, they demonstrate unequivocally that a small number of young children, on cross-sectional diagnosis, demonstrate a syndrome phenomenologically similar to schizophrenia seen in adults. This includes meeting criteria for deterioration, duration, and exclu-

TABLE 2.3
Characteristics of Schizophrenic Children in Three Centers

	Kolvin (1971) N=33	*Green et al. (1984)* N=24	*UCLA/CPRC(1988)** N=35	
Age				
Mean (SD)	11.1[a]	9.96 (±1.63)	9.54 (±2.07)	
Range	(5–15)	(6.7–11.11)	(4.9–13.3)	NS
Sex				
Male (M)	24	15	24	
Female (F)	9	9	11	NS
Ratio (M:F)	2.66:1	1.67:1	2.2:1	
Race				
Caucasian	33	4	22	Chi^2=42.63[b]
Black	0	13	7	$p < .005$
Hispanic	0	6	4	
Asian	0	1	0	
SES				
I & II	5(16%)	0	19 (54.0%)	Chi^2=31.6
III	12(37%)	4 (16.6%)	8 (23.0%)	$p < .005$
IV & V	16(47%)	20 (83.3%)	5 (14.0%)	

IQ				
N	30	24	34	NS[c]
Mean	85.9	88.5(±16.0)	94(±10.5)	
Range	<69–>110	65–125	76–114	
		Systemomatic Presentation		
Auditory hallucinations	27 (81.8%)	19 (79.2%)	28 (80.0%)	NS
Visual hallucinations	10 (30.3%)	11 (45.8%)	13 (37.0%)	NS
Delusions	19 (57.6%)	13 (54.2%)	22 (63.0%)	NS
Thought disorder	20 (60%)	24 (100%)	14 (40.0%)	$Chi^2=22.3$ $p < .005$

**Note*: From "Phenomenology of Schizophrenia Occurring in Childhood" by A. Russell, L. Bott, and C. Sammons, 1989, *Journal of the American Academy of Child and Adolescent Psychiatry*, 3, p. 405. Copyright 1989 by American Academy of Child and Adolescent Psychiatry.

[a]Estimated from tabular data "age of recognition of psyhosis"

[b]Caucasian v. other

[c]Green v. UCLA only

sion of major affective disorder. Although there may be age distinctions in the content of hallucinations, delusions, and thought disorder (i.e., simpler, less well-differentiated in younger children), the basic symptoms do occur and can be elicited at evaluation. Furthermore, the English and Bellevue studies, by employing comparison groups of autistic children, demonstrated that schizophrenia occurring in childhood is phenomenologically distinct from autism.

What questions about the DSM-III-R criteria are not answered by the aforementioned studies? Perhaps foremost is the issue of whether the current criteria are sufficiently inclusive. Although there are children who meet the narrow criteria for schizophrenia, are there also a significant number of psychotic children who cannot be appropriately classified within the available categories? This question has been partially addressed by a retrospective chart review conducted by Volkmar and colleagues (1988) at Yale. This group reviewed records of 228 children who had received a psychotic diagnosis over a 10-year period and divided them into three major groups: autistic (autism or childhood onset pervasive developmental disorder), atypical (atypical pervasive developmental disorder), or schizophreniform (schizophrenia or psychotic illness with schizophrenic features). There were 144, 42, and 42 children in the groups, respectively. The children were then blindly rediagnosed and assigned to strict DSM-III categories. Of the 42 schizophreniform children, only 14 met full DSM-III criteria for schizophrenia. The remaining 28 children presented a "complicated diagnostic picture" in which the "most appropriate DSM-III diagnosis generally appeared to be schizoid disorder of childhood" (p. 197). When examined further it was found that 20 of the 28 did not meet criteria for schizophrenia because the "onset of the illness was gradual and a period of deterioration could not be adequately documented." One can speculate that several of these children might have met the broader DSM-III-R deterioration criteria. In 12 cases the "degree of hallucinations/delusions required for the diagnosis was not apparent." These children probably would not have met the even stricter hallucination criteria for schizophrenia in DSM-III-R. Even with the changes between DSM-III and DSM-III-R criteria one can speculate that between one-half and one-third of the "schizophreniform" group would not meet DSM-III-R criteria for schizophrenia. How should these children be classified?

Volkmar and associates (1988) suggested that these children would best fit the DSM-III category of schizoid disorder of childhood. This investigator would argue that an even more appropriate category, from a phenomenological standpoint, might be the DSM-III or DSM-III-R category of schizoptypal personality disorder. This disorder requires, for the purpose of this discussion, ignoring that DSM-III views personality disorders as fixed patterns of personality traits that seldom can be diagnosed before adolescence and, instead, concentrating on the clinical criteria. These criteria, presented in Table 2.4, can be compared with the prodromal/residual criteria of schizophrenia (Table 2.2c). Volkmar described the nonschizophrenic subjects in the schizophreniform group as exhibiting long-standing disturbances in relatedness, overengagement with fantasy figures, magical thinking, subtle thought disturbance, and hallucinations or delusions of insufficient intensity to meet criteria for schizophrenia. These symptoms are all suggestive of schizotypal personality disorder.

What do we know about schizoid or schizotypal children? Not a great deal. Perhaps the most extensive study of these children has been done by Wolff and colleagues in England (Wolff & Barlow, 1979; Wolff & Chick, 1980). Wolff identified the following core characteristics: (a) solitariness, (b) impaired empathy and emotional detachment, (c) increased sensitivity, (d) rigidity of mental set, and (e) an unusual or

TABLE 2.4
DSM-III-R Criteria for Schizotypal Personality Disorder

A. A pervasive pattern of deficits in interpersonal relatedness and peculiarities of ideation, appearance, and behavior, beginning by early adulthood and present in a variety of contexts, as indicated by at least five of the following:
   (1) ideas of reference (excluding delusions of reference)
   (2) excessive social anxiety, e.g., extreme discomfort in social situations involving unfamiliar people.
   (3) odd beliefs or magical thinking, influencing behavior and inconsistent with subcultural norms, e.g., superstitiousness, belief in clairvoyance, telepathy, or "sixth sense", "others can feel my feelings" (in children and adolescents, bizarre fantasies or preoccupations)
   (4) unusual perceptual experiences, e.g., illusions, sensing the presence of a force or person not actually present (e.g., "I felt as if my dead mother were in the room with me")
   (5) odd or eccentric behavior or appearance, e.g., unkempt, unusual mannerisms, talks to self
   (6) no close friends or confidants (or only one) other than first-degree relatives
   (7) odd speech (without loosening of associations or incoherence), e.g., speech that is impoverished, digressive, vague, or inappropriately abstract
   (8) inappropriate or constricted affect, e.g., silly, aloof, rarely reciptrocates gestures or facial expressions, such as smiles or nods
   (9) suspicousness or paranoid ideation
B. Occurrence not exclusively during the course of schizophrenia or a pervasive developmental disorder.

Note: From *DSM-III-R: Diagnostic and Statistical Manual of Mental Disorders* (3rd ed., rev.) by the American Psychiatric Association, 1987, Washington, DC: Author.

"odd" style of thinking. She described groups of children with these characteristics as similar to those described by Asperger (1944) as "autistic psychopathy of childhood" (title). She also endorsed the definition of schizoid as "resembling schizophrenia phenotypically but in a dilute fashion" (Wolff & Chick, 1980, p. 96). The fact that this group of children in some ways resembles high functioning autistic children and in other ways resembles individuals with schizotypal personality disorders is at the heart of the differential diagnosis problem. In a recent review, Wolff (1989) emphasized the need to use a broad definition of this disorder until it is better studied and understood:

> The term *schizoid personality disorder* . . . is used in a broad sense to include conditions that have also been described in Asperger's syndrome, childhood-onset pervasive developmental disorders, and schizoid, paranoid, or schizotypal personality disorders. The children and people to be described most often, but by no means invariably, fulfill the criteria for schizotypal personality disorder and, unlike children with pervasive developmental disorders, they are not usually lacking in imaginative activity. (p. 213)

As the preceding quote suggests, there is some evidence to support that, despite the considerable diagnostic overlap, children meeting criteria for DSM-III-R schizotypal personality disorder may be more closely allied to schizophrenia than to autism. Wolff and Chick (1980) conducted a longitudinal study involving 22 schizoid children and controls. When followed up as young adults, two of the schizoid children and none of the controls had developed schizophrenia. Nagy and Szatmari (1986) found a similar proportion in a retrospective chart review study. Perhaps more importantly, in the Wolff study 18 of the 22 remained "schizoid" as compared to only 1 control, suggesting the chronicity and persistence of the disorder. In addition, the steadily growing high-risk literature in Schizophrenia generally supports the link between schizotypy and Schizophrenia (for a review see Asarnow, 1988). For example, Parnas, Schulsinger, Schulsinger, Sarnoff, and Teasdale (1982) and Fish (1986) found increased rates of schizophrenia and schizotypal personality disorder as compared to controls in their longitudinal studies of offspring of schizophrenic mothers. Approaching the problem from a cross-sectional perspective, Russell and colleagues (Russell, Bott, & Sammons, 1987, 1989) found striking phenomenological similarities between children meeting full criteria for DSM-III schizophrenia occurring in childhood and children meeting criteria for schizotypal personality disorder. In the course of the UCLA-CPCRC study described previously, we identified 20 children who fell short of meeting criteria for schizophrenia, but who met full criteria for DSM-III schizotypal personality disorder. When these 20 children were compared with the sample of 35 schizophrenic children, using the eight symptoms in the DSM-III schizotypal criteria set, the only significant difference between the two groups was the frequency of the symptom social anxiety/sensitivity to criticism, which was more frequent in the schizotypal group. The only major differences between the groups were the presence of full-fledged hallucinations and delusions, which of course lead to a forced diagnosis of schizophrenia. These major distinctions also became distinctions of severity (i.e., perceptual disturbances vs. frank hallucinations, bizarre preoccupations vs. firmly held delusional beliefs). Generally, the similarities between the two groups in our cross-sectional study seemed to reflect the conclusions reached by Bleuler (1950) when studying the families of schizophrenics:

> If one observes the relatives of our patients, one often finds in them peculiarities which are qualitatively identical with those of the patients themselves, so that the disease appears to be only a quantitative increase in the anomalies in the parents and siblings. (p. 238)

In summary, there clearly is an interesting group of children who are not easily classified using DSM-III or DSM-III-R. These children, as described by Asperger (1944), Wolff (1989), Nagy and Szatmari (1986), Russell and colleagues (1989), and Volkmar and associates (1988) (see also Asarnow & Ben-Meir, 1988; Wing, 1981), fall between the well-defined categories of autism and schizophrenia occurring in childhood. They currently tend to be classified in the DSM-III-R system in the categories of a pervasive developmental disorder-NOS (PDD-NOS), atypical psychosis, or schizotypal personality disorder. Within this broad heterogeneous group it would seem that two, somewhat distinct subgroups can be found. The first group more closely resembles autistic children, but tends to be higher functioning and exhibits less severe impairments in language and social interaction. The most appropriate diagnosis for this group is pervasive developmental disorder-NOS. The second group seems to resemble children with schizophrenia more closely, but lacks the florid positive symptoms of that disorder. These children, in contrast to the PDD-NOS group, often exhibit a rather bizarre and convoluted fantasy life, are suspicious of others, and may be subtly thought disordered. These children seem to fall into the "schizophrenia spectrum" and tend to be similar to adult relatives of schizophrenics who exhibit schizotypal personality disorder. Diagnosing these children as schizotypal personality disorder may be appropriate from a phenomenological standpoint, but this diagnosis certainly is awkward from developmental and, perhaps, prognostic viewpoints. Personality disorders are rarely appropriate diagnoses for young children because of the fluidity of development in this age group and the uncertainty that traits observed on cross-section will be enduring and persistent. There is also evidence from the high-risk literature that a subgroup of schizotypal children may not remain schizotypal but rather be at risk for the development of schizophrenia in adolescence or young adulthood. The difficulties in appropriately categorizing schizotypal children is an issue that should be addressed by DSM-IV.

Before completing this selective review of schizophrenia occurring in childhood, mention should be made of a recent study that once again raises the issue of the distinctiveness of autism and schizophrenia. Watkins, Asarnow, and Tanguay, 1988, in conjunction with the UCLA-CPCRC study, meticulously examined the early histories of 18 children diagnosed with schizophrenia occurring in childhood. These 18 children were recruited prior to the sample of 35 described in the Russell and colleagues (1989) study and used a different diagnostic protocol (see Watkins et al., 1988, for details). Interview and other data (e.g., past medical reports, school reports) were reviewed independently by two senior clinicians and subjects were included in the study only if there was perfect agreement on final diagnosis. Using a follow-back design and a DSM-III symptom rating scale, clinicians then rated contemporaneous evaluation data from multiple sources at each of four age ranges: 0 to 30 months, 30 months to 5 years, 6 to 8 years, and 9 to 11 years. The most surprising finding was that 7 of 18 children (39%) who developed schizophrenia before age 12 met full criteria for autism between 0 and 30 months of age. This finding has implications for the now generally accepted belief that autism and schizophrenia are separate and distinct disorders. In support of the finding, Watkins and associates (1988) cited the case report of Petty and colleagues (1984). This report described three children with a clear history of autism who later developed the full syndrome of schizophrenia. Cantor (1982) also described a number of early autistic symptoms in her sample of schizophrenic children. We provided partial support to both sides of the controversy. In our sample of 35 children, using a cross-sectional method that included extensive questioning about early autistic symptoms, 26% of the schizophrenic children exhibited a variety of symptoms of autism and/or pervasive developmental disorder prior to the onset of schizophrenia, but none met full criteria for either disorder (Russell et al., 1989) Watkins and colleagues (1988) themselves urged caution in overinterpreting their finding. They cited their own clinical experience and data from follow-up studies indicating that only a small percentage of autistic children go on to develop schizophrenia. They also pointed out that their findings do not necessarily support a continuity between autism and schizophrenia but, rather, that cross-sectional methodologies and overemphasis on age of onset (e.g., Kolvin, 1971) may have obscured the developmental course of childhood-onset schizophrenia.

Recommendations for DSM-IV

What implications does the previous selective review of our knowledge concerning schizophrenia occurring in childhood have for DSM-IV? Keeping in mind Kendler and colleagues' (1989) cogent arguments for limiting changes in diagnostic criteria to the minimum, this investigator would like to recommend the following:

1. The criteria for schizophrenia, with one exception, should remain unchanged. There is clear evidence that schizophrenia diagnosed using the present criteria occurs in childhood. The phenomenological picture in children differs only developmentally (e.g., simpler, less elaborate delusions), and not substantively, from what is seen in adults. The changes between DSM-III and DSM-III-R (e.g., broadening the definition of deterioration, tightening up on the frequency of hallucinations) have been helpful and, there is insufficient new evidence to recommend further changes at this time. However, "markedly illogical thinking" should be restored to the criteria for formal thought disorder. As noted previously, this seems to be an important component of clinically significant thought disorder, at least in children.

2. In contrast to the basic criteria, several changes are indicated for the text and/or the glossary. These changes are required to give DSM-IV a more developmental perspective and to emphasize phenomenological differences between symptoms in children, adolescents, and adults.

   a. It should be stated that, in children, true auditory hallucinations should be distinguished from normal phenomena such as imaginary companions (per Egdell & Kolvin, 1972).

   b. It should be noted that delusions in children must be distinguished from fantasy and, compared to adults, tend to be simpler, less well-developed, and may reflect developmental themes such as identity confusion.

   c. "Marked(ly)" when describing disturbance of thought should be, if possible, defined or operationalized. For example, the K-SADS-P uses as the definition of *severe* derailment: "Very frequent instances with definite impairment in understandability (>25%)." The fact that young children (under the age of 10) normally exhibit subtle forms of thought disorder should be mentioned.

3. The description of onset should include the fact that schizophrenia may occur in childhood and is typically of insidious onset, often preceded by a variety of behavioral and other prodromal symptoms.

4. The differential diagnosis section should include a discussion of multiple personality disorder and (in children) early forms of MPD. schizophrenia is now discussed as a differential for MPD, but the converse is not true.

5. Most important, a category should be established, in the childhood section, for **Schizotypal Disorder of Childhood.** The criteria could be similar to the current criteria for Schizotypal Personality Disorder with appropriate modifications to emphasize children (see Table 4.4). For example, the phrase "beginning by early adulthood" should be dropped from criterion A; criterion A3 should simply read "Bizarre fantasies or preoccupations"; a different example should be used in criterion A4. The rationale for the addition of this category has been outlined previously. It is clear that a certain number of children meet criteria for schizotypal personality disorder and need to be distinguished from children with pervasive developmental disorder-NOS. The use of a personality disorder diagnosis in young children is ill-advised because developmental patterns are not yet fixed. This is supported by the fact that some of these children, rather than going on to become schizotypal adults, may be at risk for schizophrenia. The text should cite the phenomenological and possible genetic links with schizophrenia and the differential diagnosis between schizotypal disorder and pervasive developmental disorder-NOS.

ASSESSMENT

The diagnosis of schizophrenia occurring in childhood to a large extent depends on direct interview of the child and parents. Although flat affect, disturbances of form of thought, and bizarre behavior (e.g., catatonia) can be "observed," it is only in exceptional cases that the diagnosis of schizophrenia in a child can be comfortably made on observations alone. Aside from the clinical interview, other modes of diagnostic assessment are either nonexistent or insufficiently developed. Although there is considerable interest in psychobiological correlates of schizophrenia occurring in childhood and adolescence (see

Asarnow, Sherman, & Strandberg, 1986, for review), as in adult schizophrenia, there is no consistent biological or cognitive marker that is diagnostic of the disorder. Diagnostic systems using factor analysis and related statistical techniques are also very limited in regards to schizophrenia occurring in childhood although both Quay and Peterson (1983) and Achenbach (1980) identified a "psychotic" factor (Prior & Werry, 1986). Projective psychological tests, in terms of leading to a specific diagnosis, also have limited usefulness with children (Gittelman, 1980). Finally, to the best of the author's knowledge, there are no available rating scales in common use that focus on the diagnosis of schizophrenia or schizotypal personality disorder occurring in childhood.

If one needs to rely on the psychiatric interview for the diagnosis of schizophrenia, which approach is best? The use of one of the structured or semistructured interviews now available for use with children would appear most useful at present. It is beyond the scope of this chapter to review the field of structured diagnostic interviewing and the reader is referred to Gutterman, O'Brien, and Young (1987) and Edelbrock and Costello (1988) for recent surveys of this topic. There are several DSM-III linked interview instruments that are now available including the Diagnostic Interview for Children and Adolescents (DICA), (Herjanic & Reich, 1982), the Child Assessment Schedule (CAS) (Hodges et al., 1982), the Schedule for Affective Disorders and Schizophrenia for School-Age Children—Present Episode (K-SADS-P) (Chambers et al., 1985), the Interview Schedule for Children (ISC) (Kovacs, 1978), the Diagnostic Interview Schedule for Children (DISC) (Costello, Edelbroch, & Costello, 1985), and the Interview for Childhood Disorders and Schizophrenia (ICDS) (Russell et al., 1989). Perhaps the two best suited for an in-depth clinical assessment of schizophrenia occurring in childhood are the K-SADS-P and a derivative, the ICDS. The focus of this section is to consider what little is known about diagnostic reliability and validity with these instruments when diagnosing schizophrenia and related disorders in childhood and adolescence.

Using the SADS, (Endicott & Spitzer, 1978), the adult version of the K-SADS, Strober, Green, and Carlson (1981) measured interrater diagnostic reliability on a group of 95 adolescent subjects, including 15 cases of schizophrenia. They achieved a highly satisfactory diagnostic agreement (kappa = .82) for the diagnosis of schizophrenia. Chambers and associates (1985) examined test–retest reliability of the K-SADS-P on a sample of 52 children and adolescents (age range = 6 to 17, mean age = 12.3 years). Unfortunately, the number of children exhibiting psychotic symptoms in this outpatient sample was small. However, modest agreement on types of auditory hallucinations was achieved, with 4 of 5 types of hallucinations showing an intraclass correlation coefficient of above .50. In a recent diagnostic study of hospitalized adolescents, Apter, Orvaschel, Laseg, Moses, and Tyano (1989) examined interrater, test–retest, and parent–child agreement using the K-SADS-P. Among their sample of 70 adolescents (age range = 11 to 18, mean age = 16.3 years) were 22 cases of schizophrenia. Interrater and test–retest reliabilities for the entire sample were both .78 (kappa statistic), an excellent level of agreement. More importantly for this review, 19 items that make-up the hallucinations and delusions symptom scale were examined separately for interrater and test–retest reliability. They obtained an intraclass correlation coefficient of .98 and .84, respectively, again showing high levels of reliability for these symptoms.

The previous data, although very limited in scope, suggest that schizophrenia in adolescence can be diagnosed with adequate reliability using a semistructured clinical interview that thoroughly explores a wide range of psychotic symptoms. The situation for younger children, however, is even more limited. Russell and colleagues (1989) incorporated the psychosis section of the K-SADS-P into a semistructured interview we have called the Interview for Childhood Disorders and Schizophrenia (ICDS). It differed from the standard K-SADS by the addition of detailed inquiries into autism, pervasive developmental disorders, and schizotypal personality disorder (see Russell et al., 1989, for a more complete description). In conjunction with the development of the ICDS, test–retest reliability using videotaped interviews was measured in a subsample of 23 children, all below the age of 12. The kappa agreement for principal DSM-III diagnosis for the 23 children was .88. Seven of 23 prepubertal children received a diagnosis of schizophrenia. There was independent diagnostic agreement on all seven cases. There was disagreement between schizotypal personality disorder and schizophrenia on one additional case. Although the sample was very small, we also examined kappa agreement at the DSM-III criteria level and found good to barely acceptable levels of agreement: characteristic delusions (any type), $k = 1.0$; characteristic auditory hallucinations, $k = .69$; thought disorder, $k = .86$; blunted or inappropriate affect, $k = .56$; and disorganized behavior, $k = .47$.

The more difficult to achieve test–retest reliability was not measured. This is an important qualification because Edelbrock, Costello, Dulcan, Kalas, and Conover (1985) demonstrated, using the more highly structured DISC interview, poor test–retest reliability for children under age 10, especially for schizoid/psychotic symptoms. However, the frequency of psychotic symptoms in the 70 children between 6 and 9 years of age in the study was not reported, and low rates of occurrence can influence reliability determinations (Robins, 1985).

In summary, empirical data concerning the reliability of diagnosis of schizophrenia occurring in children and adolescents using a structured interview approach is limited. There is relatively good evidence that adolescents who are severely ill (i.e., requiring hospitalization) can be reliably diagnosed using a semistructured interview such as the K-SADS. There is limited and conflicting evidence that a similar approach with younger children is also useful and reliable. Based on our experience (Russell et al., 1989), we would make the following recommendations for diagnostic evaluation of schizophrenia in childhood. First, a semistructured interview approach with extensive probes into psychotic symptomatology is a prerequisite for obtaining useful symptom data in the psychotic spectrum. We were impressed that if carefully questioned and if time is available to elicit extensive examples, even young children can report significant and useful information. If, however, the questions are not asked, or if one relies solely on indirect methods of inquiry (i.e., play, drawings), much important information is not revealed. We also learned that multiple sources of information (e.g., parents, therapists, teachers) are required to obtain necessary information. However, as demonstrated by rather poor levels of parent–child agreement (e.g., Apter et al., 1989), direct interview of the child is required. It was the rule rather than the exception that parents were often unaware of significant internal symptomatology, (e.g., hallucinations). Finally, we have become somewhat pessimistic that a strictly epidemiological approach, using lay raters and requiring word-for-word inquiries, will provide useful information concerning psychosis in young children. As noted previously, this diagnostic area requires careful and subtle distinctions between pathological psychotic symptoms and normal developmental phenomenon (e.g., imaginary friends). This is especially true for schizotypal children who present with subtle signs and symptoms, but who do not exhibit florid positive symptoms of psychosis. We feel that reliable diagnosis of these children will require a flexible, semistructured interview approach employing experienced clinicians, and will perhaps require several interviews over time to establish a valid diagnosis.

It is also becoming clear that special diagnostic techniques may be required for the adequate clinical assessment of thought disorder in children. As noted previously, two instruments, at least for research purposes, are now available: the Thought Disorder Index (TDI; Johnston & Holzman, 1989) and the Kiddie Formal Thought Disorder Scale (Caplan et al., 1989). The Thought Disorder Index is comprised of 21 different types of thought disturbance in weighted categories. The language sample used in the previously mentioned study was from a verbatim transcript of the Rorschach, although "in principle any extended verbal sample can provide the raw material for the TDI" (Arboleda & Holzman, 1985, p. 1007). Using this instrument the investigators noted a general decrease in thought disorder with age. They also found a three times greater level of thought disorder in psychotic children and in children born to a psychotic mother. Although clearly useful from a research standpoint, a high level of training is required to rate transcripts reliably with the TDI, thus precluding its use as a general clinical tool. The Kiddie Formal Thought Disorder Rating Scale (K-FTDS) and Story Game (SG) may have more potential as a clinical tool (Caplan et al., 1989). These investigators recognized that extended speech samples are often difficult to elicit from young children and tend not to occur during a structured clinical interview. To provide more extended language samples, they developed the SG, which consists of playing two tape-recorded stories and asking the child to answer open-ended questions about the stories. In addition, the child is asked to make-up their own story on one of four topics. The language samples are then rated with the K-FTDS. Over 80% of the children cooperated with the SG and, in general, produced better speech samples than on the direct clinical interview.

The results from these two studies are important from research and clinical viewpoints. As noted previously, thought disorder is a symptom that is a critical component of the DSM-III-R criteria, and it may be particularly difficult to assess in young children. These studies demonstrate that to assess this symptom properly, an indirect or "projective" approach may be required to obtain adequate examples of a child's thinking. To date, most of the more structured interviews do not incorporate such an indirect approach and may need to do so.

In conclusion, it is clear that a great deal needs to be done concerning the assessment of schizophrenia occurring in childhood. Semistructured interview techniques need to be tested in larger samples of children with relatively high rates of psychotic symptoms. A particular need is to evaluate the issue of test–retest reliability more carefully. The relative importance of multiple sources of diagnostic information also remains crucial. Special consideration needs to be given to the reliable assessment of thought disorder in children and adolescents. There is a dearth of supplementary diagnostic tools such as observational and self-report rating scales focusing on psychotic symptomatology. Such tools need to be developed and carefully tested. In this area, a particular need is for a simple and reliable screening tool for symptoms of schizophrenia and related disorders analogous to such instruments as the Childhood Depression Index (Kovacs, 1985) for assessing childhood depression. In a rare disorder such as schizophrenia occurring in childhood, the recruitment of a "high-risk" sample that then can be studied more intensively remains a critical research problem, and current screening instruments are inadequate for addressing this problem.

CONCLUSIONS

Despite a torturous history, real progress has been made in classifying children with childhood schizophrenia into more homogeneous subgroups. The critical distinctions between autism and schizophrenia occurring in childhood are now well-established and represent a major research and clinical accomplishment. Although interesting new evidence suggests that some children who develop schizophrenia in childhood may resemble high-functioning autistic children in their early stages of development (Watkins et al., 1988), it is equally clear that the majority do not. The converse is also true, that the vast majority of autistic children do not go on to develop schizophrenia. There appear to be no reasons to modify the basic distinction between autism and schizophrenia incorporated into DSM-III-R and ICD-9.

However, it is also clear that DSM-III-R does not deal as well with the group of highly disturbed children who do not meet criteria for either autism or schizophrenia. There is growing evidence that these difficult to classify children may fall into two general groups. On the one hand are children with atypical pervasive development disorder who most closely resemble autistic children, but who tend to function at a higher cognitive level and exhibit less pervasive and severe forms of impairment. On the other hand are a group of children who generally meet criteria for schizotypal personality disorder. This latter group of children seem to have a disturbance more closely related to the schizophrenic disorders. Gradually increasing data from the high-risk schizophrenia research may provide important and much needed knowledge concerning these children. Because of the awkwardness of using a personality disorder diagnosis in young children, this investigator recommends that a separate category in the childhood disorder section be incorporated into DSM-IV.

So-called psychotic symptoms are not pathognomonic of schizophrenia. Following adult research themes, a growing body of knowledge in children and adolescents has established that symptoms such as hallucinations or thought disorder occur in a variety of disorders in childhood and, in some children, may not even be indicative of psychopathology. This knowledge emphasizes the need for continuing phenomenological research in children which, in turn, requires the continued development of more reliable and useful assessment techniques.

A related issue is the effect of development on the expression of symptoms. We simply do not know enough about the expression of symptoms at different ages. Sophisticated cross-sectional assessments at multiple age points and even better, careful longitudinal studies, will be required to remedy this important gap in our knowledge of childhood psychopathology.

This leads to one final point. In reviewing our knowledge concerning schizophrenia and related disorders in childhood, it is clear that what is largely missing is a longitudinal perspective. For example, on cross-sectional assessment, there are clearly children who meet criteria for schizotypal personality disorder. Are these children at risk for the development of schizophrenia? If so, when? Although the study of Wolff and Chick (1980), suggests only a small number go on to develop schizophrenia, the high-risk literature suggests that schizotypal offspring of schizophrenic mothers are the most vulnerable for developing the full syndrome as adults. Clearly, a great deal more information is required to clarify this issue. An even more basic question is what happens to children who develop schizophrenia in childhood? Do they go on to resemble schizophrenic adults? How many recover? Do treatment interventions (e.g., neuroleptics) affect the course of the disorder? At the present time we do not have sufficient knowledge to answer these basic questions accurately.

This lack of knowledge concerning schizophrenia occurring in childhood is not a trivial matter. Although a rare disorder, when it occurs it is typically devastating to the child the child's family. Both children and parents suffer intensely. We need to be able to offer a sophisticated diagnostic assessment, an accurate prognosis, and proven treatment. We await the diagnostic, longitudinal, and treatment research that will allow us to improve our services to these children and their families.

REFERENCES

Achenbach, T. M. (1980). DSM-III in the light of empirical research on classification of childhood psychopathology. *Journal of the American Academy of Child and Adolescent Psychiatry, 19*, 395–412.

American Psychiatric Association (1980). *Diagnostic and statistical manual of mental disorders*. Washington, DC: Author.

American Psychiatric Association (1987). *Diagnostic and statistical manual of mental disorders* (3rd ėd., rev.) Washington, DC: Author.

Andreasen, N. C. (1979). Thought, language, and communication disorders. *Archives of General Psychiatry, 36*, 1325–1330.

Apter, A., Orvaschel, H., Laseg, M., Moses, T., & Tyano, S. (1989). Psychometric properties of the K-SADS-P in an Israeli adolescent inpatient population. *Journal of the American Academy of Child and Adolescent Psychiatry, 28* (1), 61–65.

Arboleda, C., & Holzman, P. S. (1985). Thought disorder in children at risk for psychosis. *Archives of General Psychiatry, 42,* 1004–1013.

Asarnow, J. R. (1988). Children at risk for schizophrenia: Converging lines of evidence. *Schizophrenia Bulletin, 14,* (4).

Asarnow, J. R., & Ben-Meir, S. (1988). Children with schizophrenia spectrum and depressive disorders: A comparative study of premorbid adjustment, onset pattern and severity of impairment. *Journal of Child Psychology and Psychiatry, 29,* 477–488.

Asarnow, R. F., Sherman, T., & Strandberg, R. (1986). The search for the psychobiological substrate of childhood onset schizophrenia. *Journal of the American Academy of Child Psychiatry, 25,* 601–604.

Asarnow, R. F., Tanguay, P. E., Bott, L., & Freeman, B. J. (1987). Patterns of intellectual functioning in non-retarded autistic and schizophrenic children. *Journal of Psychology and Psychiatry, 28,* 273–280.

Asperger, H. (1944). Die autistichen Psychopathen im Kindesalter. [Autistic Psychopathy of Childhood] *Archiv fur Psychiatic und Nerveukrankhheuen, 177,* 76–137.

Beitchman, J. H. (1983). Childhood schizophrenia: A review and comparison with adult onset schizophrenia. *Psychiatric journal of the University of Ottawa, 8*(2), 25–37.

Bender, L. (1947). Childhood schizophrenia: Clinical study of one hundred schizophrenic children. *American Journal of Orthopsychiatry, 17,* 49–56.

Bleuler, E. (1950). *Dementia praecox, or the group of schizophrenias.* (J. Zinkin, Trans.). New York: International Universities Press.

Bliss, E. L., Larson, E. M., & Nabashima, R. S. (1983). Auditory hallucinations and schizophrenia. *Journal of Nervous and Mental Disorders, 171,* 30–33.

Bradley, C., & Bowen, M. (1941). Behavior characteristics of schizophrenic children. *Psychiatry Quarterly, 15,* 298–315.

Cantor, S. (1988). *Childhood schizophrenia.* New York: Guilford Press.

Cantor, S., Evans, J., Pearce, J., & Pezzot-Pearce, T. (1982). Childhood schizophrenia: Present but not accounted for. *American Journal of Psychiatry, 139,* 758–762.

Caplan, R., Guthrie, D., Fish, B., Tanguay, P. E., & David-Lando, G. (1989). The Kiddie Formal Thought Disorder Rating Scale (K-FTDS). Clinical assessment, reliability and validity. *Journal of the American Academy of Child & Adolescent Psychiatry, 28*(3), 408–416.

Chambers, W. J., Puig-Antich, J., Hirsch, M., Paez, P., Ambrosini, P. J., Tabrizi, M. A., & Davies, M. (1985). The assessment of affective disorders in children and adolescents by semistructured interview. *Archives in General Psychiatry, 42,* 696–702.

Chambers, W. J., Puig-Antich, J., Tabrizi, M. A., & Davies, M. (1982). Psychotic symptoms in prepubertal major depressive disorder. *Archives of General Psychiatry, 39,* 921–927.

Costello, A. J., Edelbrock, C. S., & Costello, A. J. (1985). Validity of the NIMH Diagnostic Interview Schedule for Children: A comparison between psychiatric and pediatric referrals. *Journal of Abnormality in Child Psychiatry, 13,* 579–595.

Creak, M., Cameron, K., Cowie, W., Ini, S., MacKeith, R., Mitchell, G., O'Gorman, G., Orford, F., Rogers, W., Shapiro, A., Stone, F., Stroh, G., & Yudkin, S. (1961). Schizohrenic syndrome in childhood. *British Medical Journal, 2,* 889–890.

De Sanctis, S. (1971). On some varieties of dementia praecox. (M.-L. Osborn, Trans.) In J. G. Howells (Ed.), *Modern perspectives in international child psychiatry* (pp. 590–609). Brunner/Mazel. (Original work published 1906)

Despert, J. L. (1948). Delusional and hallucinatory experiences in children. *American Journal of Psychiatry, 104,* 528–537.

Edelbrock, C., & Costello, A. J. (1988). Structured psychiatric interviews for children. In: M. Rutter, A. H. Tuma, & I. Lann (Eds.), *Assessment and diagnosis in child psychopathology* (pp. 87–112). New York: Guilford Press.

Edelbrock, C., Costello, A. J., Dulcan, M. K., Kalas, R., & Conover, N. C. (1985). Age differences in the reliability of the psychiatric interview of the child. *Child Development, 56,* 265–275.

Egdell, H. G., & Kolvin, I. (1972). Childhood hallucinations. *Journal of Child Psychology and Psychiatry, 13,* 279–287.

Eggers, C. (1978). Course and prognosis of childhood schizophrenia. *Journal of Autism and Childhood Schizophrenia, 8,* 21–36.

Endicott, J., Nee, J., Fleiss, J., Cohen, J., Williams, J. B. W., & Simon, R. (1982). Diagnostic criteria for schizophrenia. *Archives of General Psychiatry, 39,* 884–889.

Endicott, J., & Spitzer, R. L. (1978). A diagnostic interview: The schedule for affective disorders and schizophrenia. *Archives of General Psychiatry, 35,* 837–844.

Feighner, J. P., Robins, E., Guze, S. B., Woodruff, R. A., Winokur, G., & Munoz, R. (1972). Diagnostic criteria for use in psychiatric research. *Archives of General Psychiatry, 26,* 57–63.

Fenton, W. S., McGlashan, T. H., & Heinssen, R. (1988). A comparison of DSM-III and DSM-III-R schizophrenia. *American Journal of Psychiatry, 145,* 1446–1449.

Fish, B. (1986). Antecedents of an acute schizophrenic break. *Journal of the American Academy of Child Psychiatry, 5,* 595–600.

Fish, B., & Shapiro, T. (1965). A typology of children's psychiatric disorders. I. Its application to a controlled evaluation of treatment. *Journal of the American Academy of Child Psychiatry, 4,* 436.

Freeman, L. N., Poznanski, E. O., Grossman, J. A., Buchsbaum, Y. Y., & Banegas, M. E. (1985). Psychotic and depressed children: A new entity. *Journal of the American Academy of Child Psychiatry, 24*(1), 95–102.

Garralda, M. (1984a). Hallucinations in children with conduct and emotional disorders: I. The clinical phenomena. *Psychological Medicine, 14,* 589–596.

Garralda, M. (1984b). Hallucinations in children with conduct and emotional disorders: II. The follow-up study. *Psychological Medicine, 14,* 597–604.

Gittelman, R. (1980). The role of psychological tests for differential diagnosis in child psychiatry. *Journal of the American Academy of Child Psychiatry, 19,* 413–438.

Goodwin, D. W., & Guze, S. B. (1989). *Psychiatric diagnosis* (4th ed.). New York: Oxford University Press.

Green, W., Campbell, M., Hardesty, A., Grega, D., Gadron-Gayol, M., Shell, J., & Erlenmeyer-Kimling, L. (1984). A comparison of schizophrenic and autistic children. *Journal of the American Academy of Child Psychiatry, 23,* (4), 399–409.

Group for the Advancement of Psychiatry (1966). *Psychopathological disorders in childhood: Theoretical considerations and a proposed classification* (Report No. 62, Vol. 6, pp. 250–259). New York: Author.

Gutterman, E. M., O'Brien, J. D., & Young, J. G. (1987). Structured diagnostic interviews for children and adolescents: Current status and future directions. *Journal of the American Academy of Child and Adolescent Psychiatry, 26,* 621–630.

Herjanic, B., & Reich, W. (1982). Development of a structured psychiatric interview for children: Agreement between child and parent on individual symptoms. *Journal of Abnormal Child Psychology, 10,* 307–324.

Hodges, K., Kline, J., Stern, L., Cytryn, L., & Mcknew, D. (1982). The development of child assessment schedule for research and clinical use. *Journal of Abnormal Child Psychology, 10,* 173–189.

Howells, J. G., & Guirguis, W. R. (1984). Childhood schizophrenia 20 years later. *Archives of General Psychiatry, 41,* 123–128.

Johnston, M. H., & Holzman, P. S. (1979). *Assessing schizophrenic thinking.* San Francisco: Jossey-Bass.

Kanner, L. (1943). Autistic disturbances of affective contact. *Nervous Child, 2,* 217–250.

Kanner, L. (1971). Childhood Psychosis: A historical over-view. *Journal of Autism and Childhood Schizophrenia, 1,* 14–19.

Kendler, K. S., Spitzer, R. L., & Williams, J. B. (1989). Psychotic disorders in DSM-III-R. *American Journal of Psychiatry, 146,* 953–962.

Kluft, R. (1985). *Childhood antecedents of multiple personality.* Washington, DC: American Psychiatric Press.

Kolvin, I. (1971). Studies in the childhood psychoses: I. Diagnostic criteria and classification. *British Journal of Psychiatry, 118,* 381–384.

Kolvin, I., Garside, R. F., & Kidd, J. S. H. (1971a). Studies in the childhood psychoses: IV. Parental personality and attitude and childhood psychoses. *British Journal of Psychiatry, 118,* 403–406.

Kolvin, I., Humphrey, M., & McNay, A. (1971b). Studies in the childhood psychoses: VI. Cognitive factors in childhood psychoses. *British Journal of Psychiatry, 118,* 415–419.

Kolvin, I., Ounsted, C., Humphrey, M., & McNay, A. (1971c). Studies in the childhood psychoses: II. The phenomenology of childhood psychoses. *British Journal of Psychiatry, 118,* 385–395.

Kolvin, I., Ounsted, C., Richardson, L. M., & Garside, R. F. (1971d). Studies in the childhood psychoses: III. The family and social background in childhood psychoses. *British Journal of Psychiatry, 118,* 396–402.

Kolvin, I., Ounsted, C., & Roth, M. (1971e). Studies in the childhood psychoses: V. Cerebral dysfunction and childhood psychoses. *British Journal of Psychiatry, 118,* 407–414.

Kovacs, M. (1978). *The Interview Schedule for Children (ISC),* form C. Unpublished manuscript, available from M. Kovacs, Western Psychiatric Institute and Clinics, Pittsburgh, PA.

Kovacs, M. (1985). The Children's Depression Inventory (CDI). *Psychopharmacological Bulletin, 21,* 995–998.

Kraepelin, E. (1919). Dementia praecox and paraphrenia. (R. M. Barclay, Trans.). From *Textbook of psychiatry* (8th German ed.). Edinburgh: Livingstone.

Kydd, R. R., & Werry, J. S. (1982). Schizophrenia in children under 16 years. *Journal of Autism and Developmental Disorders, 12,* 343–357.

Malenbaum, R., & Russell, A. T. (1987). Case report: Multiple personality disorder in an 11-year-old boy and his mother. *Journal of the American Academy of Child and Adolescent Psychiatry, 26* (3), 436–439.

Meltzer, H. Y., & Liberman, R. P. (1982). What is Schizophrenia? *Schizophrenia Bulletin, 8* (3), 433–437.

Nagy, J., & Szatmari, P. (1986). A chart review of schizotypal personality disorders in children. *Journal of Autism and Developmental Disorders, 16,* 351–367.

Parnas, J., Schulsinger, F., Schulsinger, H., Mednik, S. A., & Teasdale, T. W. (1982). Behavioral precursors of schizophrenia spectrum: A prospective study. *Archives of General Psychiatry, 39,* 658–664.

Parnas, J., Schulsinger, F., Schulsinger, H., Sarnoff, A. M., & Teasdale, T. W. (1982). Behavioral precursors of schizophrenia spectrum. *Archives of General Psychiatry, 39,* 658–664.

Petty, L. K., Ornitz, E. M., Michelman, J. D., & Zimmerman, E. G. (1984). Autistic children who become schizophrenic. *Archives of General Psychiatry, 41,* 129–135.

Potter, H. W. (1933). Schizophrenia in children. *American Journal of Psychiatry, 12,* 1253–1270.

Prior, M., & Werry, J. S. (1986). Autism, schizophrenia, and allied disorder. In H. C. Quay & J. S. Werry (Eds.). *Psychopathological disorders of childhood* (pp. 156–210). (3rd ed.). New York: Wiley.

Quay, H. C., & Peterson, D. R. (1983). *Interim manual for the revised behavior problem check list.* University of Miami: Authors.

Robins, L. N. (1985). Epidemiology: Reflecting on testing the validity of psychiatric interviews. *Archives of General Psychiatry, 42,* 918–924.

Rumsey, J. M., Rapoport, J. L., & Sceery, W. R. (1985). Autistic children as adults: Psychiatric, social, and behavioral outcomes. *Journal of the American Academy of Child Psychiatry, 24* (4), 465–473.

Russell, A., Bott, L., & Sammons, C. (1987, October) *Schizotypal disorder in childhood: A schizophrenic spectrum disorder?* Paper presented at the 34th Annual Meeting, American Academy of Child and Adolescent Psychiatry, Washington, DC.

Russell, A., Bott, L., & Sammons, C. (1989). The phenomenology of schizophrenia occurring in childhood. *Journal of the American Academy of Child and Adolescent Psychiatry, 3,* 399–407.

Rutter, M. (1972). Childhood schizophrenia reconsidered. *Journal of Autism and Childhood Schizophrenia, 2,* 315–337.

Rutter, M., & Lockyer, L. (1967a). A five to fifteen year follow-up study of infantile psychosis: I. Description of sample. *British Journal of Psychiatry, 113,* 1169–1182.

Rutter, M., & Lockyer, L. (1967b). A five to fifteen year follow-up study of infantile psychosis: II. Social and behavioural outcome. *British Journal of Psychiatry, 113,* 1183–1199.

Simonds, J. (1986). Hallucinations in children: Diagnostic considerations. In D. Pilowsky & W. Chambers (Eds.), *Hallucinations in children.* (pp. 17–49). Washington DC: American Psychiatric Press.

Spitzer, R. L., Endicott, J., & Robins, E. (1978). *Research Diagnostic Criteria (RDC) for a selected group of functional disorders* (3rd ed.). New York State Psychiatric Institute.

Strober, M., Green, J., & Carlson, G. (1981). The reliability of psychiatric diagnosis in hospitalized adolescents: Interrater agreement using the DSM-III. *Archives of General Psychiatry, 38,* 141–145.

Tanguay, P., & Asarnow, R. (1985). Schizophrenia in children. In R. Michaels & J. O. Cavenar (Eds.). *Psychiatry* (Vol. 2, chap. 29). New York: Lippincott.

Volkmar, F. R., Cohen, D. J., Hoshino, Y., Rende, R. D., & Paul, R. (1988). Phenomenology and classification of the childhood psychoses. *Psychological Medicine, 18,* 191–201.

Watkins, J., Asarnow, R., & Tanguay, P. (1988). Symptom development in childhood onset schizophrenia. *Journal of Child Psychology and Psychiatry, 29* (6), 865–878.

Werry, J. S. (1979). The childhood psychoses. In H. Quay & J. S. Werry (Eds.). *Psychopathological disorders of childhood* (2nd ed., pp. 43–89). New York: Wiley.

Werry, J. S., Methven, R. J., Fitzpatrick, & Dixon, H. (1983). The interrater reliability of DSM-III in children. *Journal of Abnormal Child Psychology, 11,* (3), 341–354.

Wing, L. (1981). Asperger's syndrome: A clinical account. *Psychological Medicine, 11,* 115–129.

Wolff, S. (1989). Schizoid disorders in childhood and adolescence. In C. G. Last & M. Hersen (Eds.), *Handbook of child psychiatric diagnosis* (pp. 209–232). New York: Wiley.

Wolff, S., & Barlow, A. (1979). Schizoid personality in childhood: A comparative study of schizoid, autistic and normal children. *Journal of Child Psychology and Psychiatry, 20,* 29–46.

Wolff, S., & Chick, J. (1980). Schizoid personality in childhood: A controlled follow-up study. *Psychological Medicine, 10,* 85–100.

World Psychiatric Association. (1983). *Diagnostic criteria for schizophrenic and affective psychoses.* American Psychiatric Press.

CHAPTER 3

Major Depression in Childhood and Adolescence

Joshua P. Newman
Amherst H. Wilder Foundation

Barry D. Garfinkel
University of Minnesota Medical School

Before embarking on a detailed analysis of major depression in children and adolescents, it will be useful to briefly review the historical debate on whether or not the syndrome exists in these populations. Freud's theories (1917/1950) stated that the mechanism of depression involves the introjection of a lost object and the turning against the self of aggressive impulses originally directed against the ambivalently loved lost object. The diathesis to depression in adults was created by interpersonal loss during early stages of development. From that time to the present, many psychoanalytically oriented authors have postulated that children could not experience mourning or depression. Many of these psychoanalytic theories of depression required a specific symptom or developmental condition to be present for the diagnosis to be established. This symptom or condition was necessary, but not sufficient, for diagnosis. For example, Rochlin (1959) noted that only ego-versus-superego conflicts were properly called depression. These depressions were characterized by guilt. Rie (1966) regarded the discrepancy between the person's self-representation and the wished-for concept of the self as the central conflict in depression. He viewed patients' verbal descriptions of their own mood as the most important symptom in depression. This type of reasoning led clinicians to infer that depression could not exist in children. Generally, the arguments stated that because young children did not have a sufficiently developed superego, or because children did not form stable self-concepts, then these children could not be truly depressed. Mendelson (1974) summarized the various arguments doubting the existence of mourning in children. These assertions follow a line of reasoning, not founded on clinical observation, used to argue against the existence of depression in children. These include that children: (a) do not have sufficiently developed egos, (b) lack object constancy, (c) have insufficiently developed reality testing, (d) feel sad only for short periods of time, (e) lack the capacity for sustained mourning, and (f) use regressive defenses too extensively. Both Mendelson (1974) and Garfinkel (1986) found that the empirical evidence from a large number of investigators refutes these positions.

The theoretical approaches that have "proved" that depression cannot exist in children appear to be based on circular reasoning. The reasoning is as follows: Observations of adults have led to the designation of certain attributes to be central to depression—children who use different or immature defenses do not conform to this central attribute model (e.g., no superego/no guilt; no object constancy/no mourning; etc.)—therefore, children cannot be truly depressed. These approaches assume that for depression to be clinically present, a specific developmental psychological milestone had to be achieved. A number of secondary questions were directed at this premise. For example, would mentally retarded individuals experience depression because they may not progress through these psychological mechanisms? Are all adults who experience depression examined to see that they have achieved these mental mechanisms? Needless to say, mentally retarded individuals do indeed suffer depression (Sovner & Hurley, 1983) and many adults who are depressed have not achieved object constancy (Greenacre, 1971) or specific superego development. Mendelson (1974), referring to the arguments against the existence of depression in children, noted: "Reading their arguments, one has the same kind of bemused feeling that one might have reading a well-reasoned text arguing against the possibility of heavier-than-air machines while flying across the Atlantic" (p. 160).

PSYCHOLOGICAL THEORIES

Problems associated with the recognition of childhood depression arose from other sources as well. One source of these problems involved etiology. There are a number of biological theories of causation, as well as several, for lack of a better term, psychological theories. Two of the psychological theories of depression, the learned helplessness and cognitive models, are reviewed here. The biological theories are discussed in a subsequent section.

The phenomenon of learned helplessness was first observed in dogs subjected to inescapable electric shocks (McKinney, 1984). The animals learned that no response prevented the shocks and, subsequently, they stopped trying altogether. According to Lennerlof (1988), Abramson, Seligman, and Teasdale (1978) reformulated the theory because it did not account for self-esteem loss, or the chronicity and generalization of depressive symptoms. In the revised theory, an individual makes a causal attribution to explain negative life experiences. These attributions can be perceived by the individual as specific or global; personal or universal; transient or chronic helplessness. According to the revised theory, these attributions lead to decreased self-esteem and depression. Brewin (1985) noted "associations between self-esteem and self-blame for failure in the predicted direction" (p. 298).

However, Brewin (1985) found only limited empirical support for learned helplessness as a cause of depression. Brewin reviewed five models exploring the relationship between negative attributions and depression. These models had different cause-and-effect relationships between the cognitions and the mood state, as well as the role of stressful life events in producing depression. Brewin found good support for depressive attributions leading to the *maintenance* of depression, but conflicting data supporting attributions leading to the *onset* of depression. In particular, negative attributions frequently disappeared with the resolution of the depression (Hamilton & Abramson, 1983; Lewinsohn, Steinmetz, Larson, & Franklin, 1981). In addition, studies demonstrating the feasibility of models involving negative attributions leading to depression have a design flaw—the studies do not rule out the possibility that depression causes negative attributions (Brewin, 1985).

Similar to the learned helplessness theory is the cognitive model as originally proposed by Beck (1970). Eelen and Van Den Bergh (1986) summarized the key features of the model, noting that central to depression is the cognitive triad: (a) negative views of the self, the world, and the future, (b) stable cognitive patterns or schemata, and (c) cognitive errors. These ways of thinking lead to dysphoria that, in turn, causes behavioral symptoms.

Hammen, Adrian, and Hiroto (1988) tested this etiological theory by investigating 79 children at risk for depression with an initial and 6-month follow-up. Initially, children of unipolar depressed women were found to have significantly more depression and negative explanatory styles than children of medically ill or normal mothers. At follow-up, one third of all children had a diagnosable disorder. Initial diagnostic status was the strongest predictor of depression at follow-up. However, neither the negative attributional style nor the interaction of attributions and stress were predictive of depression at follow-up.

The psychological theories, which are perhaps the most widely studied, have attempted to define the central features of depression based on theory alone. In addition, these hypotheses imply a specific etiology of depression with their own cardinal mechanism initiating a chain reaction of symptoms, resulting in the depressive symptom complex. Furthermore, the learned helplessness and cognitive models, by defining the etiology of the syndrome, suggest a certain type of treatment that would be directed specifically to this pathogenic mental mechanism. Unfortunately, the various reductionist models have oversimplified the problem of etiology. The contradiction of these theories by other explanations and empirical observations are evidence to this assertion. However, though these theories are not complete working models of depression, they are windows into specific aspects of the syndrome. The models form a framework from which certain assumptions about depression may be studied. Negative self-attributions may not be causal in depression, though they appear to play a major role in its perpetuation (Brewin, 1985). The theories emphasize the need for a clearer definition of what symptoms constitute depression and have led to therapies that appear to be effective for some types of depression—cognitive-behavioral therapy perhaps providing the best example.

DIAGNOSIS OF DEPRESSION IN CHILDHOOD AND ADOLESCENCE

Cantwell (1983c) described four hypotheses on the existence of depression in childhood:

1. Depression does not exist in childhood.
2. Depression in children "consists of certain unique characteristics and symptoms which occur in addition to those that indicate depression."
3. Depression in children presents as other symptom complexes, such as conduct or attention deficit disorder, which completely mask the designated criteria (i.e., "masked depression" or "depressive equivalents").
4. Depression in children manifests with the same symptoms as seen in adults.

The first hypothesis, suggesting that depression does not exist in this age group, was reviewed earlier and is not based on clinical observations, but rests on fitting children into a theory. The third hypothesis, the masked depression hypothesis, has been challenged by a number of authors. Carlson and Cantwell (1979) studied 28 children who were found to meet criteria for depression. Although 14 of the 28 had a preexisting psychiatric disorder, the symptoms of these coexisting disorders did not completely mask the symptoms of depression.

The second and fourth hypotheses presented by Cantwell (1983c) are very similar. Carlson and Kashani (1988) examined depressive symptoms from infancy to adulthood by compiling the data of Baker, Dorzob, Winokur, and Cadoret (1971) (N = 100 adult psychiatric inpatients), Ryan, Puig-Antich, Ambrosini, Rabinovich, Robinson, Nelson, Iyengar, and Twomey (1987) (N = 187 children ages 6-18), and their own data (N = 1,000 preschool-age children). They found that: (a) anhedonia, (b) diurnal mood variation, (c) hopelessness, (d) psychomotor retardation, and (e) delusions increased in frequency with increasing age. Depressed appearance, low self-esteem, somatic complaints and hallucinations decreased in frequency as they grew older. Only depressed mood, decreased concentration, sleep disturbance, and suicidal ideation were seen with approximately the same frequency at each age group. The study demonstrates that the presentation of depressive symptoms in patients who are still maturing changes, depending on the age and development of the individual. Nonetheless, many diagnostic criteria utilized in recent years employ the same symptom lists to establish the diagnosis of depression for patients of any age—consistent with Cantwell's fourth hypothesis.

DESCRIPTION

The use of diagnostic criteria has evolved over time. These diagnostic systems date back to Feighner (1972) and include DSM-III, Weinberg, and Research Diagnostic Criteria. DSM-III-R criteria have subsequently evolved from these four original classification systems. These diagnostic schemes represent the general consensus for what constitutes a major depressive episode. These criteria, unfortunately, have important distinctions. The Feighner and Research Diagnostic Criteria were developed for research to help select more homogeneous samples, whereas DSM-III and DSM-III-R were designed to be used clinically to avoid false negatives (Cantwell, 1983c). The latter clinical schemes attempt to use strict criteria to identify all "true" clinical cases and not to miss someone who is actually depressed. The use of different criteria often identified different populations.

In Table 3.1, the Feighner, Research Diagnostic Criteria, DSM-III, and DSM-III-R criteria for major depression are displayed to highlight their similarities and differences. There is a major difference between the first two classification systems and DSM-III and DSM-III-R. The latter two systems require fewer symptoms for the diagnosis to be made.

TABLE 3.1
Diagnostic Criteria

Criteria	*Feighner*	*Research Diagnostic Criteria*	*DSM-III*	*DSM-III-R*
Mood disturbance	Dysphoric mood—depressed, sad, discouraged, despondent, irritable	One or more periods of dysphoric mood, pervasive loss of interestor pleasure	Dysphoric mood or loss of interest or pleasure in all or almost all usual activities	*DSM-III-R* lists dysphoric mood and loss of interest in usual activities symptoms as part of the symptom list [see Table 2.2c]. However, either (a) depressed mood or (b) loss of interest symptoms are required.
Other symptoms	Five of eight:	Five of eight:	Four of eight including three of the first four in children under age 6	Five of nine:
Appetite/Weight	Poor appetite and weight loss	Increase or decrease appetite, weight	Poor appetite or weight loss—failure to make expected weight gain; or increased appetite or weight	>5% weight loss or gain, or failure to make expected gains; or change in appetitie nearly every day
Sleep	Insomnia or hypersomnia	Insomnia or hypersomnia	Insomnia or hypersomnia	Insomnia or hypersomnia
Energy	Loss of energy	Loss of energy or fatigability	Loss of energy or fatigue	Loss of energy or fatigue

Agitation or retardation	Agitation or retardation	Psychomotor agitation or retardation	Observable psychomotor agitation or retardation —hypoactivity in children <6	Observable psychomotor agitation or retardation
Loss of interest or pleasure	Loss of interest in usual activities—including sex drive	Loss of interest in social contact or sex	Loss of interest or pleasure in usual activities or decrease in sex drive—apathy in children <6	Subjective or objective markedly diminished interest or pleasure in all or almost all activities
Guilt	Self-reproach or guilt	Self-reproach or guilt	Worthlessness, self-reproach, or excessive guilt—may be delusional	Worthlessness or inappropriate guilt—may be delusional
Concentration	Diminished ability to think or concentrate	Diminished ability to think or concentrate	Complaints or evidence of diminished ability to think or concentrate	Subjective or objective diminished ability to think or concentrate
Suicide	Recurrent thoughts of death or suicide	Recurrent thoughts of death or suicide	Recurrent thoughts of death or suicide; or suicide attempt	Recurrent thoughts of death—not simply fear of dying, suicidal thoughts, suicidal plan or attempt
				Subjective or objective depressed mood—may be irritability in children and adolescents

(Continued)

TABLE 3.1
(Continued)

Criteria	*Feighner*	*Research Diagnostic Criteria*	*DSM-III*	*DSM-III-R*
Duration	1 month	1 week	2 weeks	2 weeks
Functional impairment		Sought help, medicated, functional impairment		
Delusions, hallucinations, or thought disorder	Must diagnose as Schizoaffective	May have mood congruent psychotic features with depressive symptoms, but not thought disorder, auditory hallucinations, or delusions or hallucinations discordant for depression	Neither mood incongruent delusions nor hallucinations dominate the clinical picture in the absence of depressive symptoms	Delusions or hallucinations have not been present for 2 weeks in the absence of depressive symptoms
Other exclusions			Not superimposed on schizophrenia, schizophreniform disorder, or a paranoid disorder, not due to any organic mental disorder or uncomplicated bereavement	An organic factor has not intitiated or maintained the disturbance. Symptoms not due to uncomplicated bereavement, not superimposed on schizophrenia, schizophreniform disorder, delusional disorder or psychotic disorder NOS

Note: Adapted from "Depression in Childhood: Clinical Picture and Diagnostic Criteria" by D. Cantwell, 1983, in D. Cantwell & G. Carlson (Eds.), *Affective Disorders in Childhood and Adolescence* (pp. 10–11), New York: Spectrum. Adapted by permission.

(Note that DSM-III and DSM-III-R criteria are basically the same.) The Feighner and Research Diagnostic Criteria produce a more homogeneous sample, but exclude patients that would qualify for a DSM-III-R diagnosis of depression. The Feighner and Research Diagnostic Criteria have a lower sensitivity for diagnosing major depression than DSM-III or DSM-III-R. Another difference in these classification systems relates to the degree to which DSM-III and DSM-III-R criteria for depression indicate how children may meet specific criteria in mood, appetite/weight, psychomotor agitation/retardation, and anhedonia symptom areas. This allows for more diagnoses of depression to be made in these ages and thus greater sensitivity of diagnosis. The Feighner criteria require that symptoms be present for 1 month, whereas DSM-III and DSM-III-R criteria demand 2 weeks. Finally, DSM-III and DSM-III-R allow for the diagnosis of depression to be made as long as delusions, hallucinations, bizarre behavior, or thought disorder are not present for 2 weeks in the absence of the constellation of depressive symptoms. Feighner and Research Diagnostic Criteria handle these symptoms differently, as shown in Table 3.1. In summary, DSM-III and DSM-III-R criteria create a more heterogeneous sample because they require fewer associated symptoms for depression than Feighner or Research Diagnostic Criteria. However, these systems have the advantage of being more sensitive for identifying clinical cases of depression, resulting in fewer false negatives.

To make the diagnosis of major depression, all four of these classification systems rely on five or six of the same nine symptoms along with requiring some type of depressed mood symptom. Children who have been irritable, waking frequently at night, lethargic, not making their expected weight gain, and isolative for several weeks, as well as adults who have been sad with profound diurnal mood variation, sleeping and eating more than usual, pacing constantly, and commanded by auditory hallucinations to kill themselves, could both be diagnosed as having a major depressive episode by DSM-III-R criteria. Obviously, these two cases must be subtypes of major depression that have vastly different criteria.

CLASSIFICATION

Various subclassifications of major depressive disorder have been proposed and studied to demonstrate their construct validity. The *International Classification of Diseases, Injuries and Causes of Death* (ICD-9), a system used by the World Health Organization, has 17 subclassifications of affective disorders. A special category of depression exists (i.e., disturbance of emotions specific to childhood and adolescence—misery and unhappiness disorder) to distinguish adult and nonadult diseases. DSM-III-R distinguishes major depressions for the presence of psychotic features, melancholia, association with bipolar affective states, and seasonal pattern. The DSM-III-R criteria for melancholia, a subtype of depression, are five of the following: (a) loss of interest in activities, (b) lack of reactivity to pleasurable stimuli, (c) worse depression in the morning, (d) early morning awakening, (e) psychomotor agitation or retardation, (f) anorexia or weight loss, (g) no significant personality disturbance prior to the first major depressive episode, (h) at least one previous episode followed by a complete recovery, and (i) previous good response to specific and adequate antidepressant therapy. Although melancholia is commonly observed in elderly patients, it has been recognized as occurring in young children as well.

Other classification systems have been proposed for adult and childhood depression. Two are reviewed briefly here and involve the primary versus secondary and the endogenous versus reactive concepts. Cantwell and Carlson (1983) reported the results of a study in which they subgrouped 28 children and adolescents meeting DSM-III criteria for depression into primary (i.e., without pre-existing psychiatric or medical illness) and secondary groupings. Subjects with secondary depression were more chronically disturbed, but there were no significant differences in the presence or absence of depressive symptoms between the two groups. The 5-year follow-up data on half of the sample revealed that while depressive symptoms resolved in those with secondary depression, there was a persistence of their "primary" problems. Most of the primary depressive group, however, were doing well on follow-up. Though the classification system may prove helpful, the authors concluded that "data are insufficient to draw conclusions about the validity of the primary/secondary distinction in childhood depression" (p. 36).

The endogenous versus reactive distinction in depression also is important because of its highlighting the nature versus nurture argument. Endogenous depression corresponds to psychotic and melancholic subgroupings. These depressions are typically more acute, have a better prognosis, and respond better to antidepressant therapy. Reactive depression corresponds to the old "neurotic" classification of DSM-II (Cantwell & Carlson, 1983). According to Cantwell and Carlson (1983), factor analysis has shown:

> As with endogenous depressions, there is a characteristic set of symptoms that tend to occur in those individuals with the neurotic-reactive type depression. These include a precipitating factor, a sudden onset, a

clinical picture of irritability, mood that is responsive to the environment, and features such as self-pity, hysterical personality features, and immaturity. (p. 27)

Winokur (1986) described two possible examples of environmental events potentially causing a depressive episode: (a) complicated bereavement and (b) early parental loss. Winokur found that one third of bereaved persons meet criteria for major depression. He also noted that the causal role of early parental loss reported in many studies is in question because most of the studies did not control for depression in the deceased parent. He noted that this "may indicate a familial (genetic) factor just as much as an environmental factor" (p. 69).

Because of the aforenoted studies, major depression, as a diagnosis, has evolved from the psychoanalytically oriented entity with implied etiology to the heterogeneous syndrome defined by various modern classification systems. The effort to find subcategories of major depression has met with limited success. Although the subclassification dichotomies, such as primary/secondary and endogenous/reactive, have not been shown to be generally useful in classifying all major depressive episodes, the use of these systems may help delineate aspects of depression and guide research and treatment in specific areas.

BIOLOGICAL BASIS OF CHILDHOOD DEPRESSION

The research on major depression has extended to include biological factors. Included are neurochemical, neuroendocrine, sleep, and genetic data.

Neurotransmitters

The research on the role of various neurotransmitters in the etiology of depression has yielded conflicting data. Norepinephrine (NE) and its principle breakdown product 3-methoxy-4-hydroxyphenylglycol (MHPG) along with epinephrine (EPI) have been shown to be altered in some patients with Major Depression. Schildkraut (1965) hypothesized that depressed patients had decreased levels of NE available at important synapses in the brain. The decreased level of normetanephrine—another breakdown product of NE—in the urine of psychomotorically retarded depressed patients, which corrected with administration of imipramine, a tricyclic antidepressant, helped Schildkraut support the hypothesis. However, although Christensen, Vestergaard, Sorensen, and Rafaelsen (1980) noted decreased levels of EPI in the cerebral spinal fluid (CSF) of depressed patients compared to controls, the investigators did not find changes in CSF NE. Garver and Davis (1979) noted that some depressed subjects had decreased levels of MHPG in their urine.

Evidence supporting increased levels of NE in the etiology of depression has also been collected. Wyatt, Portnoy, Kupfer, Snyder, and Engelman (1971) noted increased levels of NE and EPI in the plasma of depressed patients. Koslow and colleagues (1983) noted increased levels of MHPG in the CSF of depressed patients. Roy, Pickar, De Jong, Karoum, and Linnoila (1988) found similar results in their sample of cortisol-nonsuppressor depressed subjects. Finally, Bunney and Davis (1965) and Roy et al. (1988) found increased urinary excretion of NE in their samples of depressed patients.

Animal models have also been used for NE research. Hughes and associates (1984) noted that rats, exposed to inescapable shock in a learned helplessness paradigm, had decreased levels of NE and serotonin in the locus ceruleus (LC)—the major location of noradrenergic cell bodies in the brain. However, direct electrical stimulation of the LC or use of alpha-2 adrenergic antagonists—which would be expected to produce elevated levels of NE—produced anxiety, hypervigilance, and an inhibition of exploratory behavior in rats (Redmond & Huang, 1979).

Serotonin has also been postulated to be altered in depression. Garver and Davis (1979) noted decreased CSF 5-hydroxyindoleacetic acid (5-HIAA)—the principle breakdown product of serotonin—in 26%–29% of depressed subjects who did not have decreased urinary levels of MHPG. This supported the authors' hypothesis of NE- and serotonin-type depressions. Quintana (1988) found that platelet monoamine oxidase activity was higher in depressed subjects than in controls, presumably leading to a lower availability of serotonin. The enzyme activity was significantly decreased by imipramine—a tricyclic antidepressant—administration. This finding is supported by observations that decreased CSF 5-hyxdroxyindoleacetic acid (5HIAA), the major metabolite of serotonin, correlates with suicide, aggression, and high impulsivity. In contrast, Koslow et al., (1983) showed that there are some depressed patients who have elevated 5HIAA in the CSF. However, neither Roy et al. (1988) nor Christensen and colleagues (1980) found any difference in CSF levels of 5-HIAA in depressed subjects compared to controls.

To make matters more complicated, other neurotransmitters have been reputed to be altered in depression, including acetylcholine (Kasper, Moises, & Beckman, 1981), gamma aminobytyric acid (GABA) (Lloyd, Morselli, & Bartholini, 1987), and dopamine (Kashani & Cantwell, 1983). Furthermore, Seifert, Foxx, and Butler (1980) noted that CSF concentrations of the primary breakdown products of dopamine and serotonin are much higher in children than adults. If the relative balance of neurotransmitters changes as a function of age, it seems plausible that the neurochemistry of depression in children might differ from that of adolescents or adults.

A hypothesis emerges from the neurotransmitter research on depression suggesting that subtypes of depression have different underlying neurochemical alterations. For example, one type of depression might have elevated levels of several neurotransmitters, including NE and serotonin, whereas another subtype might be characterized by diminished levels of serotonin only. Alternatively, or adding to the complexity of this hypothesis, the neurochemical alterations may change as a function of the stage of the depressive illness. An example might be a depressive illness that involved an initial drop in the levels of serotonin followed by chronic variations in the levels of several neurotransmitters. Although no simple etiologic model of depression emerges from existing neurotransmitter research, studies of neurotransmitters in carefully diagnosed subgroups of depressed children followed into adolescence and adulthood could clarify our understanding of the underlying neurochemistry of depression.

Neuroendocrine Changes—Growth Hormone

Research concerning neuroendocrine changes in depression has also been undertaken (Puig-Antich, 1987). The hypothalamic-pituitary axis is thought to be involved in the regulatory of many symptoms of depression, including sleep and appetite (Gold, Goodwin, & Chrousos, 1988). This system receives input from a number of neurotransmitters, including norepinephrine, acetylcholine, serotonin, and dopamine. Growth hormone, produced in the anterior pituitary, has been measured following a number of pharmacological challenges in depressed and normal subjects. These changes in growth hormone appear to change depending on the age of the subjects tested (Jensen & Garfinkel, 1990). In 50% of unipolar endogenous depressions, Puig-Antich (1987) noted a blunted increase in growth hormone in response to insulin-induced hypoglycemia (GH-ITT) compared to normals. Puit-Antich, Novacenko, and associates (1984) found significantly more blunting of GH-ITT in prepubertal endogenous depressives compared to nonendogenously depressed children and psychiatric controls. The effect seems to be most pronounced in those individuals with low levels of circulating sex hormones, particularly prepubertal or postmenopausal subjects. Prepubertal depressives (Puig-Antich, Goetz, et al., 1984), but not depressed adolescents (Puig-Antich, 1987), were noted to hypersecrete growth hormone in the first one-third of sleep. Puig-Antich (1987) further noted that stimulation of growth hormone by desmethylimipramine (DMI) did not distinguish between depressed and nondepressed prepubertal subjects, though adolescents with endogenous or nonendogenous depression have a blunted GH-DMI. Jensen and Garfinkel (1990) examined the growth hormone response of depressed children and adolescents to clonidine and L-Dopa. Postpubertal adolescent depressives were not different from normal adolescents or published normative values for growth hormone response to either clonidine or L-Dopa. However, Tanner stage I and II depressed children had significantly decreased growth hormone peak responses to clonidine.

As with the neurotransmitter research, data collected on growth hormone regulation identifies biological differences across various age and developmental groups. Growth hormone is influenced by a number of neurotransmitter systems that may change as a function of age. In addition, the sex hormone status of the individual may account for the differential response of growth hormone to a variety of challenges in depressed subjects. Whatever the particular mechanism, biological differences are observed across age groups. The disparate findings in prepubertal children and older subjects may be explained by a number of separate or co-existing hypotheses. Growth hormone regulation may be different in younger children. Alternatively, the biochemical changes in adults and children with depression may be different. Irrespective, the growth hormone responses in childhood or adult depression do not support the notion that these depressive illnesses are identical in every possible way.

Cortisol

Considerably more research has been done on the cortisol system in depressed patients. Cortisol is involved in stress responses and, like growth hormone, is regulated in part by the hypothalamus (corticotropin releasing hormone, CRH) and anterior pituitary (adrenocorticotropic hormone, ACTH). Puig-Antich (1987) noted that only 10% of the sample of the endogenously depressed prepubertal children that he studied hypersecreted cortisol. Overall, there were no differences observed in the 24-hour cortisol secretion of endogenously or nonendogenously depressed children, psychiatric controls, or normal controls. Cortisol secretion appeared to vary directly with age and activity, and may be related to stress.

Another method of investigating the cortisol system is the Dexamethasone Suppression Test (DST). Roy and colleagues (1988) found that post-dexamethasone levels of cortisol were correlated with CSF MHPG levels in depressed adult subjects. He stated "these significant correlations from studies of CSF, plasma and urine suggest that dysregulation of the noradrenergic system and the hypothalamic-pituitary-adrenal axis occur together in depression" (p. 852). In prepubertal children with Major Depression, there are considerable differences across studies concerning DST sensitivity and specificity. While Livingston and Martin-Cannici (1987), Petty, Asarnow, Carlson, and Lesser (1985), and Weller, Weller, Fristad, Preskorn, and Teare (1985) all showed sensitivities greater than 80% in their inpatient depressive samples, other investigators have noted much lower rates. For example, Geller, Rogol, and Knitter (1983) found only 2 of 14 outpatient subjects with depression were DST escapers, and Puig-Antich (1987) reported no difference between depressed children, nondepressed psychiatric controls and normal controls on the DST. Furthermore, the specificity observed by Preskorn, Weller, Hughes, Weller, and Bolle (1987) (i.e., 0% of normal controls and 15% of psychiatric controls were nonsuppressors on the DST) has not been universally replicated. For example, Livingston and Martin-Cannici (1987) had 8 of 12 patients with anxiety disorders with cortisol hypersecretion on the DST, and Petty and colleagues (1985) found no differences between Major Depression and dysthymia on the DST.

In adolescents, Puig-Antich (1987) noted that an outpatient sample had very low rates of DST nonsuppression. Evans, Nemeroff, Haggerty, and Pedersen (1987) found 43% of nonmelancholic depressed adolescents hypersecreted cortisol, whereas 16% of nondepressed adolescents with other psychiatric diagnoses were nonsuppressors. Four of the five subjects in the latter group were found to be depressed on follow-up. Klee and Garfinkel (1984) found 40% sensitivity and 92% specificity in a sample of 33 inpatient children and adolescents. Nonsuppressors were noted to have trends toward less appetite loss and more suicidal ideation. Nonsuppressors also had significantly more family members with depression, and all had experienced one or more previous episodes of depression. Cortisol suppression was associated with significantly more conduct problems, as measured on the Minnesota Multiphasic Personality Inventory (MMPI).

As with growth hormone research, no definitive etiologic model of depression involving cortisol was identified by the research completed thus far. Cortisol secretion in depressed subjects appears to vary with age (Puig-Antich, 1987). DST research has shown that diagnoses, other than depression, may have elevated cortisol levels after dexamethasone administration. Furthermore, lower rates of DST escape in children with depression are observed compared to those seen in adults (Geller, Rogol, & Knitter, 1983; Puig-Antich, 1987). Although the DST may be a useful measure in specific groups of depressed children, at this time it does not appear to be a biological marker for depression.

Malatonin

There are fewer studies in adults and children concerning changes in melatonin secretion. Melatonin is secreted by the pineal gland, and it appears to be very important in the regulation of wake–sleep cycles. Cavallo, Holt, Hejazi, Richards, and Meyer (1987) noted that the pineal gland "is intimately related to the endogenous pacemaker and functions in a rhythmic manner, whereas affective illness is accompanied by disruption of various biological rhythms" (p. 395). Cavallo and colleagues (1987) studied the secretion of melatonin in 9 depressed male children, ages 7 to 13, and 10 normal controls. Nocturnal melatonin secretion was found to be significantly decreased in children with major depression or dysthymia compared to controls. The pattern of nocturnal secretion was noted by the investigators to be different than that noted by Nair, Hariharasubramanian, and Pilapil (1983) in adults with major depression. In that study, depressed patients were found to have an earlier onset of the nocturnal melatonin surge and an earlier peak melatonin secretion than controls. Although these results further support the hypothesis that the underlying neurochemical changes in children and adults with depression are probably not the same, the conclusions that can made are limited by the paucity of data in children.

Sleep

Sleep studies in depressed children have also been investigated. This type of study is relevant because sleep disturbance is one of the cardinal symptoms used in establishing the diagnosis of major depression. The regulation of sleep may involve the same neurotransmitters that mediate major depression. Cholinergic supersensitivity may mediate shortened rapid eye movement (REM) latency (Puig-Antich, 1987).

The use of sleep EEGs in adults, adolescents, and children has yielded more data suggesting that the underlying neurochemistry of major depression in these age groups is different. Emslie, Roffwarg, Rush, Weinberg, and Parkin-Feigenbaum (1987) noted no differences on any sleep measures between 10 pre- and 7 postpubertal depressed inpatients. However, these children, ages 9 to 14, had a significantly increased number of arousals, increased REM latency, increased REM time, increased REM activity, and an increased number of REM periods when compared with normal controls. Whereas these findings are similar to those observed in adults, Puig-Antich (1987) found, in a series of studies, different results. Prepubertal children with major depression were not found to be significantly different than nondepressed neurotic children or normal controls on any sleep EEG measure. There was no evidence of shortened REM latency, increased REM density, decreased slow wave sleep, or decreased sleep efficiency—various characteristics of adult Major Depressive Disorder. Puig-Antich (1987) concluded:

> It is therefore likely that the lack of sleep findings during major depressive episodes in youngsters is secondary either to maturational factors that modify the first NREM period, or the neurobiology of the initiation or maintenance of the depressive episode in predisposed individuals, or in the higher genetic loading characteristic of very early onset affective illness. (p. 512)

Puig-Antich and colleagues (1983) examined the sleep EEG data in 28 prepubertal children during episodes of major depression, after 4 months of full recovery, and at least 1 month off medications. Recovered depressive children showed significantly shorter first REM period latency and greater numbers of REM periods when compared to controls or when compared with themselves during their depressive episodes. Overall, sleep continuity was found to be improved in recovered subjects.

Although it may be argued that some data on sleep EEGs indicate similar changes across age groups, there are ample data that appear to refute that hypothesis. The observations of REM latency shortening in recovered depressive children is in the opposite direction from what the adult data predict. Though further studies would be helpful to clarify some of the conflicting results, it appears that sleep EEG measures will yield different results in children and adults because of the maturational difference inherent in the underlying neurochemistry. It is also likely that only a small proportion of depressed children continue in their adult life to have depression.

GENETICS

There have been a number of studies that have supported a genetic transmission of some affective disorders. These studies are of three types: (a) twin studies, which attempt to demonstrate a higher concordance rate for an illness or trait in monozygotic (MZ) as compared to dizygotic (DZ) twins, (b) adoption studies, which compare the incidence of an illness or trait in the biologic versus the adoptive parents, and (c) family aggregation studies, which show a higher incidence of an illness or trait in the families of affected probands as compared to the families of normal probands. Twin studies of affective disorders have involved bipolar probands more than unipolar index cases. Kringlen (1985) showed higher concordance rates for bipolar disorder in monozygotic (67%) than in dizygotic twins (9%). It is noteworthy that the concordance in MZ twins is not 100%, suggesting that other factors besides genetics are involved in the etiology of affective disorder. Torgersen (1986) studied 151 same-sex pairs of twins in which 10 index subjects had bipolar disorder, 92 had major depression, 35 had dysthymic disorder, and 14 had adjustment disorders; by design, relatively few psychotically depressed subjects were included. There was a 75% concordance rate for bipolar disorder in MZ twins compared to a 0% rate in the DZ co-twin of a bipolar proband. There was a nonsignificant difference in the concordance rates for major depression in MZ (27%) and DZ (12%) twins. However, when all affective disorders (i.e., bipolar, unipolar, etc.) were considered in the co-twin of the proband with major depression, there was a significant difference in MZ (45%) versus DZ (22%) subjects. When the depressed probands are divided into psychotic versus nonpsychotic depressions, the psychotic depression group approaches significance for concordance rates for MZ (40%) and DZ (15%) co-twins. This difference would likely become significant with a larger number of subjects. The study supported the hypothesis that unipolar and bipolar affective disorder are distinct illnesses, as very few co-twins of unipolar disorder had bipolar diagnoses. There was no significant difference in the concordance rates of MZ and DZ twins with respect to dysthymia or adjustment disorder. Data from twin studies supports a genetic transmission of bipolar and severe forms (i.e,., psychotic) of unipolar affective disorder. No support for a genetic basis of milder forms of depression, dysthymia, or adjustment disorders was obtained.

Mendelwich and Rainer (1977) found that 31% of the biological parents of 29 bipolar adoptees had affective disorders, most of which were major depression. However, only 12% of the adoptive parents had affective disorders. Normal adoptees had low rates of affective disorders in both biological (2%) and adoptive (10%) parents. Cadoret (1978) noted more unipolar depression in children whose biological mothers had affective disorders (i.e., 3 of the children of 8 mothers) compared to children of biological mothers with nonaffective psychiatric disturbances (i.e., 4 of the children of 75 mothers). In contrast, Von Knorring, Clonigen, Bohman, and Sigvardsson (1983) found that 5 of the 98 biological parents of 56 depressed children had been treated at some time in their lives for affective disorder. This was not significantly different compared to the biological parents of normal controls of whom 11 of 203 had, at some time, been treated for affective disorders. In fact, the study noted a stronger relationship between affective disorder in the adoptees and their adoptive parents than with the biological parents. Overall, the contradictory data are equivocal for a purely genetic etiology for depression.

Family aggregation studies do not necessarily imply a genetic basis of transmission, as environmental factors contributing to affective illness may also be important. Careful evaluation demonstrates that affective disorders are not the only ones that aggregate in families. Puig-Antich (1987) noted an age-corrected morbidity of .5 for first-degree relatives over 16 years of age for depressed prepubertal probands. Keller and associates (1986) found depression in 24% of the children from 37 families in which at least one of the parents was depressed, usually with major depression. More severe or chronic depression in the parent was associated with greater impairment in the children. In addition, depression in the mother, but not in the father, was associated with greater impairment in the children. This latter observation could support X-linked transmission of depression and/or environmental factors being important in the etiology of depression.

Hammen and colleagues (1987) looked at 84 children, ages 8 through 16, or 58 mothers with affective disorder, chronic medical illness, or no illness. Children of affectively ill mothers had higher lifetime rates of psychopathology and higher lifetime rates of affective disorders than those from parents with medical illness or normal control parents. When both biological parents had affective disorders, the risk of affective disorder in their offspring was 80%, whereas the rate was 67% to 70% if only one parent was affected. Hierarchical multiple regression analysis was then used to assess relative contributions to outcome measures. Though marital status and socioeconomic status were not significant contributors to the outcome of the children in the study, a measure of chronic strain did contribute to the prediction of follow-up diagnosis at 6 months as well as follow-up depression scores. Furthermore, the lifetime diagnostic status of the mother added to the prediction of lifetime diagnostic status in the children. The mother's current mood contributed to the prediction of the child's current and lifetime diagnostic status, as well as behavior at school. This study supports both genetic and environmental etiological factors of affective disorder in children.

Weissman and associates (1987) found that the early (i.e., less than age 20) onset of depressive symptoms were noted to be associated with increased family loading among relatives. In addition, the lifetime prevalence of major depression in the 125 children of 56 depressed proband parents was 37.6%. This figure is 1.6 times higher than that of the 95 children of 35 normal control parents. The children of depressed probands had a peak age of onset of 12.0 and a mean age of onset of 12.7 for depression. Children of normal probands had a peak onset of depression after age 15.0 and a mean age of onset of depression at 16.8.

Depression was not the only diagnosis found to be increased in the children of depressed probands. Alcoholism was found in 16.8% of these children, a rate 2.3 times that seen in children of normal probands. Overall, children with a depressed parent had 1.4 times as many DSM-III diagnoses as those of control subjects. This study supports the comorbidity findings of other studies and demonstrates a difference in familial aggregation based on age. However, the effects of the environment cannot be ruled out, as 25% of the fathers in the depressed proband group were widowed, divorced, or separated, compared to only 7% of the fathers of the control population.

Livingston, Nugent, Rader, and Smith (1985) studied the relatives of inpatient depressed and anxious children, and found that only 28% of the relatives of depressed children and 29% of the relatives of the anxious children had no psychiatric diagnoses. There was no difference in the types of psychopathology between the two groups, with depression and alcoholism being the two most common diagnoses.

The role of the environment and genetics in the transmission of depression is far from being completely understood. Existing evidence indicates that something is inherited, though it does not appear to be depression alone. A vulnerability or diathesis to psychopathology of a nonspecific type may be what is inherited. Depressive illness in children appears to have a different pattern of inheritance, though this appears only to be by a matter of degree. Environmental effects cannot be minimized and should not be overlooked when explaining etiology. More behavioral genetic studies in this area could clarify these early findings.

COMORBIDITY

Another important aspect of affective disorders in childhood is comorbidity. Comorbidity is the coexistence of more than one axis I diagnosis or disorder simultaneously observed in a specific patient. The coexistence of the two disorders does not in any way suggest etiology or the order of occurrence.

Dysthmic Disorder

Kovacs, Feinberg, Crouse-Novak, Paulauskas, and Finkelstein (1984) found that 79% of the children, ages 8 to 13, with major depression in their follow-up studies had other concurrent psychiatric diagnoses.

Over three-quarters of the depressed children in the study had other prominent symptoms. A question that arises is whether "pure" major depressive disorder (MDD) is a common enough entity that it should be diagnosed separately from its associated nondepressive symptoms. Kovacs found more children had both MDD and dysthymic disorder (DD) than MDD alone. Kovacs also observed that the onset of the symptoms of these other diagnoses are as likely to occur before, as during or after, the onset of the depressive symptoms. This refutes the notion that the depression, when it exists with other symptom clusters, needs to be a reaction to the stress of the other "primary" diagnoses, and that the depressive symptoms are more or less central or predominant when compared with the nonaffective comorbid symptomatology. The most common comorbid diagnosis Kovacs found in those children with MDD with dysthymic disorder.

Thirty-eight percent of the MDD children met criteria for DD. In addition, 93% of the children with DD had other concurrent psychiatric diagnoses, including MDD in 57% of them. Kovacs questioned whether MDD and DD might, in the preadult years, represent variations of the same illness. Table 3.2 lists the DSM-III-R criteria for dysthymic disorder.

TABLE 3.2
DSM-III-R Criteria for Dysthymia

A. Depressed mood (or can be irritable mood in children and adolescents) for most of the day, more days than not, as indicated either by subjective account or observation of others, for at least two years (one year for children and adolescents)
B. Presence, while depressed, of at least two of the following:
   1. Poor appetite or overeating
   2. Insomnia or hypersomnia
   3. Low self-esteem
   4. Poor concentration or difficulty making decisions
   5. Feelings of hopelessness
C. During a two-year period (one year for children and adolescents) of the disturbance, never without the symptoms in A for more than two months at a time
D. No evidence of an unequivocal major depressive episode during the first two years (one year for children and adolescents) of the disturbance
E. Has never had a manic episode or an unequivocal hypomanic episode
F. Not superimposed on a chronic psychotic disorder, such as schizophrenia or delusional disorder
G. It cannot be established that an organic factor initiated and maintained the disturbance

Note: From *Diagnostic and Statistical Manual of Mental Disorders* (3rd. ed., rev., p. 232) by American Psychiatric Association, 1987, Washington, DC: Author.

Anxiety Disorders

Another group of disorders commonly found in children with MDD are the anxiety disorders. Kovacs, Feinberg, Crouse-Novak, Paulauskas, and Finkelstein (1984) found that 33% of the MDD children and 36% of the DD group had anxiety disorders. Related evidence for the depressive and anxiety disorder overlap comes from work with school phobics or school refusers. Tisher (1983) found that 75% of her 40 school phobic children, ages 9 to 16, had separation problems. The author noted that school refusers had significantly more anxiety and depression than attenders. Waldron, Shrier, Stone, and Tobin (1975) noted the same percentage of separation problems in 35 school phobic children, ages 5 to 12, compared to 32% in a group of neurotic controls. In addition, 42% of the school refusers had low self-esteem and 64% were rated to have at least moderate anxiety. Bernstein and Garfinkel (1986) used depression and anxiety rating scales to help evaluate 26 chronic, treatment-resistant school refusers. There were 13 children with MDD, and 5 with adjustment disorder with depressed mood, with the latter children differing from the MDD children only by virtue of an identifiable precipitating stressor. Sixteen of the children had anxiety disorders, with 13 of these patients having concurrent affective disorders. Six children had conduct disorder; of these six, two had only conduct disorder, two had an affective disorder concurrently, and two had affective and anxiety disorders concurrently with conduct disorder. Depressed children had elevated scores on depression and anxiety rating scales, while anxious patients had high scores on only the anxiety scales. When children were divided into low and high anxiety groups for data analysis, children with high anxiety were indistinguishable from depressed children.

These studies offer support for the large overlap in affective and anxiety disorder diagnoses. The high proportion of school refusers with MDD also raises the possibility that school phobia may represent a subgroup of major depression, or at least a behavioral marker for major depressive disorder.

Conduct Disorder

Conduct Disorder has also been seen as a frequent concurrent diagnosis with MDD. Puig-Antich (1982) found that 16 of 43 prepubertal males with MDD met criteria for Conduct Disorder. Eleven of 13 of the MDD conduct disordered patients who were treated with imipramine had resolution of their conduct symptoms after "adequate antidepressant response." Kovacs, Feinberg, Crouse-Novak, Paulauskas, and Finkelstein (1984) found conduct disorder predating depressive symptoms in 7% of the MDD and 11% of the DD children. Welner, Welner, and Fishman (1979) found that 4 of 9 secondarily depressed children had antisocial personality disorder. Finally, Jensen, Burke, and Garfinkel (1988) cited 11 studies showing either increased behavior problems in depressive children or depressive symptoms in children with disruptive behavioral disorders.

Attention Deficit-Hyperactivity Disorder

The data supporting the overlap between Attention Deficit-Hyperactivity Disorder (ADHD) and affective disorders are not as convincing. Comings and Comings (1987) found no depression in a sample of pure ADHD children. Kovacs, Feinberg, Crouse-Novak, Paulauskas, and Finkelstein (1984) found that no child with MDD had ADHD, but did find that 14% of those with DD and 9% of those with adjustment disorder with depressed mood had concurrent diagnoses of ADHD. Jensen, Burke, and Garfinkel (1988) looked at 35 male subjects, ages 8 through 18. Twelve subjects had MDD, 12 had ADHD, and 11 were normal controls. Subjects were selected so that they would not have both MDD and ADHD or meet criteria for another diagnosis, such as conduct disorder or oppositional defiant disorder. Children were rated on depression, conduct, and hyperactivity rating scales. On the Children's Depression Rating Scale (CDRS), only the depressed group was noted to have elevated overall scores. The ADHD children, however, scored significantly higher than normal controls on a cluster of four symptoms: social withdrawal, guilt, weeping and depressed affect. Depressed children scored higher than controls, but lower than ADHD subjects on the Connors Parent Questionnaire (CPQ). Finally, the MDD and ADHD groups had significantly elevated scores compared to controls on the Jesness Manifest Aggression Scale, a self-report measure rating conduct disordered symptoms. The study demonstrated that there is significant overlap in conduct, ADHD and depressive symptoms even when samples are selected to minimize this effect.

There are other comorbid diagnoses that have been described less frequently in the literature. Chemical dependency was noted by Welner and colleagues (1979) in 1 of 12 bipolar adolescents and 2 of 16 unipolar adolescents at the time of their 10-year follow-up as young adults. Weissman, Beck, and Kovacs (1979) noted that drug addiction was associated with high rates of suicide and depression. Of 384 suicide attempters, ages 17 to 63, 86 were dependent on drugs. Hopelessness was the main determinant of suicide in the abusers and nonabusers. Anorexia nervosa has also been noted to overlap with depression. Eckert and Mitchell (1986) noted that "anorexia nervosa may be an atypical affective disorder occurring in adolescent females at a time in their lives when body image issues are important" (p. 172). They noted family history, follow-up, and biological marker studies that supported this premise. They also observed that anxiety and depression were frequently observed in anorectic patients. Welner and colleagues (1979) noted 1 of 9 secondary depressions was associated with anorexia. Finally, Tourette Syndrome (TS) has been shown to coexist with affective symptoms. Comings and Comings (1987) noted that 22.9% of TS patients had elevated scores on a depression scale compared to 2.1% of controls. As mentioned previously, ADD children were not found to have elevations on this scale, though 20% of subjects with ADD associated with TS had elevated scores. Similar results were noted with a manic symptom scale and the Beck Depression Inventory. The investigators noted that the severity of the TS was directly associated with higher depression scores, although the depression was not thought to be a secondary reaction to vocal or motor tics.

PREVALENCE/INCIDENCE

The prevalence and incidence of MDD have been carefully examined in several large studies in adults. Robins and associates (1984) found that the lifetime risk for MDD in relatives of psychiatrically well surgical patients in Iowa is 8.1%, with a threefold greater risk seen in women. In Weissman and Meyer's study (1978) in New Haven, the lifetime risk was 18.0%, with females having twice the risk. The point prevalence (i.e., all those in a population who have the diagnosis at any one point in time) of MDD has been reported to be between 1.0% and 10.8% by Boyd and Weissman (1981) in their review. Finally, Winokur (1986) found that the annual incidence (i.e., the number of new cases per year) of MDD varies between 247 and 7,800 cases per 100,000 people per year.

The same type of data has, to a lesser degree, been collected in children. According to Kaplan and Sadock (1985), 10-year-olds have depression or dysthymia at 1.7% rate, 15% of adolescents have affective disorders by a general psychiatric survey, and only 5% of prepubertal children have various affective disorders. Rutter (1971) found a 1-year prevalence of 1.4 per every 1,000 young individuals. Rutter also noted that the risk of MDD at 14 years of age is three times greater than the risk at age 10. Nissen (1971) noted 1.8% of 6,000 German children had severe depression. Kashani and Simonds (1979) observed major affective disorder in 1.9% of 103 children. Finally, Kashani and colleagues (1983) noted major affective disorder in 1.8% of 641 New Zealand 9-year-olds.

LIFETIME COURSE

Evidence presented thus far indicates that depressive illness occurs rarely in children, but more commonly postpubertally. The symptom criteria in children and adolescents can be identified in the same way as that in adults. One question remains, however: Is childhood MDD a harbinger of adult MDD? There are some long-term follow-up studies of MDD in childhood and adolescence that provide data that can help determine whether MDD in childhood is continuous with adult depressive illness. Rutter (1971) noted, "The matter requires further investigation but so far the findings all indicate that it is quite uncommon for child psychiatric disorders of any type to develop into depressive illness in adult life" (pp. 13–14). Twelve years later, Cantwell (1983b) concluded: "In general, there does not seem to be evidence of a specific 'predepressive' disorder occurring in childhood, that does not manifest itself as adult-like depression, which can identify a group of children who are likely to develop depression later in life any more than there seems to be a pre-schizophrenic picture" (p. 276).

Four years later, Puig-Antich (1987) observed that "no study has yet followed prepubertal depressive children up into adulthood, the key test of the continuity hypothesis" (p. 509). Not all investigators have reached the same conclusions. Poznanski, Kraheneuhl, and Zrull (1976) showed that one half of the 10 prepubertal children with MDD she followed 6½ years later had depression; the clinical picture resembled that found in adults. Kovacs, Feinberg, Crouse-Novak, Paulauskas, and Finkelstein (1984; Kovacs et al., 1984) followed children, ages 8 to 13, for up to 9 years. Twenty-six children had MDD, 19 DD, 9 MDD-DD, and 11 adjustment disorder with depressed mood (ADDM). Controls were selected to have diagnoses similar to the non-affective comorbid diagnoses of the study sample and included 15 with ADD, 5 with conduct disorder, 7 with oppositional defiant disorder, and 3 with anxiety disorders. The MDD group improved maximally by 5 to 18 months following the initial episode. The remission rate was not related to sex of the subject, nor the presence of concurrent anxiety or dysthymic disorder. Early age of onset of MDD was associated with longer recovery times. Interestingly, recovery rates varied in the opposite direction from what one might predict with regard to the presence or absence of treatment; that is, subjects treated for their symptoms took longer to recover, on average, than untreated patients. Perhaps most significant, the study found that 69% of the children with DD developed their first MDD episode within 5 years of diagnosis, and 72% of children with MDD had recurrent episodes of depression within 5 years. No MDD developed in $5\frac{1}{2}$ years of follow-up in the ADDM group, and only one control subject developed a depressive episode in 9 years of follow-up.

Several other studies addressed the continuity of childhood depression into adulthood. Herjanic (1976) found only 2 of 20 children with previous diagnoses of depression showed affective disorders at follow-up. Penot (1971), though finding a favorable course in the follow-up of 17 depressed children, found no continuity of depressive diagnoses over time. Chess, Thomas, and Hassibi (1983) conducted a prospective study of 133 infants followed to young adulthood, of whom only 6 had clinical depression that continued into adulthood. It appears likely that only a small number of children with childhood depression will continue to have depression over a long follow-up period. Although there may be many types of childhood depression, only some will be a chronic remitting type. At this time, there are no distinguishing features among the various types of childhood depression that would indicate those that will not progress and those that will extend into adulthood.

The outcome in adolescent MDD was investigated by Strober and Carlson (1982), who followed 60 patients for 3 to 4 years. Subjects were hospitalized for MDD for the first time between the ages of 13 to 16. Twelve subjects developed mania in the interval from the initial hospitalization to the time of follow-up. Of the 48 nonbipolar outcomes, 10 had repeat episodes and 1 failed to recover. The nonbipolar group had more suicidality, weight gain, irritability, self-pity, and demanding behavior. The bipolar outcome group tended to have rapid onset of symptoms, psychomotor retardation, delusions and hallucinations, self-reproach, bodily concerns, and diminished concentration. Tricyclic antidepressant response was rated as unequivocally positive in 53% of the unipolar versus 18% of the bipolar group. Bipolar outcomes were associated with more familial loading, more three-generational histories of affective disorder, and a greater risk in first- and second-degree relatives than the nonbipolar outcomes.

Similarly, Welner and colleagues (1979) reported on the 10-year follow-up of 110 adolescents who were hospitalized with psychiatric diagnoses at ages 12 to 19. Seventy-seven subjects were available for follow-up. The 33 subjects who were not available for interview did not have significantly different initial diagnoses than the study sample. Twelve of the 77 subjects had bipolar diagnoses at follow-up. Initial diagnoses in this group were 4 with unipolar depression, 7 with bipolar depression, and 1 undiagnosed with a mean age of onset of symptoms for the group of 15 years. One patient was alcoholic, 3 committed suicide, 9 were socially disabled, and all had poor work histories. Sixteen of the 77 subjects had unipolar diagnoses at follow-up. Fifteen of the 16 had the same diagnosis initially. The mean age of onset of the symptoms was age 15. Five subjects had only the initial episode of depression, 1 had seven hospitalizations with reportedly normal baseline functioning between episodes, 10 had only partial remissions, 2 became alcoholic, and 1 committed suicide.

Kandel and Davies (1986) followed-up 1,004 adolescents 9 years after being surveyed as a public high school sample from New York state. Elevated depressed mood in adolescence did not predict psychiatric problems in males, but it did for females. High depressive symptom rating scores in adolescence did predict high symptom scores, less closeness with spouses and parents, delinquent behavior, and health problems in male and female subjects at follow-up. Female subjects with high depressive symptom scores had an increased propensity to contact a mental health professional and did so 1½ years sooner on the average than students with normal scores. Female subjects with high scores were also more likely to drop out, more likely to divorce, less likely to be working, and more likely to be parents. Male subjects with high depressive score were found to be less likely to be employed.

Though these studies do not completely answer questions about the continuity of MDD from childhood to maturity, there appear to be at least some depressions in children that are predictive of similar symptoms in adulthood. The risk of *bipolar* affective disorder seems to be increased significantly, as does depressive recurrence rates for *early-onset* MDD. Finally, affectively ill children have profound emotional and social consequences from their affective disorders, although the relative contribution of comorbid diagnoses is unclear.

SUICIDE

Another aspect of depressive disorders in children is rate of suicide. Suicidal behavior includes those who succeed in killing themselves and those who make attempts with and without lethal intent. Though there are important distinctions between suicide attempters and suicide completers, they are often arbitrary. Suicidal gestures can be "accidentally" fatal and, conversely, attempts at self-destruction can fall short. In addition, Otto (1971) and Dahlgren (1977) demonstrated that 1 in 10 attempters will ultimately succeed. Garfinkel (1986) suggested that the extent of suicide is underestimated in children, especially those who are younger. Garfinkel, Froese, and Hood (1982) noted higher mortality rates in a group of children and adolescents who had attempted suicide than in a control population of medically and surgically ill children.

Carlson (1983) reported that in 1975 there were 12.2 suicides per 100,000 people, ages 15 to 24, and the rate of suicide in those under 15 is 0.8 per 100,000, with males having higher rates than females for all age groups. Carlson reported that there are many more attempts than completed suicides and females have a lifetime prevalence of attempts twice that of males. Garfinkel (1986) noted:

> The unique features of completed suicide in children and adolescents not only distinguish it from suicide in adults, but also provide specific characteristics that allow clinicians to identify the young individual at risk for self-destructive behavior. . . . The identification of a successful plan is a critical factor that is both intelligence and age dependent and explains the steep increase in the suicide rate according to age. (pp. 318–319)

Garfinkel further described a number of features of suicide in children and adolescents including: (a) familial clustering of suicide and suicide attempts, (b) ability to use abstract reasoning, (c) much lower unemployment, (d) higher socioeconomic status, (e) marital breakdown, and (f) psychiatric disorders not limited to affective disorders.

Suicide and suicidal behavior are not exclusively depressive phenomena. As was previously mentioned, Weissman, and colleagues (1979) found that hopelessness was the key predictor of suicide in drug abusers versus nonabusers. Cantwell (1983b) observed that affective disorders account for 50% of suicides and alcoholism for another 25%. Carlson (1983) reported on the outcome of psychiatrically referred children with respect to suicidal issues. It was noted that suicidal ideation increased as a function of age. Of the 12 children who felt seriously suicidal, 83% met criteria for major depressive disorder. These children tended to have more familial loading for depression and alcoholism, and tended to have higher scores on a depression rating scale. Forty-five children denied suicidal ideation and met few criteria for major depression. Forty-five children only thought about suicide, with one third of these children having depressive disorders, one third having behavioral disorders, and the other third having other psychiatric disorders. The investigators concluded that "the intensity of suicidal ideation was usually a reflection of the *severity* of depression but that many youngsters who thought about suicide were not depressed at all" (p. 346).

Suicide completion and attempts are possible outcomes of several illnesses in children, adolescents, and adults, depression being the most common. Suicidal thoughts and attempts may be symptoms of affective disorders, behavioral disorders, psychotic disorders, personality disorders and substance abuse disorders, although in DSM-III-R only affective disorders and borderline personality have suicidal ideation/attempts in their diagnostic criteria. Suicidal behavior and thinking may represent different psychopathological disorders in children compared to adults. More often, depression in adults is a precursor of suicide (Murphy, 1983). Thus, the investigation of suicidal thoughts or behaviors must include a wide range of psychiatric symptoms, not just affective symptoms. The maturation of the patient and the influence of that person's particular environment are also very important.

ASSESSMENT

The assessment of psychiatric disorders in children should include multiple sources of information, when available, and encompass a broad range of children's psychopathology, even if the presence of certain symptoms (e.g., suicidal ideation, dysphoria) suggests a specific diagnosis. The various sources include parental reports, teacher reports, peer or other family reports, and clinician assessments. Self-reports, even in prepubertal children, are a key part of the assessment. Puig-Antich, Chambers, and Tabrizi (1983) observed that "most clinical researchers interested in prepubertal and/or adolescent depression strongly emphasize the diagnostic importance of the interview with the child" (p. 161). However, Cantwell (1983a) noted:

> There are certain symptoms that tend to be reported more by parents and likewise certain symptoms that tend to be reported more by children. Thus, when using the semi-structured interviews with parents and children, it is not surprising that different results will be obtained, and some clinical judgment must be used in assessing where the weight should be put with each individual child-parent combination. (p. 149)

In addition, the motivation of the child or parent to report symptoms may be lacking. For example, children or adolescents, invested in not staying overnight in a hospital, may deny even incapacitating symptoms that they may be experiencing. Therefore, an evaluation using information obtained from a variety of sources is more likely to result in an accurate clinical picture of the patient.

Though data from dynamic formulations may be therapeutically useful, this type of assessment does not address specific symptoms. In the case of childhood depression, Puig-Antich, Chambers, and Tabrizi, (1983) noted that "although the assessment of psychodynamic constellations and symbolic meanings through play is an important part of the general psychiatric assessment of children, it has only a minor, if any, role to play in the clinical process of arriving at a diagnosis of major depression" (p. 160). In addition, special attention should be given to identifying comorbid diagnostic symptoms. A selection of tests listed in Table 3.3 would meet the requirements for an adequate work-up, such as the following.

TABLE 3.3
Instruments used to Assess Childhood Depression

Instrument	*Source*	*Comment*
Diagnostic Interview for Children and Adolescents (DICA)	Herjanic, Herjanic, Brown, & Wheatt (1975)	Lifetime assessment of psychopathology with the child as the source—Puig-Antich, Chambers & Tabrizi (1983)
Diagnostic Interview Schedule for Children (DISC)	Costello, Edelbrock, Dulcan, Kalas, & Klaric (1984)	Very structured interview made for use for non-clinician with the child as the source—Cantwell (1983a)
Schedule for Affective Disorders and Schizophrenia for School-Age Children (Present Episode) (K-SADS-P)	Puig-Antich & Chambers (1978)	Data from the parent and child is included for assessment of current psychopathology—Puig-Antich, Chambers, & Tabrizi (1983)
(K-SADS-E)	Puig-Antich, Orvaschel, Tabrizi, & Chambers (1980)	Epidemiological version which measures past and present episodes—Orvaschel, Puig-Antich, Chambers, Tabrizi, & Johnson (1982)
Interview Scheduled for Children (SCI)	Kovacs (1978)	Lifetime psychopathology is assessed and a separate parent form is available—Puig-Antich, Chambers, & Tabrizi (1983)
(DISC-P)		Parent form of (DISC)
(DICA-P)		Parent form of (DICA)

TABLE 3.3
(Continued)

Instrument	*Source*	*Comment*
Self-Reports		
Children's Depression Scale (CDS)	Lang & Tisher (1978)	48 items
Children's Depression Inventory (CDI)	Kovacs & Beck (1977)	Ages 7–17
Birleson	Birleson (1981)	18 items
Parent Reports		
Children Behavior Checklist	Achenbach & Edelbrock (1979)	Symptoms grouped by factor analysis rather than presorted by diagnostic criteria
(CDS-P)		Parent version of (CDS)
Personality Inventory for Children	Wirt, Lachar, Klinedinst, & Seat (1977)	
Teacher Reports		
Children Behavior Checklist	Achenbach & Edelbrock (1979)	
Clinician Reports		
Children's Depression Rating Scale (CDRS)	Poznanski, Cook, & Carroll (1979)	Items similar to Hamilton scale used in adults
Other		
Peer Nomination Inventory of Depression (PNID)	Lefkowitz & Tesini (1981)	

Note. Adapted from "Major Affective Disorders in Children and Adolescents" by B. Garfinkel, 1986, in G. Winokur & P. Clayton (Eds.), *The Medical Basis of Psychiatry* (p. 315), New York: Saunders Publishing.

These instruments have been selected because they sample a number of perspectives, including child, parent, and teacher, and employ clinical judgment as well. These instruments have been extensively used, thus there are norms for many, allowing for the clinician to compare a particular child to others. Clinicians cannot, at this time, rely on psychometric methods in making the diagnosis of major depression. Such methods can, however, tell a clinician whether or not a particular child is highly symptomatic for affective symptoms. These instruments represent a marked advance over the era when highly projective tests (e.g., Rorschach, etc.) were used to diagnose disorders in children and adolescents.

A number of criticisms about these methods of symptom identification rest on the fact that they rely too heavily on the cognitive component of depression (e.g., Beck Depression Inventory). They also demonstrate a gender bias, with girls finding it easier to self-disclose their personal problems and symptoms. Furthermore, there is observer bias, with parents and others are being good identifiers of internalizing disorders, such as affective and anxiety symptoms. Nevertheless, as clinicians, we routinely rely on a *self-report* (BDI or Birleson), a *parent* report (DISC-P), and a *clinician* scale (CDRS). These measures would be regarded as a minimum sampling of symptoms necessary to formulate a diagnosis of affective disorder.

CONCLUSION

This chapter has outlined evidence suggesting that depression in childhood and adolescence exists and does so in a form that is recognizable, meeting largely the same criteria observed in adults. Diagnostic criteria, such as DSM-III-R, outline a number of symptoms that constitute major depressive disorder in children, adolescents, and adults. These criteria allow for some variability in the presentation of the depression. There are several different subclassifications in adult depression that may predict treatment response. Less is known about types of depression in children. One major problem that remains is determining whether the illness in children corresponds to or predicts the same illness in adults.

There is biological evidence from neurochemical, endocrinological, sleep, and genetic transmission studies of children that does not replicate data obtained from adult depressives. In addition, data from treatment studies, a thorough review of which is beyond the scope of this chapter, fail to replicate the results of treatment studies in adults. In a review of this literature, Puig-Antich (1987) found that 30 out of 50 double-blind studies of adults with major depression demonstrated superiority of imipramine to placebo. In contrast, though some studies of antidepressants in children showed positive benefits when compared to placebo (Frommer, 1967; Preskorn, Weller, & Weller, 1982; Geller, Perel, Knitter, Lycaki, & Farocki, 1983; Petti & Connors, 1983), other studies with double-blind, placebo controls did not support the benefits of tricyclic antidepressants in prepubertal children (Puig-Antich 1987) and adolescents with major depression (Ryan et al., 1986). In general, the response to antidepressants is less profound and the rates of placebo response higher (e.g., 68% in Puig-Antich's 1987 study) than the response found in adults.

These differences in childhood and adult depression may indicate that depression, although phenomenologically similar, affects children in unique ways. Any discrepancy in the clinical presentation or response to treatment may be caused by differences in the underlying substrate, developmental level, and selected individual differences. A certain genotype or predisposition to depressive illness may lead to several phenotypes, all with sufficient symptoms in common, so that they all meet DSM-III-R criteria for depression (i.e., a single disease entity in this model).

There is an alternative explanation for the biological differences between childhood and adult depression; depression in childhood is a different disease entity (or entities), bearing only a phenotypic or behavioral relationship with its adult counterpart. Different genotypes may lead to a common or similar phenotype. If one expands this concept further, depression might be a final common pathway for a number of psychopathological processes. A person with severe chronic environmental stress, another with a medical illness, a third with three generations of familial loading for depression, and one who suffered the death of an ambivalently loved parent all might exhibit the behavioral criteria for depression. This diagnosis would be descriptive, but not necessarily predictive of treatment response or outcome.

One method of differentiating these underlying models would be to follow youngsters longitudinally. Do childhood depressives later become depressed adults? Do recurrent or chronic depressive episodes in children lead to personality disorders in adult patients? There is not, unfortunately, enough data to answer these questions at this time.

Are there psychopathological states in children, although not defined as affective disorder by DSM-III-R, which may be precursors of the adult form of major depression? This possibility, along with the high incidence of comorbid diagnoses in childhood depression, raises another possible model of depressive disorders in children. If the majority of children with depression have more diagnoses than simply major depression, should these other diagnoses determine the most common symptom pictures? Does the subclassification of affective disorders have different etiological, biological, treatment response, and outcome correlates? This model would allow different genotypes to correspond to different phenotypes, some of which may be recognizable by DSM-III-R diagnostic criteria.

One patient might meet diagnostic criteria for depression in childhood but, as an adult, the natural history of the disease would have caused a change in symptoms such that the patient no longer satisfies criteria for major depression (i.e., recurrent childhood depressive episodes leading to a personality disorder or bipolar affective disorder in its adult form). Other patients might have various depression/comorbid diagnoses symptom pictures that might lead to readily recognizable depressive episodes in adults with different features, depending on the childhood comorbid diagnosis (e.g., children with depression and school phobia might become adults with major depression and panic attacks; children with depression and conduct disorder might become adults with major depression and antisocial personality disorder). Other patients might have psychopathology that does not meet criteria for major depression (e.g., dysthymic disorder, school phobia, conduct disorder), but that results in major depressive disorder in adulthood. Finally, a patient could have an illness related to depression but that never manifests itself as major depression in the patient's lifetime, such as anorexia nervosa, dysthymia, or borderline personality disorder. This model might be made more complicated by allowing for each genotype and childhood phenotype to have multiple potential adult outcomes.

Until there is sufficient evidence from studies that follow carefully diagnosed children through adulthood, it is unlikely whether any model explaining the relationship and continuity of childhood and adult depression will be established. There is an advantage to focusing on comorbid diagnoses as a potential method of subclassifying childhood depression because it relies on the same type of data as is needed to make the diagnosis of major depression. In addition, there is a degree of face validity for a hypothesis that children with major depression and conduct disorder will have different natural histories than children with major depression alone or with other comorbid diagnoses.

Future research with childhood depression should strive for complete and accurate diagnostic procedures utilizing *multiple sources* of informants and *standardized and normed instruments*. Special attention should be given to *nonaffective* symptomatology. Diagnostic groups used in studies should be made as homogeneous as possible and control groups should be chosen carefully. Research comparing subgroups of depressed children could explain the inconsistent results found in all areas of childhood depression studies. Finally, when these comparisons are made, subgroupings may be validated and thus included or not included in future diagnostic systems. For example, it may be necessary to recognize and give special diagnostic attention to common comorbid conditions, such as conduct disorder/affective disorder and anxiety/affective disorder. Eventually, there may be some utility in having a separate diagnostic number and category for these combinations.

DSM-III-R and DSM-III should be viewed as advances over all other conceptual frameworks in understanding affective disorders. This advantage is based on the use of observable behaviors with specific developmental deviation and impairment criteria. The three basic limitations of these diagnostic schema are that the same names are used for adult and childhood disorders, giving the false impression to clinicians that they are the same disorder and that the childhood version will continue into the adult form. This occurs infrequently. Second, it does not take into account frequent comobid (i.e., coexisting) diagnoses (e.g., conduct disorder/affective disorder). Third, there are individuals who have very intense brief depressions that would not meet duration criteria (Angst & Dobler-Mikola, 1985). Unfortunately, people who get depressed do not fit into all the categories as they have been presently constructed. It may be necessary to add additional entities. These criticisms must be viewed as not taking away from a very advanced classification system—far better than anything previously available.

This chapter has attempted to make a number of points regarding the diagnosis of major depression in children and adolescents. First, the core group of symptoms that constitute depression in childhood are very similar to those in adults. In addition, biological studies in depressed children have yielded more discrepant results than studies in depressed adults that may reflect different processes and/or different underlying biological substrates, depending on age. Moreover, there is value in understanding comorbid diagnoses as a potentially key factor in the understanding of etiology, biology, natural history, treatment response, and subclassification of major depressive disorder in childhood. Finally, following carefully diagnosed children into adulthood will be the ultimate test of any model of depression in children and adolescents.

REFERENCES

Abramson, L. Y., Seligman, M., & Teasdale, J. D. (1978). Learned helplessness in humans: Critique and reformulation. *Journal of Abnormal Psychology, 87*, 49–74.

Achenbach, T., & Edelbrock, C. (1979). The child behavior profile: II Boys aged 12–16 and girls aged 6–11 and 12–16. *Journal of Consulting Clinical Psychology, 47*, 223–233.

American Psychiatric Association (1987). *Diagnostic and statistical manual of mental disorders* (3rd ed., rev.) Washington, DC: Author.

Angst, J., & Dobler-Mikola, A. (1985). The Zurich study: A prospective epidemiological study of depressive, neurotic and psychosomatic syndromes: IV. Recurrent and non-recurrent brief depression. *European Archives of Psychiatry and Neurological Sciences, 234*, 408–416.

Baker, M., Dorzob, J., Winokur, G., & Cadoret, R. (1971). Depressive disease: classification and clinical characteristics. *Comprehensive Psychiatry, 12*, 354–365.

Beck, A. T. (1970). Cognitive therapy: Nature and relation to behavior therapy. *Behavior Research and Therapy, 7,* 184–200.

Bernstein, G., & Garfinkel, B. (1986). School phobia: The overlap of affective and anxiety disorders. *Journal of the American Academy of Child Psychiatry, 25,* 235–241.

Boyd, J., & Weissman, M. (1981). Epidemiology of affective disorders: A re-examination and future directions. *Archives of General Psychiatry, 38,* 1039–1046.

Birleson, P. (1981). The validity of depressive disorders in childhood and the development of a self rating scale: A research report. *Journal of Child Psychology and Psychiatry, 22,* 73–88.

Brewin, C. (1985). Depression and causal attributions: What is their relation? *Psychological Bulletin, 98,* 297–309.

Bunney, W. E., & Davis, J. M. (1965). Norepinephrine in depressive reactions: A review. *Archives of General Psychiatry, 13,* 483–494.

Cadoret, R. S. (1978). Evidence for genetic inheritance of primary affective disorder in adoptees. *American Journal of Psychiatry, 135,* 463–466.

Cantwell, D. (1983a). Assessment of childhood depression: An overview. In D. Cantwell & G. Carlson (Eds.), *Affective disorders in childhood and adolescence* (pp. 146–156). New York: Spectrum.

Cantwell, D. (1983b). Childhood depression: Issues regarding natural history. In D. Cantwell & G. Carlson (Eds.), *Affective disorders in childhood and adolescence* (pp. 266–278). New York: Spectrum.

Cantwell, D. (1983c). Depression in childhood: Clinical picture and diagnostic criteria. In D. Cantwell & G. Carlson (Eds.), *Affective disorders in childhood and adolescence* (pp. 3–18). New York: Spectrum.

Cantwell, D., & Carlson, G. (1983). Issues in clarification. In D. Cantwell & G. Carlson (Eds.), *Affective disorders in childhood and adolescence* (pp. 19–38). New York: Spectrum.

Carlson, G. (1983). Depression and suicidal behavior in children and adolescents. In D. Cantwell & G. Carlson (Eds.), *Affective disorders in childhood and adolescence* (pp. 335–352). New York: Spectrum.

Carlson, G., & Cantwell, D. (1979). A survey of depressive symptoms in a child and adolescent psychiatry population. *Journal of the American Academy of Child Psychiatry, 18*(4), 857–599.

Carlson, G., & Kashani, J. (1988). Phenomenology of major depression from childhood through adulthood: Analysis of three studies. *American Journal of Psychiatry, 145,* 1222–1225.

Cavallo, A., Holt, K., Hejazi, M., Richards, G. E., & Meyer, W. J. (1987). Melatonin circadian rhythm in childhood depression. *Journal of the American Academy of Child and Adolescent Psychiatry, 26*(3), 395–399.

Chess, S., Thomas, A., & Hassibi, M. 1983). Depression in childhood and adolescence: A prospective study of six cases. *Journal of Mental and Nervous Disease, 171,* 411–420.

Christensen, N. J., Vestergaard, P., Sorensen, T., & Rafaelson, O. J. (1980). Cerebrospinal fluid adrenaline and noradrenaline in depressed patients. *Acta Psychiatrica Scandinavica, 61,* 178–182.

Comings, B., & Comings, D. (1987). A controlled study of Tourette Syndrome. V. Depression and mania. *American Journal of Human Genetics, 41,* 804–821.

Costello, A., Edelbrock, C., Dulcan, M., Kalas, R., & Klaric, S. (1984). "Report on the NIMH Diagnostic Interview Schedule for Children (DISC-C)" National Institute of Mental Health, Washington, DC.

Dahlgren, K. G. (1977). Attempted suicides—35 years afterward. *Suicide Life Threatening Behavior, 7,* 75–79.

Eckert, E., & Mitchell, J. (1986). Anorexia nervosa and bulimia. In G. Winokur & P. Clayton (Eds.), *The medical basis of psychiatry* (pp. 171–181). New York: Saunders.

Eelen, P., & Van Den Bergh, O. (1986). Cognitive-behavioral models of depression. *Acta Psychiatrica Belgica, 86,* 748–759.

Emslie, G., Roffwarg, H., Rush, A., Weinberg, W. A., & Parkin-Feigenbaum, L. (1987). Sleep EEG findings in depressed children and adolescents. *American Journal of Psychiatry, 144,* 668–670.

Evans, D., Nemeroff, C., Haggerty, J., & Pedersen, C. (1987). Use of the dexamethasone suppression test with DSM-III criteria in psychiatrically hospitalized adolescents. *Psychoneuroendocrinology, 12*(3), 203–209.

Feighner, J. P., Robins, E., Guze, S. B., Woodruff, R., Winokur, G., & Munoz, R. (1972). Diagnostic criteria for use in psychiatric research. *Archives of General Psychiatry, 26,* 57–63.

Freud, S. (1950). *Mourning and melancholia in collected papers* (Vol. 4, 6th ed., pp. 152–170). London: Hogarth. (original work published 1917)

Frommer, E. (1967). Treatment of childhood depression with antidepressant drugs. *British Medical Journal, 1,* 729–732.

Garfinkel, B. (1986). Major affective disorders in children and adolescents. In G. Winokur & P. Clayton (Eds.), *The medical basis of psychiatry* (pp. 308–330). New York: Saunders.

Garfinkel, B., Froese, A., & Hood, J. (1982). Suicide attempts in children and adolescents. *American Journal of Psychiatry, 139,* 1257–1261.

Garver, D. L., & Davis, J. M. (1979). Biogenic amine hypotheses of affective disorders. *Life Sciences, 24,* 383–394.

Geller, B., Perel, J., Knitter, E., Lycaki, H., & Farocki, Z. Q. (1983). Nortriptyline in major depressive disorder in children: Response, steady-state plasma levels, predictive kinetics, and pharmacokinetics. *Psychopharmacology Bulletin, 19*(1), 62–68.

Geller, B., Rogol, A., & Knitter, E. (1983). Preliminary data on the dexamethasone suppression test in children with major depressive disorder. *American Journal of Psychiatry, 140,* 620–622.

Gold, P., Goodwin, F., & Chrousos, G. (1988, August 18). Clinical and biochemical manifestations of depression: Second of two parts. *New England Journal of Medicine, 319,* 7.

Greenacre, P. (1971). *Emotional growth: Psychoanalytic studies of the gifted and a great variety of other individuals* (Vol. 2, pp. 776–806). New York: International Universities Press.

Hamilton, E. W., & Abramson, L. Y. (1983). Cognitive patterns and major depressive disorder: A longitudinal study in a hospital setting. *Journal of Abnormal Psychology, 92,* 173–184.

Hammen, C., Adrian, C., Gordon, D., Burge, D., Jaenicki, C., & Hiroto, D. (1987). Children of depressed mothers: Maternal strain and symptom predictors of dysfunction. *Journal of Abnormal Psychology, 96*(3), 190–198.

Hammen, C., Adrian, C., & Hiroto, D. (1988). A longitudinal test of the attributional vulnerability model in children at risk for depression. *British Journal of Clinical Psychology, 27,* 37–46.

Hammen, C., Gordon, D., Burge, D., Adrian, C., Jaenicke, C., & Hiroto, D. (1987). Maternal affective disorders, illness, and stress: Risk for children's psychopathology. *American Journal of Psychiatry, 144,* 736–741.

Herjanic, B. (1976). *Follow-up study of 20 children given a discharge diagnosis of depression: St. Louis Children's Hospital.* Paper presented at the American Psychiatric Association Meeting, Miami, FL.

Herjanic, B., Herjanic, M., Brown, F., & Wheatt, T. (1975). Are children reliable reporters? *Journal of the Association of Child Psychology, 3*, 41–48.

Hughes, C., Kent, T., Campbell, J., Oke, A., Croskell, H., & Preskorn, S. (1984). Cerebral blood flow and cerebrovascular permeability in an inescapable shock (learned helplessness) animal model of depression. *Pharmacology, Biochemistry and Behavior, 21*, 891–894.

Jensen, J., Burke, N., & Garfinkel, B. (1988). Depression and symptoms of attention deficit disorder with hyperactivity. *Journal of the American Academy of Child and Adolescent Psychiatry, 27*(5), 742–747.

Jensen, J., & Garfinkel, B. (1990). Growth hormone dysregulation in prepubertal major affective disorder children. *Journal of the Academy of Child and Adolescent Psychiatry, 29*, 295–301.

Kandel, D., & Davies, M. (1986). Adult sequelae of adolescent depressive symptoms. *Archives of General Psychiatry, 43*, 255–262.

Kaplan, H., & Sadock, B. (1985). Modern synopsis of comprehensive textbook of psychiatry—IV (4th ed., pp. 83, 253, 264). Baltimore, MD: Williams & Wilkins.

Kashani, J., & Cantwell, D. (1983). Etiology and treatment of childhood depression: A biopsychological perspective. *Comprehensive Psychiatry, 24*(5), 476–486.

Kashani, J. H., McGee, R. O., Clarkson, S. E., Anderson, J. C., Walton, L. A., Williams, S., Silva, P. A., Robins, A. J., Cytryn, L., & McKnew, D. H. (1983). Depression in a sample of 9-year-old children. *Archives of General Psychiatry, 40*, 1217–1223.

Kashani, J. H., & Simonds, J. F. (1979). The incidence of depression in children. *American Journal of Psychiatry, 136*, 1203–1205.

Kasper, S., Moises, H. W., & Beckman, H. (1981). The anticholinergic biperiden in depressive disorders. *Pharmacopsychiatry, 14*, 195–198.

Keller, M., Beardslee, W., Dorer, D., Lavori, P. W., Samuelson, H., & Klerman, G. R. (1986). Impact of severity and chronicity of parental affective illness on adaptive functioning and psychopathology in children. *Archives of General Psychiatry, 43*, 930–937.

Klee, S., & Garfinkel, B. (1984). Identification of depression in children and adolescents: The role of the DST. *Journal of the American Academy of Child Psychiatry, 4*, 410–415.

Koslow, J. H., Maas, J. W., Bowden, C. L., Davis, J. M., Hanin, I., & Javoid, J. (1983). CSF and urinary biogenic amines and metabolites in depression and mania: A controlled, univariate analysis. *Archives of General Psychiatry, 40*, 999–1010.

Kovacs, M. (1978). Interview Schedule for Children, unpublished document. Pittsburgh, University of Pittsburgh.

Kovacs, M., & Beck, A. (1977). An empirical-clinical approach toward a definition of childhood depression, in J. Schulterbrandt, and Alan Raskin (Eds.), *Depression in childhood: Diagnosis, treatment, and conceptual models* (pp. 1–25.) New York: Raven.

Kovacs, M., Feinberg, T., Crouse-Novak, M., & Paulauskas, S. L., & Finkelstein, R. (1984). Depressive disorders in childhood I. *Archives of General Psychiatry, 41*, 229–237.

Kovacs, M., Feinberg, T., Crouse-Novak, M., Paulauskas, S. L., Pollock, M., & Finkelstein, R. (1984). Depressive disorders in childhood II. *Archives of General Psychiatry, 41*, 643–649.

Kringlen, E. (1985). Depression research: A review with special emphasis etiology. *Acta Psychiatrica Scandinavica, Supp. 319*(71), 117–130.

Lang, M., & Tisher, M. (1978). Children's Depression Scale. Victoria, Australia, Australian council for educational research.

Lefkowitz, M., & Tesini, E. (1981). Assessment of childhood depression. *Journal of Consulting Clinical Psychology, 48*, 43–51.

Lennerlof, L. (1988). Learned helplessness at work. *International Journal of Health Services, 18*(2), 207–221.

Lewinsohn, P. M., Steinmetz, J. L., Larson, D. W., & Franklin, J. (1981). Depression-related cognitions: Antecedent or consequence? *Journal of Abnormal Psychology, 90*, 213–219.

Livingston, R., & Martin-Cannici, C. (1987). Depression, anxiety and the dexamethasone suppression test in hospitalized prepubertal children. *Hillside Journal of Clinical Psychiatry, 9*(1, Spring/Summer), 55–63.

Livingston, R., Nugent, H., Rader, L., & Smith, R. (1985). Family histories of depressed and severely anxious children. *American Journal of Psychiatry, 142*, 1497–1499.

Lloyd, K., Morselli, P., & Bartholini, G. (1987). GABA and affective disorders. *Medical Biology, 65*, 159–165.

McKinney, W. (1984). Animal models of depression: An overview. *Psychiatric Developments, 2*, 77–96.

Mendelson, M. (1974). *Psychoanalytic concepts of depression* (2nd ed.). New York: Spectrum.

Mendelwich, J., & Rainer, J. D. (1977). Adoption study supporting genetic transmission in manic-depressive illness. *Nature, 268*, 327–329.

Murphy, G. E. (1983). Problems in studying suicide. *Psychiatric Developments, 4*, 339–350.

Nair, N., Hariharasubramanian, N., & Pilapil, C. (1983). Circadian rhythm of plasma melatonin in endogenous depression. *Progress in Neuro-Psychopharmacology and Biological Psychiatry, 8*, 715–718.

Nissen, G. (1971). Symptomatik und prognose depressive vertimmungszustande in kindes und jungendelter. In A. L. Annell (Ed.), *Depressive states in childhood and adolescence* (pp. 517–524). Stockholm: Almquist & Wiskell.

Orvaschel, H., Puig-Antich, J., Chambers, W., Tabrizi, M. A., & Johnson, R. (1982). Retrospective assessment of prepubertal major depression with the Kiddie-SADS-E. *Journal of the American Academy of Child Psychiatry, 21*(4), 392–397.

Otto, U. (1971). Suicidal attempts in childhood and adolescence—today and after 10 years: A follow-up study. In A. L. Annel (Ed.), *Depressive states in childhood and adolescence* (pp. 357–366). Stockholm: Almquist & Wiskell.

Penot, D. (1971). Caracteristiques et devenir des depressions de la deuxieme enfance. In A. Annel (Ed.), *Depressive states in childhood and adolescence* (pp. 525–533). Stockholm: Almquist & Wiskell.

Petti, T., & Connors, C. K. (1983). Changes in behavior ratings of depressed children treated with imipramine. *Journal of the American Academy of Child Psychiatry, 22*(4), 355–360.

Petty, L., Asarnow, J., Carlson, G., & Lesser, L. (1985). The dexamethasone suppression test in depressed, dysthymic, and nondepressed children. *American Journal of Psychiatry, 142*, 631–633.

Pozanski, E., Cook, S., & Carroll, B. (1979). A depression rating scale for children. *Pediatrics, 64*, 442–450.

Poznanski, E., Kraheneuhl, V., & Zrull, J. (1976). Childhood depression—A longitudinal perspective. *Journal of the American Academy of Child Psychiatry, 15*, 491–501.

Preskorn, S., Weller, E., & Weller, R. (1982). Depression in children: Relationship between plasma imipramine levels and response. *Journal of Clinical Psychiatry, 43*, 450–453.

Preskorn, S., Weller, E., Hughes, C., Weller, R. A., & Bolle, K. (1987). Depression in prepubertal children: Dexamethasone nonsuppression predicts differential response to imipramine vs. placebo. *Psychopharmacology Bulletin, 23*(1), 128–133.

Puig-Antich, J. (1982). Major depression and conduct disorder in prepuberty. *Journal of the American Academy of Child Psychiatry, 21*, 118–123.

Puig-Antich, J. (1987). Psychobiologic markers of prepubertal major depression. *Journal of Adolescent Health Care, 8*, 505–529.

Puig-Antich, J., & Chambers, W. (1978). "The schedule for Affective Disorders and Schizophrenia for school aged children (Kiddie-SADS)." New York State Psychiatric Institute, New York.

Puig-Antich, J., Chambers, W., & Tabrizi, M. (1983). The clinical assessment of current depressive episodes in children and adolescents: Interview with parents and children. In D. Cantwell & G. Carlson (Eds.), *Affective disorders in childhood and adolescence* (pp. 157–179). New York: Spectrum.

Puig-Antich, J., Goetz, R., Davies, M., Tabrizi, M. A., Novacenko, H., Hanlon, C., Sachar, E., & Weitzman, E. (1984, May). Growth hormone secretion in prepubertal depression II. *Archives of General Psychiatry, 41*, 463–466.

Puig-Antich, J., Goetz, R., Hanlon, C., Tabrizi, M. A., Davies, M., & Weitzman, E. D. (1983). Sleep architecture and REM sleep measures in prepubertal major depressives: Studies during recovery from a major depressive episode in a drug free state. *Archives of General Psychiatry, 40*, 187–192.

Puig-Antich, J., Navacenko, H., Davies, M., Chambers, W. J., Tabrizi, M. A., Krawiec, V., Ambrosini, P. J., & Sachar, E. J. (1984, May). Growth hormone secretion in prepubertal children with major depression I. *Archives of General Psychiatry, 41*, 455–460.

Puig-Antich, J., Orvaschel, H., Tabrizi, M., & Chambers, W. (1980). "The Schedule for affective disorders and schizophrenia for school aged children–epidemiologic version (Kiddie-SADS-E) Ed. 3. New York State Psychiatric Institute and Yale University School of Medicine, New York.

Puig-Antich, J., Perel, J., Lupatkin, W., Chambers, W. J., Tabrizi, M. A., King, J., Goetz, R., Davies, M., & Stiller, R. L. (1987). Imipramine in prepubertal major depressive disorders. *Archives of General Psychiatry, 44*, 81–89.

Quintana, J. (1988). Platelet MAO deamination of serotonin in depressed patients. *Biological Psychiatry, 23*, 44–52.

Redmond, D. E., & Huang, Y. H. (1979). New evidence for a locus ceruleus—Norepinephrine connection with anxiety. *Life Sciences, 25*, 2149–2162.

Rie, H. (1966). Depression in childhood: A survey of some pertinent contributors. *Journal of the American Academy of Child Psychiatry, 5*, 653–685.

Robins, L., Helzer, J., Weissman, M., Overaschel, H., Gruenberg, E., Burke, J., & Regier, D. (1984). Lifetime prevalence of specific psychiatric disorders in three sites. *Archives of General Psychiatry, 41*, 949–958.

Rochlin, G. (1959). The loss complex. *Journal of the American Psychoanalytic Association, 7*, 299–316.

Roy, A., Pickar, D., De Jong, J., Karoum, F., & Linnoila, M. (1988). Norepinephrine and its metabolites in cerebrospinal fluid, plasma, and urine. *Archives of General Psychiatry, 45*, 849–857.

Rutter, M. (1971). Relationships between child and adult psychiatric disorders. *Acta Psychiatrica Scandinavica, 48*(1), 3–21.

Ryan, N. D., Puig-Antich, J., Ambrosini, P., Rabinovich, H., Robinson, D., Nelson, B., Iyengar, S., & Twomey, J. (1987). The clinical picture of major depression in children and adolescents. *Archives of General Psychiatry, 44*, 854–861.

Ryan, N., Puig-Antich, J., Cooper, T., Rabinovich, H., Ambrosini, P., Davies, M., King, J., Torres, D., & Fried, J. (1986). Imipramine in adolescent major depression: Plasma level and clinical response. *Acta Psychiatrica Scandinavica, 73*, 275–288.

Schildkraut, J. J. (1965). The catecholamine hypothesis of affective disorders: A review of supporting evidence. *American Journal of Psychiatry, 122,* 509–522.

Seifert, W. E., Foxx, J. L., & Butler, I. J. (1980). Age effect on dopamine and serotonin metabolite levels in CSF. *Annals of Neurology, 8,* 38–42.

Sovner, R., & Hurley, A. D. (1983). Do the mentally retarded suffer from affective disorders? *Archives of General Psychiatry, 40,* 61–67.

Strober, M., & Carlson, G. (1982). Bipolar illness in adolescents with major depression. *Archives of General Psychiatry, 39,* 549–555.

Tisher, M. (1983). School refusal: A depressive equivalent? In D. Cantwell & G. Carlson (Eds.), *Affective disorders in childhood and adolescence* (pp. 129–144). New York: Spectrum.

Torgerson, S. (1986). Genetic factors in moderately severe and mild affective disorders. *Archives of General Psychiatry, 43,* 222–226.

Von Knorring, A. L., Clonigen, C. R., Bohman, M., & Sigvardsson, S. (1983). An adoption study of depressive disorders and substance abuse. *Archives of General Psychiatry, 40,* 943–950.

Waldron, S., Shrier, D., Stone, B., & Tobin, F. (1975). School phobia and other childhood neuroses: A systematic study of the children and their families. *American Journal of Psychiatry, 132*(8), 802–808.

Weissman, A., Beck, A., & Kovacs, M. (1979). Drug abuse, hopelessness, and suicidal behavior. *International Journal of the Addictions, 14*(4), 451–464.

Weissman, M., Gammon, D., John, K., Merikangas, K. R., Warner, V., Prusoff, B. A., & Sholomskas, D. (1987). Children of depressed parents. *Archives of General Psychiatry, 44,* 847–853.

Weissman, M., & Meyers, J. (1978). Affective disorders in a U.S. urban community: The use of research diagnostic criteria in an epidemiological survey. *Archives of General Psychiatry, 35,* 1304–1311.

Weissman, M., Prusoff, B., Gammon, G., Merikangas, K. R., Leckman, J. F., & Kidd, K. F. (1984). Psychopathology in the children (ages 6–18) of depressed and normal parents. *Journal of the American Academy of Child Psychiatry, 23*(1), 78–84.

Weller, E., Weller, R., Fristad, M., Preskorn, S. H., & Teare, M. (1985). The dexamethasone suppression test in prepubertal depressed children. *Journal of Clinical Psychiatry, 46,* 511–513.

Welner, A., Welner, Z., & Fishman, R. (1979). Psychiatric adolescent inpatients. *Archives of General Psychiatry, 36,* 698–700.

Winokur, G. (1986). Unipolar depression. In G. Winokur & P. Clayton (Eds.), *The medical basis of psychiatry* (pp. 60–79). New York: Saunders.

Wirt, R., Lachar, D., Klinedinst, J., & Seat, P. (1977). Multidimensional description of child personality, Manual for the Personality Inventory for Children, Los Angeles, Western Psychological Services.

Wyatt, R. J., Portnoy, B., Kupfer, D. J., Snyder, F., & Engelman, K. (1971). Resting plasma catecholamine concentrations in patients with depression and anxiety. *Archives of General Psychiatry, 24,* 65–70.

CHAPTER 4

Conduct Disorder

Donald K. Routh
Timothy K. Daugherty
University of Miami

Conduct disorder is one of the most widely recognized and most thoroughly validated kinds of psychopathology seen among children and adolescents. In assessing this problem, the clinician commonly seeks information from various sources, which may include: parent interview or checklist, child interview or questionnaire, teacher checklist, behavioral observations in different settings, peer nominations and ratings, and others. However, the information from these different sources is quite often discrepant. Thus, a group of children who would be identified as having conduct disorder on the basis of a parent interview is not the same group that would be identified on the basis of a teacher checklist or an interview with the youngsters themselves. The issues addressed in this chapter are: (a) a critique of DSM-III and DSM-III-R criteria for conduct disorder from a research standpoint and (b) a discussion of how to integrate different sources of information in the assessment and diagnosis of conduct disorder in children and adolescents. There seem to be four different models in the current literature as to how different sources of information might be integrated in the assessment of conduct disorder. These could be named the *gold standard* model, the *actuarial* model, the *clinical judgment* model, and the *hypothetical construct* model. Our own views at present favor the use of the hypothetical construct model.

VALIDITY OF CONDUCT DISORDER AS A FORM OF CHILD AND ADOLESCENT PSYCHOPATHOLOGY

Current Diagnostic Criteria

The definition of conduct disorder (see Table 4.1) given in the DSM-III-R (American Psychiatric Association, 1987) has not yet been subjected to extensive formal validation, but is probably as well accepted as any current definition of conduct disorder. Like its predecessor, the DSM-III, the DSM-III-R was devised by committees of experienced consultants, most of whom were psychiatrists. Though they attempted to be sensitive to empirical findings, these committees often resolved controversies by polling their members. In the absence of studies on the revision, some data pertaining to DSM-III bear discussion.

In the DSM-III, conduct disorders were divided into four subcategories based on the presence or absence of adequate social bonds and aggressive behavior. Quay (1986) reviewed 61 studies spanning the previous four decades, finding that conduct disorder is a ubiquitous pattern found throughout the multivariate literature. Support was particularly strong for the undersocialized aggressive pattern, and ample support was found for the socialized aggressive pattern (particularly among older children and adolescents), but no support was forthcoming for the two nonaggressive categories. Thus, recent studies confirm the original research of Hewitt and Jenkins (1946), who did the earliest factor analysis of a behavior checklist on delinquent youngsters, in supporting two, rather than four categories, of conduct disorder.

Werry, Methven, Fitzpatrick, and Dixon (1983) evaluated the reliability of the DSM-III, based on 195 admissions to a child psychiatric inpatient unit who were diagnosed independently by two to four clinicians. conduct disorder fell into the moderately unreliable category (kappa = .53), and appeared to have been impaired by subcategorization and by the use of oppositional disorder, construed by Werry and colleagues (1983) to be a milder form of conduct disorder.

In the DSM-III-R, two primary subtypes of conduct disorder are outlined: solitary aggressive type and group type. Solitary aggressive corresponds roughly to undersocialized aggressive, whereas group type collapses the socialized aggressive and nonaggressive types. The nature and direction of these changes appear consistent with the findings of Quay (1986) and Werry and colleagues (1983). A third type, undifferentiated, manifests qualities of both solitary and group types and might correspond to the "versatile" conduct disordered child studied by

TABLE 4.1
DMS-III-R Criteria for Conduct Disorder

A. A disturbance of conduct lasting at least six months, during which at least three of the following have been present:
  (1) has stolen without confrontation of a victim on more than one occasion (including forgery)
  (2) has run away from home overnight at least twice while living in parental or parental surrogate home (or once without returning)
  (3) often lies (other than to avoid physical or sexual abuse)
  (4) has deliberately engaged in fire-setting
  (5) is often truant from school (for older person, absent from work)
  (6) has broken into someone else's house, building, or car
  (7) has deliberately destroyed others' property (other than by fire-setting)
  (8) has been physically cruel to animals
  (9) has forced someone into sexual activity with him or her
  (10) has used a weapon in more than one fight
  (11) often initiates physical fights
  (12) has stolen with confrontation of a victim (e.g., mugging, purse-snatching, extortion, armed robbery)
  (13) has been physically cruel to people.
  (Note: The above items are listed in descending order of discriminating power based on data from a national field trial of the *DMS-III-R* criteria for Disruptive Behavior Disorders.)

B. If 18 or older, does not meet criteria for Antisocial Personality Disorder

Note. From *Diagnostic and Statistical Manual of Mental Disorders* (3rd ed., rev., p. 55) by American Psychiatric Association, 1987, Washington, DC: Author.

Loeber (1982). However, as noted earlier, the reliability and validity of the new criteria are as yet unknown.

Oppositional defiant disorder has a new name and slightly revised criteria in the revision. Reeves, Werry, Elkind, and Zametkin (1987) examined conduct disordered and opposition disordered children and found no significant differences between the two groups on a number of variables. The new name and revised criteria do not address opposition disorder's lack of support in the research literature, and the maintenance of the disorder in the taxonomy is likely to create diagnostic noise (see Werry et al., 1983) whenever conduct disorder is studied.

The new severity ratings, to be given along with the diagnosis of disruptive behavior disorders, are a move toward dimensionalizing the taxonomy and, as such, may serve both clinical and research interests. Severity ratings, for instance, could facilitate the comparison of clinical diagnoses with psychometric assessment.

From the standpoint of the present chapter, note that the DSM-III-R definition of conduct disorder makes no statement about the exact source(s) of information on which the clinician's judgments are to be based, let alone how information from different sources is to be combined. In the case of conduct disorder, the authors of the manual appear to assume that information exists independent of its source. With respect to certain other disorders, in contrast, the DSM-III-R does specify sources of information in some detail and states how the information should be combined. In the diagnosis of mental retardation, for example, general intellectual functioning may be estimated by an individually administered intelligence test, and adaptive functioning by a standardized scale of adaptive behavior. A subnormal score on both of these dimensions is required for the diagnosis of mental retardation.

Proposed Diagnostic Criteria

We favor a continuous dimensional approach to the definition of conduct disorder, rather than the categorical approach advocated in the DSMs. Edelbrock and Costello (1988) studied the relationship between dimensional syndromes and DSM-III diagnoses. Parents of 270 clinically referred children were administered the Child Behavior Checklist (producing behavior problem dimensions) and the Diagnostic Interview Schedule for Children (producing DSM-III diagnoses). A very strong linear relation emerged between scores on the Delinquent subscale of the CBCL and the diagnosis of conduct disorder, with no "diagnostic threshold" below which children do not receive a diagnosis and above which they are labeled conduct disordered. Approximately 7% of subjects with *T* scores of 55 were diagnosed, compared with 85% of those having *T* scores above 86.

Edelbrock and Costello (1988) argued that the categorical approach of the DSM is arbitrary and ignores potentially important information about how far above or below the cutoff the child falls—information likely to be predictive of clinical course and treatment response. Currently, we believe the most valid and useful definition of conduct disorder flows from the work of Fergusson and Horwood (1987a, 1987b), whose model consists of an equally weighted combination of maternal and teacher ratings of conduct disorder. This model and the empirical support for it is discussed further later in the chapter.

Principles for Determining Validity

Quay, Routh, and Shapiro (1987) voiced the need to go beyond description to validation of syndromes of child psychopathology. In a recent elaborating on Quay and associates' views, Routh (1989) stated:

> Within the field of child psychopathology, validating a diagnostic category means investigating whether inferences based on it are correct or incorrect. The diagnostic category should convey some clinically important information about a child's condition beyond what was known before the category was assigned. What this new information might be depends on the particular diagnostic construct and how much solic scientific information there is about it, but typically clinicians are most concerned about: (1) the prognosis of the condition (its natural history and outcome in the absence of any particular intervention); (2) its etiology (known antecedents or causes); and (3) its response to various possible treatments. (p. 41)

Prognosis

A significant minority of children with conduct disorder go on to become adults with antisocial personality and various other problems. In fact, the DSM-III-R requires evidence of conduct disorder before age 15 for the diagnosis of antisocial personality disorder in adults. It is thus of interest to uncover factors predicting which children will have such unfortunate outcomes. The poor prognosis for those with conduct disorder includes not only such outcomes as continued antisocial behavior and alcoholism. Rydelius (1988) showed that antisocial adolescents were also at greater risk of sudden violent death (e.g., via suicide or motor vehicle accidents) than individuals the same age in the general population. Robins (cited by West, 1987) also reported that for females, childhood conduct disorder predicts not only adult antisocial behavior and substance abuse, but also depression, phobias, and obsessive compulsive disorder. Another part of the natural history of antisocial personality is the "burn out" phenomenon in which criminal activity of many, but not all, psychopaths lessens after age 40 (Hare, McPherson, & Forth, 1988).

In discussing the validity of the concept of conduct disorder or aggression, Routh (1989) specifically mentioned evidence about its prognosis. For example, Robins' (1966) 30-year-follow-up study showed that a significant number of patients presenting at a child guidance center with antisocial behavior went on to manifest antisocial personality disorder as adults, compared to children presenting with nonantisocial complaints or neighborhood control subjects. Similarly, Eron and his colleagues (Walder, Abelson, Eron, Banta, & Laulicht, 1961) obtained peer-rated measures of aggression for a sample of 8-year-old children. In their most recent follow-up study 22 years later, Huesmann, Eron, Lefkowitz, and Walder (1984) found that peer-rated aggression in childhood predicted adult Minnesota Multiphasic Personality Inventory

(MMPI) scores (they used Scales F + 4 + 9 as their composite measure of aggression), trouble with the law, spouse abuse, and other such outcome measures, even after IQ was controlled statistically. Reviews of over a dozen longitudinal studies in the literature by Olweus (1979, 1980) suggest that measures of conduct disorder or aggression are as stable as measures of intelligence. Despite the stability of conduct disorder, over half of the youngsters considered antisocial at any one time no longer are so when followed up years later (Loeber, 1982). According to Loeber (1982), one of the most robust predictors of long-term outcome of conduct disorder is the early onset of symptoms.

Recent research on conduct disorder has uncovered an additional prognostic factor, namely the simultaneous presence of attention deficit-hyperactivity disorder (ADHD). Children with conduct disorder and ADHD seem to have more severe conduct disorder and a worse outcome than those with conduct disorder alone (Stewart & Kelso, 1987). These findings are specific to the combination of the two disorders, because ADHD alone does not have a particularly bad outcome (Milich & Loney, 1979). Walker, Lahey, Hynd, and Frame (1987) also reported that children with both conduct disorder and ADHD had an earlier onset of their behavioral problems, engaged in more physical aggression, and showed a greater variety and severity of antisocial behaviors than children with conduct disorder alone. Lahey and colleagues (1988) found that children with conduct disorder, but not those with ADHD, tended to have fathers who were substance abusers and mothers who manifested depression, antisocial personality disorder, substance abuse, or somatization disorder. Children with both conduct disorder and ADHD were particularly likely to have fathers with a history of aggression, arrest, and imprisonment.

The distinction between conduct disorder and ADHD as overlapping but distinct disorders by now seems to be well accepted (e.g., Hinshaw, 1987). Milich, Widiger, and Landau (1987) presented information on the value of various symptoms in the differential diagnosis of conduct disorder and ADHD. Taylor, Schachar, Thorley, and Wieselberg (1986) found that conduct disorder ("defiance") but not hyperactivity, was associated with impaired family relationships and adverse social factors. In a companion study, Taylor and associates (1986) found that their sample of hyperactive children had a lower IQ, younger age of onset, more neurological signs, more family problems, a higher accident rate, and a significantly better response to stimulant medication than a comparison group with conduct disorder.

There has also been research suggesting that high IQ may be a factor protecting against the development of antisocial behavior among men with severely criminal fathers (Kandel et al., 1988). On the other hand, poor cognitive functioning in the sense of a "broad deficiency in acculturational learning" has been implicated as a causal factor in a longitudinal study of the development of conduct disorder in 17-year-olds (Schonfeld, Shaffer, O'Connor, & Portnoy, 1988).

Conduct disorder can also coexist with various other types of psychopathology and may turn out to have some interesting connections with them. Russell, Bott, and Sammons (1989), for example, studied 35 youngsters 4 to 13 years of age who met strict modern diagnostic criteria for schizophrenia with childhood onset. interestingly, the most common co-diagnosis for this group (10/35) was conduct disorder, and a premorbid history of ADHD was common.

A long-standing but unresolved issue is the relation of conduct disorder to depression in children. At present, the evidence for an association of the two is relatively slight (e.g., McGee & Williams, 1988). Nevertheless, many adults who are clinically depressed show irritability. Perhaps a similar phenomenon may occur in children. Thus, there could be at least a subset of children with symptoms of conduct disorder whose antisocial behavior could be a manifestation of depressive affect. They might show episodic patterns of aggressive behavior correlated with their mood swings. This possibility is certainly worthy of future investigation.

Antecedents and Response to Treatment

Recently, Routh (1989) reviewed the existing data concerning antecedents or response to treatment and did not consider it to add much to the evidence for the validity of the concept of conduct disorder. Those incarcerated in prisons and other correctional institutions, who often manifest antisocial personality and a history of conduct disorder in childhood, include many more males than females, more adolescents and young adults than persons in other age groups, and a disproportionate number of lower socioeconomic status (SES) and racial minority individuals; but, none of these demographic facts are unequivocal antecedents of conduct disorder. Similarly, the "broken homes" found to be a correlate of delinquency may turn out to be a proxy for other variables more related to the quality of family life (Lahey et al., 1988; Van Voorhis, Cullen, Mathers, & Garner, 1988). Causal theories focus on correlated factors, such as the presence of an antisocial parent in the home (or in the child's biological background), on models for aggressive and antisocial behavior in the child's environment, and on coercive patterns of interaction with other family members. In line with the present uncertainty of our knowledge about its causes, conduct disorder is generally presented, as in the DSM-III-R, as a descriptive concept only.

A number of investigators have pursued a biological approach to conduct disorders. Cadoret, Troughton, and O'Gorman (1987), for example, have emphasized the importance of genetic factors in the causation of antisocial personality and its usual childhood precursor, conduct disorder. These investigators also noted the importance of genetic factors to the related disorders of alcoholism and, mostly in relatives of alcoholics and antisocial individuals, somatization disorder. Cadoret and associates (1987) recently presented data from an adoption study in support of the specificity of inheritance of factors predisposing to alcohol abuse and antisocial personality. Their data, consisting of adoption records and interviews with adopted adult males, suggested that alcohol problems in the biologic family predicted alcohol abuse in the adoptee while antisocial behavior in the biologic family increased the probability of antisocial personality in the adoptee.

Quay (1988) viewed conduct disorder from the perspective of Gray's neurophysiological theory. According to Quay's ideas, conduct disorder involves an overactive *reward* system in the central nervous system, whereas ADHD involves an underactive *behavioral inhibition* system in the central nervous system (CNS). A recent experiment published by Shapiro, Quay, Hogan, and Schwartz (1988) supports the hypothesis of an overactive reward system in boys who were chosen on the basis of relatively high conduct disorder scores on the Revised Behavior Problem Checklist. These basic findings were replicated in recent work by Daugherty and Quay (1989).

Treatment of conduct disorders is known to be difficult (see Kazdin, 1987, for a review). The most rigorously studied treatments have generally been behavioral ones, but behavioral researchers often do not document the diagnostic status of children in their studies. Thus, knowledge about the *differential* response of conduct disorder to various interventions is still sparse. Despite the findings of Taylor and colleagues (1986) already mentioned, pharmacological approaches of the kind used with ADHD (e.g., methylphenidate) do not always seem to be differentially effective in cases with or without co-existing conduct disorder (Klorman et al., 1988). Cognitively oriented treatment research (for example, Arbuthnot & Gordon's [1986] interesting attempt to intervene with delinquents by teaching them better moral reasoning) also did not use very rigorous selection criteria, leaving its implications for differential treatment response very uncertain. Clearly, more precision in the assessment process can help to improve this situation.

SOURCES OF INFORMATION FOR ASSESSMENT AND DIAGNOSIS

A large number of particular procedures have been suggested for the assessment of conduct disorder. It is beyond the scope of the present chapter to review each of these in detail, but the more commonly used procedures are mentioned briefly.

Parent Measures

The parent interview is usually considered the single most valuable source of information concerning child psychopathology. At one time it was common practice to use unstructured parent interviews, even for research purposes. The first modern structured parent interview was developed by Rutter and his colleagues for use in the Isle of Wight study (Graham & Rutter, 1968). At present, a large number of structured interviews have been developed for use in both epidemiological and clinical research that contain questions concerning symptoms of conduct disorder. These include the Children's Assessment Schedule (CAS; Hodges, Kline, Stern, Cytryn, & McKnew, 1982), the Diagnostic Interview Schedule for Children–Parent version (DISC-P; Costello, Edelbrock, Dulcan, Kalas, & Klaric, 1984), the Diagnostic Interview for Children and Adolescents–Parent version (DICA-P; Herjanic & Campbell, 1977), and others. The most popular choice for use in epidemiological studies, at least in the United States, seems to be the DISC-P, but it is presently being revised once more. Therefore, it is unclear how long it will take to develop a structured parent interview that will merit use by all major research centers. Meanwhile, new standardized parent interview procedures continue to be introduced. For example, Kazdin and Esveldt-Dawson (1986) reported preliminary reliability and validity data on a new procedure, the Interview for Antisocial Behavior (IAB).

There are a number of behavior checklists or questionnaires that have been developed for use by parents. The best known of these are probably the Conners Parent Rating Scale (Goyette, Conners, & Ulrich, 1978), the Quay-Peterson Revised Behavior Problem Checklist (RBPC; Quay & Peterson, 1983), and the Achenbach Child Behavior Checklist (CBCL; Achenbach, 1978; Achenbach & Edelbrock, 1979, 1983). The parent version of the CBCL, probably the most commonly used of the parent rating scales, consists of 118 behavior problem items to which parents respond based on their child's behavior during the past 6 months. The three-step response scale (0, 1, 2) corresponds to *not true*, *somewhat or sometimes true*, and *very true or often true* of their child. The Conners, RBPC, and CBCL each include conduct disorder factors with slightly different names (e.g., aggressive, conduct disorder, conduct problem, delinquent). The three investigators have recently pooled their items to form a single consensual checklist, the "ACQ" (for Achenbach, Conners, and Quay), which is currently being field tested.

Parents may also provide more detailed information in the form of diaries or other reports on their children's behavior over short intervals of time. An example of this approach is the Parent Daily Report (PDR; Chamberlain & Reid, 1987), which consists of a list of 19 negative and 19 prosocial behaviors commonly exhibited by children. This information may be reported in writing or by telephone. The PDR has been shown to have a good test–retest reliability and to correlate significantly with concurrent home observations. The research of Rapoport and Benoit (1975) suggests that parent diaries might be more accurate and less biased than parent ratings concerning the same child behaviors. In their study, parent diaries correlated better with the reports of other informants than did parent ratings.

Like other informants, parents are influenced by their own feelings as well as the child's actual behavior. For example, Griest, Wells, and Forehand (1979) found that mothers' depression, as measured by the Beck Depression Inventory, was the best predictor of their perception of their children's maladjustment. In contrast, direct observations of the children's behavior did not contribute to a multiple regression equation predicting maternal perceptions of the children's maladjustment.

Child Interviews and Questionnaires

At one time, it was common to interview children only informally, perhaps in a playroom setting, and to depend almost entirely on information from the parent interview for actual clinical diagnosis. Again, in the Isle of Wight study Rutter and his colleagues (Rutter & Graham, 1968) were pioneers in devising and validating a standardized psychiatric interview with the child. They did not find the child interview to be as valuable a source of information as the interview with the parents, but definitely considered it a worthwhile addition.

Recent research has confirmed that children can be reliable reporters. Herjanic, Herjanic, Brown, and Wheatt (1975) interviewed a group of 50 children attending a mental health clinic and their mothers, using the same structured interview, and found 80% average agreement on the questions, especially factual ones (e.g., age, address, reason for referral). Children themselves are uniquely valuable sources of information about their own private experiences, including affects such as anxiety, depression, and pain; perceptual and cognitive phenomena such as hallucinations and obsessions; and, most important in the assessment of conduct disorders, covert behaviors such as theft, firesetting, and vandalism. In cases where the children have not told their parents about such events, and the parents have not observed them, the child's self-report is really the only possible information source the clinician could obtain. As an example of the unique value of self-report data from children, Kashani, Orvaschel, Burk, and Reid (1985) interviewed 50 children and adolescents of parents with affective disorders using standardized procedures. Diagnoses based on the children's reports suggested a high prevalence of depression. Information from parent interviews, in contrast, suggested a high prevalence of oppositional and attention problems in their offspring.

At this time, a number of standardized child interviews exist. For example, the Children's Assessment Schedule (CAS; Hodges, Kline, Stern, Cytryn, & McKnew, 1982), Diagnostic Interview Schedule for Children (DIS; Costello et al., 1984), the Diagnostic Interview for Children and Adolescents (DICA; Herjanic & Campbell, 1977; Welner, Reich, Herjanic, Jung, & Amado, 1987), Interview Schedule for Children (ISC; Kovacs, 1978), the Schedule for Affective Disorders and Schizophrenia for School Age Children (K-SADS; Puig-Antich & Chambers, 1978), and others are available for use. The DISC is currently the best known and most often used in epidemiological research but, like the DISC-P, it is currently being revised. The DISC is a highly structured interview that has demonstrated adequate reliability with children at or above 10 years of age (Edelbrock, Costello, Dulcan, Kalas, & Conover, 1985). With younger children, a semistructured interview, such as the CAS, may be more appropriate as it allows for the matching of the task demands and pacing to the child's developmental level (Hodges & Cools, 1990). The K-SADS, DICA, and CAS have been shown to have good concordance for child-reported conduct disorder (Carlson, Kashani, Thomas, Vaidya, & Daniel, 1987; Hodges, McKnew, Burbach, & Roebuck, 1987).

Self-report questionnaires are rarely used with preschool children and are not commonly used with children under about a third-grade level (i.e., about 8 years old). Achenbach and Edelbrock (1987) developed a Youth Self-Report (YSR) questionnaire intended to serve as a supplement to checklist information from parents and teachers. The YSR, designed for use with 11- to 18-year-olds, includes most of the behavior problem items from the CBCL, changed to first-person wording. As with the CBCL, a three-step response scale (0, 1, 2) is used. The validity of the YSR has not yet been fully explored.

Teacher Ratings and Measures of School Behavior

One of the most widely cited measures in the literature of behavioral science is Conners' (1969) Teacher Rating Scale, which in various versions (e.g., Goyette, Conners, & Ulrich, 1978) has been for many years the standardized procedure for assessing what is now called attention deficit-hyperactivity disorder (ADHD). All versions of the Conners scales also contain items tapping the overlapping condition of conduct disorder. The traditional classroom setting where a child must stay seated and carry out relatively tedious teacher-directed tasks seems to elicit many of the difficulties of the ADHD child to a unique degree. Also, teachers may have a better perspective than parents on what behaviors are typical or unusual for children of a given age.

Other teacher instruments include Quay and Peterson's Revised Behavior Problem Checklist, which is often used to obtain teacher reports of children's behavior. The RBPC has 89 items grouped into six scales including conduct disorder. Responses to each item are on a three-point scale (0 = does not constitute a problem, 1 = mild problem, 2 = severe problem). Achenbach has recently devised a Teacher Report Form (TRF) of his Child Behavior Checklist to supplement symptom reports from the child's parents. It has 113 items and uses the same three-point response alternatives as the CBCL. The scale most closely related to conduct disorder is labeled aggressive.

Teacher reports of children's behavior seem important on theoretical grounds because the classroom and the school playground provide the context for many behaviors characteristic of conduct disorder: truancy (of course), physical fights, extortion from classmates, and so forth. Shinn, Ramsey, Walker, Stieber, and O'Neill (1987) used school as a setting in which to study two groups of fifth-grade children, one that had been identified as being at-risk for antisocial behavior and the other a normal control group. Group assignment was based on a weighted combination of measures derived from home observations, child and teacher interviews, and peer nominations, as well as the Aggression scales of the CBCL and TRF (Achenbach & Edelbrock, 1983). The risk group was significantly less engaged with academic tasks and displayed higher rates of negative verbal behavior in school. This group was perceived by teachers as lower in social skills and less well socialized in the school environment. This group also had records of poor discipline in school.

Peer Nominations and Ratings

In the past, peer nomination and rating procedures have been used mainly for research purposes rather than by clinicians, who often do not consider it feasible to obtain peer ratings. Even in research, peer ratings are sometimes not approved by human subjects committees because the procedures inherently seem to require children to say negative things about their peers (i.e., to name children that they dislike). Research has, however, not confirmed the supposition of negative effects from such sociometric procedures (e.g., Bell-Dolan, Foster, & Sikora, 1989).

There is increasing evidence of the value of peer ratings, notably in predicting long-term outcomes (e.g., Huesman et al., 1984). In a follow-up study by Cowen, Pederson, Babigian, Izzo, and Trost (1973), it was found that peer ratings, notably in predicting long-term outcomes (e.g., Huesman et al., 1984). In a follow-up study by Cowen, Pederson, Babigian, Izzo, and Trost (1973), it was found that peer ratings (i.e., choices of classmates to play negative roles in a class play) were the best single predictor of future membership on a community psychiatric register 11 to 13 years later. These ratings were better than self-report questionnaires, school records, or teachers' ratings. Olweus (1977) also reported longitudinal research supporting the discriminant validity of peer ratings of children's aggressive behavior as well as the stability of such measures over time.

A recent study by Asarnow (1988) even demonstrated the feasibility of obtaining peer ratings from a group of child psychiatric inpatients who know each other from interaction on the hospital ward rather than in school. These ratings were found to reproduce a number of findings well known from sociometric studies in community settings, such as the rejection of children with conduct disorder and ADHD by their peers. It may not be so difficult to obtain clinically useful sociometric data as once seemed to be the case.

Behavioral Observations

Behavioral observations often seem more cumbersome, time-consuming, and expensive to obtain than other measures. Like peer ratings, they have also been available in the past mostly for research purposes. The pioneer in collecting detailed behavioral observations of aggressive children in the natural setting of their families was Patterson (1977). One unique value of behavioral observations lies in their relative freedom from bias, at least on the part of the observer. If observers agree that Johnny hits another child in the classroom on the average of five times a day, clinicians may feel more confidence that this in fact has actually happened (compared with a teacher's circling "a lot" next to the "hitting" item on the checklist for Johnny).

Yet, bias can exist in behavioral observations, as exemplified by the problem of reactivity to observation. Children who know when they are being observed may inhibit misbehaviors at such times. In an interesting attempt to reduce such reactivity, Johnson, Christensen, and Bellamy (1976) used a concealed wireless transmitter to detect verbal interactions between children with conduct disorder and their parents in the home. The youngsters and their parents knew the transmitter was there, but they were unaware of the particular times that were randomly selected for recording. In addition to the randomly selected times, the parents could select typically problematic times (e.g., bedtime) for taping. The tape data from parent-selected times were highly consistent with parent-reported behavioral observations, while the tape data from random times were less consistent perhaps due to lower base rates of child deviant behavior picked up at random times (versus key problematic times).

One procedure that may be used for home observation of behavior is the Dyadic Parent–Child Interaction Coding System (DPICS; Robinson & Eyberg, 1981). One of its composite codes, for example, is labeled "total child deviance" and combines the frequencies of the following behaviors: whine, cry, physical negative, smart talk, yell, destructive, and noncompliant. DPICS behaviors have been shown to discriminate clinic from nonclinic families (Forehand, King, Peed, & Yoder, 1975; Lobitz & Johnson, 1975; Webster-Stratton, 1985).

In assessing conduct disorder, there is one limitation with observational data because many of the behaviors to be observed have rather low base rates, especially in older children. Coie and Dodge (1988), for example, found that teacher and peer ratings had better intermethod agreement than observer data, partly because so little aggression was observed among the older boys they studied. The act of severely injuring another child or setting a fire may occur "only" once over a number of months or years, so that it would not be feasible to record such behaviors by direct observation. Reports by the youngster or by knowledgeable informants seem more worthwhile in the case of low frequency antisocial behaviors.

Other Sources of Information

The literature on conduct disorder overlaps to a considerable extent with that on delinquency and crime. Serious conduct disorder is often the subject of actions by the legal system, including arrest, detention, adjudication, and incarceration, and public records are kept on these matters. Information obtained from law enforcement and correctional officials is often used in both predicting and evaluating outcomes.

Although such information is important (e.g., in evaluating the long-term outcomes of children with conduct disorder and the efficacy of interventions), certain caveats must be stated concerning its use. First of all, there is a good deal of socioeconomic and ethnic bias in official records of crime and delinquency. For a given level of antisocial activity, people of low SES and Blacks are significantly more likely than high SES persons or whites to be arrested, charged, and convicted of crime (Quay, 1987). Also, it appears that most crimes that are committed are not detected, and of those detected, only a small proportion lead to arrest, trial, or incarceration (Empey, 1982). Another problem is the heterogeneity of delinquent and criminal groups. Many researchers, therefore, do not regard "delinquency" as a useful psychopathological construct. Conduct disorder and delinquency are overlapping but quite distinct entities.

Within the domain of psychopathology there is an important distinction to be made between *overt* and *covert* antisocial behavior (Loeber & Schmaling, 1985a, 1985b). DSM-III-R distinguishes between solitary aggressive conduct disorder (corresponding to overt antisocial behavior, fighting) and group conduct disorder (which aligns with covert antisocial behavior, stealing). In terms of Patterson's theory (Snyder & Patterson, 1987), the fighters are more involved in coercive interactions with other family members, whereas stealers are largely in need of closer parental monitoring. Children whose conduct disorders are the most severe and long-lasting tend to show both overt and covert antisocial behavior. DSM-III-R refers to this pattern as the undifferentiated type of conduct disorder.

DISCREPANCIES ACROSS SOURCES OF INFORMATION

Achenbach, McConaughy, and Howell (1987) conducted a meta-analysis of 119 studies of different informants' reports of children and adolescents' behavioral and emotional problems. On the average, correlations between all types of informants were statistically significant, thus providing some evidence of convergent validity of different sources of information. In many cases, however, the correlations were rather low. Between similar informants, such as parents, the average correlation was .60. Between different types of informants, such as parents and teachers, the average correlation was .28, and between self-report measures (i.e., from the subjects themselves) and other informants, the average correlation was only .22. The correlations were somewhat higher for under-controlled problems such as conduct disorder. Nevertheless, the sources by no means provided identical information. If information from parents was used to identify a group of youngsters with conduct disorder, one could generate quite a different group than if information from teachers was used.

The influence of various kinds of method variance is such that in a factor analysis of assessment data from different informants such as parents, teachers, and clinicians, one is liable to emerge with factors representing substantive dimensions of psychopathology (e.g., Langhorne, Loney, Paternite, & Bechtoldt, 1976).

MODELS FOR COMBINING DIFFERENT SOURCES OF INFORMATION

Recently, Routh (1990) argued that definitions of categories of psychopathology should go beyond simply listing symptoms to specify the sources of information to be used in assessing the symptoms and should state how these sources of information should be combined. In the case of conduct disorder, there appear to be four different models of how this might be done: the *gold standard model*, the *actuarial model*, the *clinical judgment model*, and the *hypothetical construct model*.

Gold Standard Model

As its name suggests, this model looks for a single diagnostic procedure to use as a "gold standard" for validating all other sources of information. In simpler times, the U.S. government minted gold pieces and backed up every paper dollar with gold bullion in the treasury. The nostalgic may feel that in those days people really had assurance that their money was "worth something." Similarly, in the earlier history of the behavioral sciences, teacher judgments were used as the "gold standard" against which to validate IQ tests, psychiatrists' diagnoses were used for the initial validation of scales on the Minnesota Multiphasic Personality Inventory, and the legal criterion of divorce was used to validate measures of marital adjustment. It was hoped that by starting with a somewhat imprecise "criterion" measure, it would ultimately be possible to generate a "bootstrap" effect. What was initially only a screening measure can, itself, turn out to be a more refined measure of the construct than the initial criterion. Thus, in physics, the human temperature sense may have been the initial definition of heat and cold.

The mercury thermometer was "validated" against that as a criterion, and eventually thermometer readings came to be regarded as the more valid measure of temperature than human sensory mechanisms.

Is there a "gold standard" in the diagnosis or assessment of conduct disorder? Most clinicians, if pressed to use only a single source of information in their diagnosis, would no doubt fall back on the use of a standardized interview with a parent, or perhaps a parent behavior checklist such as the Child Behavior Checklist (Achenbach & Edelbrock, 1983). However, there is little evidence at present that diagnoses based on information from parents is of superior validity to all other sources of information.

In fact, one could make a case, empirically, that if there is going to be a "gold standard" for the assessment of conduct disorder, it should be peer ratings of aggression rather than a parent interview. For example, Huesmann and associates (1984) found that they could significantly predict outcome 22 years later from peer ratings at age 8. No comparable data exist for parent interviews or checklists.

Actuarial Model

The actuarial model is atheoretical. It acknowledges, first of all, the fact that various purported measures of conduct disorder (or any other type of child psychopathology) are not highly correlated with each other. Therefore, the model states that these measures may be related to different antecedents and outcomes and may not be affected in the same way by different interventions. Therefore, to combine different measures by either adding them or weighting them unequally in a single formula is simply to lose valuable information. If one wishes to use the measures to predict a certain outcome variable (e.g., the recidivism of a group of incarcerated delinquents), the best way to do so is to calculate the appropriate regression equation, taking care to cross-validate it to avoid an inflated estimate of the efficacy of prediction. The statistical side of the long debate between clinical and statistical prediction (e.g., Meehl, 1954) would argue that one simply cannot get any better prediction than this. It goes without saying that such prediction would work best if it made use of continuous variables rather than artificial dichotomies as predictors.

Achenbach (1985) is the principal spokesman for the actuarial approach to diagnosis and assessment of all aspects of child psychopathology. He suggested the use of parent ratings, teacher ratings, youth self-reports, and standardized observations as a series of different axes in a profile. In Achenbach's system, Axis I would be based on parent perceptions, Axis II on teachers' perceptions, Axis III on cognitive assessment, Axis IV on biomedical conditions, and Axis V on the clinician's assessment via behavioral observations or the self-reports of the child. McConaughy, Achenbach, and Gent (1988) explored the relationship between the first axis (parent perceptions profile derived from the CBCL) and three of the remaining four axes (biomedical conditions were not considered). Results revealed six CBCL profile patterns that were significantly related to different patterns on the three other axes studied (teacher report, cognitive assessment, and self-report). McConaughy and associates (1988) concluded that the results indicate the importance of studying higher order patterns of functioning that extend across sources of data.

Clinical Judgment Model

In the clinical judgment model, the diagnostician obtains information from various sources and tries to resolve discrepancies between them by deciding, perhaps symptom by symptom, which report is the more credible. Thus, if a child denied stealing, but parents, peers, or teachers were sure that the child had stolen something, the diagnostician might end up believing the purported victims of theft. On the other hand, if the only one reporting that the child stole was his brother (who might have been trying to justify the fact that he stole something from the child in retaliation), the diagnostician might give the child the benefit of the doubt.

Reich and Earls (1987) developed a more formalized version of this model. They obtained data from 32 mother–child pairs from a study of families who had been exposed to severe flooding in Missouri. Parallel interviews were used for the mothers and children; namely, the DICA and DICA-P, and the Home Environment Interview for Children (HEIC) and the corresponding parent interview (HEIC-P). One rule stated that the child's age was to be taken into account in judging the credibility of the information (i.e., older children were viewed as more credible). A second rule stated that information from the HEIC, the HEIC-P, and from the teacher's report was to be used for evidence of the child's impairment in school and social adjustment. In the case of conduct disorder, a third rule stated that a summary diagnosis could be assigned only when there were two or more symptoms from either the parent or the child report and at least one other source reporting delinquent behavior on the part of the child. The following detailed comparison was made between the maternal and child interviews:

> In cases where children reported sufficient symptoms for a diagnosis and parents did not, we believed that the parents were unaware of the extent of their child's delinquent behavior. In cases where parents reported conduct disorder and their children did not, it was assumed that the children were not telling the truth. It did not seem reasonable to assume that many parents would be reporting that their children had been suspended from school, or had been in trouble with the police, if these events had not occurred. The concrete and serious nature of conduct disorder symptoms makes them believable enough to be accepted as true, even if only one person, the parent or the child, acknowledges that they are present. In all cases in which a summary diagnosis of conduct disorder was made, evidence from the teacher's report and the HEIC/HEIC-P supported the decision. (pp. 608–609)

Out of the 32 children in the study, 8 were given in a summary diagnosis of conduct disorder. Two of these diagnoses would have been possible on the basis of maternal information alone, four of them on the basis of child information alone, and two if complete concordance of mother and child had been required. Considering all diagnoses, Reich and Earls (1987) felt their most important finding was the fact that, in most cases, diagnoses could be made on the basis of the child's reports alone, and that other sources such as parent and teacher information usually served only to confirm it. This statement appears to be discrepant from the findings of the Achenbach and colleagues (1987) meta-analysis already mentioned. Achenbach and his associates reported that the average correlation between self-reports and the ratings of others was only .22.

Typically, the outcome of the clinical judgment model is a "yes–no" decision as to whether the child fits the criteria for the diagnosis, in this case, conduct disorder. The difference between this categorical approach and the dimensional approach implied by the other three models can be appreciable. For example, Shekim and associates (1986) applied both categorical and dimensional approaches to diagnosing ADHD in a sample of 114 community children. Of the 14 children diagnosed as having ADHD by using a standardized parent interview and DSM-III criteria, only two would have been so "diagnosed" by using a cut-off score on the corresponding scale of the Child Behavior Checklist completed by the parents.

Hypothetical Construct Model

Philosophers at least from the time of Plato onward have argued that beneath the surface flux of phenomena there may be some underlying realities not immediately observable by the naked eye. In psychological jargon, such entities are often referred to as "hypothetical constructs" (MacCorquodale & Meehl, 1948).

The history of science contains many examples where the initial assumption of a hypothetical construct has paid large dividends. In ancient times, Democritus spoke of matter as consisting of tiny "atoms," and his views were in a sense strongly confirmed by the emergence of modern atomic physics, including nuclear technology. Mendel spoke of hypothetical entities called "genes" as controlling heredity underlying such characteristics as smooth versus rough surfaces of peas; genes turned out to be real in the form of DNA with its templates for the enzymes serving as catalysts for all of the reactions within plant and animal cells.

Campbell and Fiske (1959) seemed to be thinking of the problem of measuring such hypothetical constructs in the behavioral sciences when they described the multitrait-multimethod matrix as a way of ordering psychometric data. The idea here is to obtain measures not just on the construct ("trait") of interest (e.g., conduct disorder), but on other distinct constructs as well (e.g., IQ, anxiety-withdrawal). Each trait is then measured by several alternative methods. These methods could correspond to what we have labeled in this chapter as sources of information (i.e., parent interview, child interview, teacher ratings, peer ratings, and behavioral observations). In this approach, no one source of information need be regarded as a "gold standard," but the correlation of measures of a particular trait across any pair of methods (e.g., parent interview and direct behavioral observations) is seen as evidence of "convergent validity." If the particular traits under study are supposed to be independent of each other, any traits measured by the same method should be uncorrelated. In fact, there tends to be a sizable correlation of supposedly different traits measured by the same method. For example, teachers who rate children as having conduct disorder will also tend to rate these same children as less intelligent than others, thus yielding a "negative halo" effect. This is known as "method" variance and is the most common impediment to "discriminate validity" as Campbell and Fiske described (1959) it.

The application of the multitrait-multimethod matrix to defining a hypothetical construct such as conduct disorder would first evaluate each purported measure of the construct, retaining only those that demonstrated evidence of at least some convergent validity. Measures using different methods or sources then might be combined in the hope that the different kinds of method variance would cancel out each other. In the absence of any further knowledge concerning the differential validity of the measures, they might be transformed into standard scores and simply averaged into a composite measure of the trait. An alternative procedure would be to weight the measures differentially in relation to the amount of convergent validity they had shown.

Whether such entities exist in the field of child psychopathology is at this time a matter of conjecture. Perhaps it is foolish to hope that a construct such as conduct disorder "really" underlies the patterns of misbehavior manifested by some youngsters. Yet, however it is measured, conduct disorder seems remarkably stable over time. It is more traitlike than just about any other attribute uncovered so far in psychology, with the exception of IQ.

Recent attempts to define conduct disorder as a hypothetical construct have involved a relatively new mathematical technique known as structural equation modeling (Dwyer, 1983). Within this framework, it has been considered as a "latent variable," not directly observable but, rather, indexed by a number of diverse measures (Patterson, 1986; Fergusson & Horwood, 1987a, 1987b). As Patterson noted, the use of structural equation modeling requires the investigator to specify a model of the constructs and their relationships in advance and to use multiple indicators to define each construct. Patterson noted that this "multimode, multiagent" approach was in keeping with the injunctions of MacCorquodale and Meehl (1948), and Cronbach and Meehl (1955) concerning the need to use multiple indicators in defining complex concepts in the social sciences. Patterson's (1986) construct of Antisocial (i.e., overt and clandestine), for example, was defined by a combination of a teacher questionnaire including 20 items selected a priori from the teacher form of the Child Behavior Checklist (Achenbach & Edelbrock, 1979), peer nominations, six different parent measures including questionnaires and telephone interviews, and telephone interviews with the child. Expanded versions of Patterson's model implicated inept discipline by parents (also a composite variable made up of information from multiple sources) as a causal factor in the child's antisocial behavior. A further model then implicated child antisocial behavior itself as a possible cause of low peer acceptance, self-esteem, and academic performance on the part of the child (all composite variables also).

Fergusson and Horwood's (1987a, 1987b) model is simpler than Patterson's and consists of an equally weighted combination of maternal and teacher ratings of conduct disorder in young children. In a birth cohort sample of 1,103 New Zealand children, the Rutter Behavior Questionnaire (Rutter, Tizard, & Whitmore, 1970) and Conners questionnaire (Conners, 1969) were completed by the teacher and mother. These investigators found that maternal ratings at ages 6 and 7 years correlated .65, and teacher ratings at ages 6 and 7 correlated .53. The composite measure correlated .92 between the 2 years and was considered to be an estimate of the trait components of the measures as distinct from the components that were method specific. Indeed, a measure of maternal depression correlated .26 and .28 with the maternal ratings of child conduct disorder at ages 6 and 7, respectively. This later finding was essentially a replication of the findings of Griest and associates (1979) that parental ratings might reflect more about the parents than about the children. In contrast, correlations of maternal depression with the composite ("trait") measure of conduct disorder were only .09 at 6 years and .12 at 7 years. In a multiple regression analysis maternal depression did not significantly predict the trait components of conduct disorder. In other words, use of the composite measure appeared to overcome the problem of method variance. Similar findings were reported with respect to maternal neuroticism and life events: "These variables were correlated with the method component of the maternal scores and when this spurious correlation was taken into account the correlation between these variables and the trait component of the score tended to decline" (Fergusson & Horwood, 1987b, p. 266).

CONCLUSIONS

There is reasonably good agreement at this time as to the types of behaviors to be included in the concept of conduct disorder (e.g., the DSM-III-R definition). Furthermore, a number of single measures of conduct disorder appear to enjoy some level of consensual validation (e.g., the CBCL).

However, there is at present little agreement in the field on how to combine information from different sources in order to arrive at agreement as to which particular children are conduct disordered, and how severely. This situation means that research will continue to be conducted on populations that are not strictly comparable, and this may slow our progress in developing further understanding of one of the most severe disorders in child psychopathology. Unfortunately, this problem is not one that can be solved simply by a thorough review of the literature, nor by the meeting of any professional committee. All four models outlined in this chapter appear to be in use today, and no clear resolution appears on the horizon.

The use of a single measure (gold standard or not) to define Conduct Disorder has simplicity to recommend it. It may be a relatively efficient way for some research programs to proceed. For example, the recent successful work of Quay and his associates (Daugherty & Quay, 1989; Shapiro et al., 1988) in applying Gray's theory to conduct disorder has used teacher ratings on the Revised Behavior Problem Checklist as its main selection criterion. The disadvantage of this single measure approach is its excessive method variance. For example, teacher measures may identify children whom teachers just do not like as well as those with conduct disorder.

If the concept of conduct disorder is merely an arbitrary one contrived for the temporary convenience and communication of persons working in this field, the actuarial model will probably prevail, as well it should. Achenbach's active research program and his effective dissemination of his work will surely encourage others to use his actuarial profile method in assessment. As noted already, Meehl (1954) and his followers demonstrated in many domains the superiority of actuarial over clinical prediction. Yet, despite the fact that he has been a consistent champion of the actuarial method, Meehl seemed to believe in the reality of some entities of psychopathology (e.g., Meehl's 1962 paper on schizotaxia, schizotypy, and schizophrenia).

If a "real" conduct disorder exists, it could be approached as a category or as a continuous dimension. The clinical judgment method described by Reich and Earls (1987) seems to be a refined version of the categorical, "medical model" of diagnosis in child psychopathology in the spirit of DSM-III-R. Therefore, this kind of approach may be common among practitioners and in many ways appeals to common sense to sort through the statements of various informants to find the "truth." Using categories, however, throws out information that continuous dimensions preserve, yet one cannot quarrel with the scientific success or at least the predominance of the medical model in this century.

The hypothetical construct method will continue to be used by those, such as Patterson and his colleagues, who are committed to a particular construct. Fergusson and Horwood (1987a, 1987b) showed how composite measures can efficiently overcome method variance even in the absence of an a priori theory. Obviously, by using Democritus in physics and Mendel in biology as examples of the hypothetical construct approach, we have indicated that we are most sanguine about its potential. We favor defining conduct disorder as a continuous dimension, and espouse Fergusson and Horwood's (1987a, 1987b) model for assessment of it. Whether the hypothetical construct method or another model will ultimately prevail probably depends on future research evaluating the models' ability to preserve and convey reliable information regarding the etiology, response to treatment, and prognosis of conduct disorder.

REFERENCES

Achenbach, T. M. (1978). The Child Behavior Profile: I. Boys aged 6–11. *Journal of Consulting and Clinical Psychology, 46,* 478–488.

Achenbach, T. M. (1985). *Assessment and taxonomy of child and adolescent psychopathology.* Beverly Hills, CA: Sage Publications.

Achenbach, T. M., & Edelbrock, C. S. (1979). The Child Behavior Profile: Boys aged 12 to 16 and girls aged 6 to 11 and 12 to 16. *Journal of Consulting and Clinical Psychology, 47,* 223–233.

Achenbach, T. M., & Edelbrock, C. S. (1983). *Manual for the Child Behavior Checklist and Revised Child Behavior Profile.* Burlington, VT: University Associates in Psychiatry.

Achenbach, T. M., & Edelbrock, C. S. (1987). *Manual for the Youth Self-Report and Profile.* Burlington, VT: University of Vermont, Department of Psychiatry.

Achenbach, T. M., McConaughy, S. H., & Howell, C. T. (1987). Child/adolescent behavioral and emotional problems: Implications of cross-informant correlations for situational specificity. *Psychological Bulletin, 101,* 213–232.

American Psychiatric Association. (1987). *Diagnostic and statistical manual of mental disorders* (3rd ed., rev.). Washington, DC: Author.

Arbuthnot, J., & Gordon, D. A. (1986). Behavioral and cognitive effects of a moral reasoning development intervention for high-risk behavior disordered adolescents. *Journal of Consulting and Clinical Psychology, 54,* 208–216.

Asarnow, J. R. (1988). Peer status and social competence in child psychiatric inpatients: A comparison of children with depressive, externalizing, and concurrent depressive and externalizing disorders. *Journal of Abnormal Child Psychology, 16,* 151–162.

Bell-Dolan, D. J., Foster, S. L., & Sikora, D. M. (1989). Effects of sociometric testing on children's behavior and loneliness in school. *Developmental Psychology, 25,* 306–311.

Cadoret, R. J., Troughton, E., & O'Gorman, T. W. (1987). Genetic and environmental factors in alcohol abuse and antisocial personality. *Journal of Studies on Alcohol, 48,* 1–8.

Campbell, D. T., & Fiske, D. W. (1959). Convergent and discriminant validation by the multitrait-multimethod matrix. *Psychological Bulletin, 56,* 81–105.

Carlson, G., Kashani, J., Thomas, M., Vaidya, A., & Daniel, A. (1987). Comparison of two structured interviews on a psychiatrically hospitalized population of children. *Journal of the American Academy of Child and Adolescent Psychiatry, 26,* 645–648.

Chamberlain, P., & Reid, J. B. (1987). Parent observation and report of child symptoms. *Behavioral Assessment, 9,* 97–109.

Coie, J. D., & Dodge, K. A. (1988). Multiple sources of data on social behavior and social status in the school: A cross-age comparison. *Child Development, 59,* 815–829.

Conners, C. K. (1969). A teacher rating scale for use in drug studies with children. *American Journal of Psychiatry, 126,* 884–888.

Costello, A. J., Edelbrock, C., Dulcan, M. K., Kalas, R., & Klaric, S. (1984). *Report on the NIMH Diagnostic Interview Schedule for Children (DISC).* Washington, DC: National Institute of Mental Health.

Cowen, E. L., Pederson, A., Babigian, H., Izzo, L. D., & Trost, M. A. (1973). Long-term follow-up of early detected vulnerable children. *Journal of Consulting and Clinical Psychology, 41,* 438–446.

Cronbach, L. J., & Meehl, P. E. (1955). Construct validity in psychological tests. *Psychological Bulletin, 52,* 281–302.

Daugherty, T. K., & Quay, H. C. (1989). *Response perseveration and delayed responding in childhood behavior disorders.* Manuscript submitted for publication.

Dwyer, J. H. (1983). *Statistical models for the social and behavioral sciences.* New York: Oxford University Press.

Edelbrock, C., & Costello, A. J. (1988). Convergence between statistically derived behavior problem syndromes and child psychiatric diagnoses. *Journal of Abnormal Child Psychology, 16,* 219–231.

Edelbrock, C., Costello, A. J., Dulcan, M., Kalas, R., & Conover, N. C. (1985). Age differences in the reliability of the psychiatric interview of the child. *Child Development, 56,* 265–275.

Empey, L. T. (1982). *American delinquency: Its meaning and construction.* Homewood, IL: Dorsey Press.

Fergusson, D. M., & Horwood, L. J. (1987a). The trait and method components of ratings of conduct disorder: Part I. Maternal and teacher evaluations of conduct disorder in young children. *Journal of Child Psychology and Psychiatry, 28,* 249–260.

Fergusson, D. M., & Horwood, L. J. (1987b). The trait and method components of ratings of conduct disorder: Part II. Factors related to the trait component of conduct disorder scores. *Journal of Child Psychology and Psychiatry, 28,* 261–272.

Forehand, R. L., King, H. E., Peed, S., & Yoder, P. (1975). Mother–child interactions: Comparison of a non-compliant clinic group and a non-clinic group. *Behaviour Research and Therapy, 13,* 79–84.

Goyette, C. H., Conners, C. K., & Ulrich, R. F. (1978). Normative data on Revised Conners Parent and Teacher Ratings Scales. *Journal of Abnormal Child Psychology, 6,* 221–236.

Graham, P., & Rutter, M. (1968). The reliability and validity of the psychiatric assessment of the child: II. Interview with the parent. *British Journal of Psychiatry, 114,* 581–592.

Griest, D., Wells, K. C., & Forehand, R. (1979). An examination of predictors of maternal perceptions of maladjustment in clinic-referred children. *Journal of Abnormal Psychology, 88,* 277–281.

Hare, R. D., McPherson, L. M., & Forth, A. E. (1988). Male psychopaths and their criminal careers. *Journal of Consulting and Clinical Psychology, 56,* 710–714.

Herjanic, B., & Campbell, W. (1977). Differentiating psychiatrically disturbed children on the basis of a structured interview. *Journal of Abnormal Child Psychology, 5,* 127–134.

Herjanic, B., Herjanic, M., Brown, F., & Wheatt, T. (1975). Are children reliable reporters? *Journal of Abnormal Child Psychology, 3,* 41–48.

Hewitt, L. E., & Jenkins, R. L. (1946). *Fundamental patterns of maladjustment.* Springfield, IL: State of Illinois.

Hinshaw, S. P. (1987). On the distinction between attention deficits/hyperactivity and conduct problems/aggression in child psychopathology. *Psychological Bulletin, 101,* 443–463.

Hodges, K., & Cools, J. N. (1990). Structured diagnostic interviews. In A. M. LaGreca (Ed.), *Through the eyes of the child* (pp. 109–149). Boston: Allyn & Bacon.

Hodges, K., Kline, J., Stern, L., Cytryn, L., & McKnew, D. (1982). The development of a child assessment interview for research and clinical use. *Journal of Abnormal Child Psychology, 10,* 173–189.

Hodges, K., McKnew, D., Burbach, D. J., & Roebuck, L. (1987). Diagnostic concordance between the Child Assessment Schedule (CAS) and the Schedule for Affective Disorders and Schizophrenia for School-Age Children (K-SADS) in an outpatient sample using lay interviewers. *Journal of the American Academy of Child and Adolescent Psychiatry, 26,* 654–661.

Huesmann, L. R., Eron, L. D., Lefkowitz, M. M., & Walder, L. J. (1984). The stability of aggression over time and generations. *Developmental Psychology, 20,* 1120–1134.

Johnson, S. M., Christensen, A., & Bellamy, G. T. (1976). Evaluation of family intervention through unobtrusive audio recordings: Experiences in "bugging" children. *Journal of Applied Behavior Analysis, 9,* 213–219.

Kandel, E., Mednick, S. A., Kirkegaard-Sorensen, L., Hutchings, B., Knop, J., Rosenberg, R., & Schulsinger, F. (1988). IQ as a protective factor for subjects at high risk for antisocial behavior. *Journal of Consulting and Clinical Psychology, 56,* 224–226.

Kashani, J. H., Orvaschel, H., Burk, J. P., & Reid, J. C. (1985). Informant variance: The issue of parent–child disagreement. *Journal of the American Academy of Child Psychiatry, 24,* 437–441.

Kazdin, A. E. (1987). Treatment of antisocial behavior in children: Current status and future directions. *Psychological Bulletin, 102,* 187–203.

Kazdin, A. E., & Esveldt-Dawson, K. (1986). The Interview for Antisocial Behavior: Psychometric characteristics and concurrent validity with child psychiatric inpatients. *Journal of Psychopathology and Behavioral Assessment, 8,* 289–303.

Klorman, R., Brumaghim, J. T., Salzman, L. F., Strauss, J., Borgstedt, A. D., McBride, M. C., & Loeb, S. (1988). Effects of methylphenidate on attention-deficit hyperactivity disorder with and without aggressive/noncompliant features. *Journal of Abnormal Psychology, 97,* 413–422.

Kovacs, M. (1978). *The Interview Schedule for Children (ISC).* Pittsburg, PA: University of Pittsburgh School of Medicine.

Lahey, B. B., Hartdagen, S., Frick, P. J., McBurnett, K., Connor, R., & Hynd, G. W. (1988). Conduct disorder: Parsing the confounded relation to parental divorce and antisocial personality. *Journal of Abnormal Psychology, 97,* 334–337.

Lahey, B. B., Piacentini, J. C., McBurnett, K., Stone, P., Hartdagen, S., & Hynd, G. (1988) Psychopathology in the parents of children with conduct disorder and hyperactivity. *Journal of the American Academy of Child and Adolescent Psychiatry, 27,* 163–170.

Langhorne, J. E., Jr., Loney, J., Paternite, C. E., & Bechtoldt, H. P. (1976). Childhood hyperkinesis: A return to the source. *Journal of Abnormal Psychology, 85,* 201–209.

Lobitz, G. K., & Johnson, S. M. (1975). Normal versus deviant children: A multimethod comparison. *Journal of Abnormal Child Psychology, 3,* 353–374.

Loeber, R. (1982). The stability of antisocial and delinquent childhood behavior. *Child Development, 53,* 1431–1446.

Loeber, R., & Schmaling, K. B. (1985a). The utility of differentiating between mixed and pure forms of antisocial child behavior. *Journal of Abnormal Child Psychology, 13,* 315–335.

Loeber, R., & Schmaling, K. B. (1985b). Empirical evidence for overt and covert patterns of antisocial conduct problems: A metaanalysis. *Journal of Abnormal Child Psychology, 13,* 337–352.

MacCorquodale, K., & Meehl, P. E. (1948). On a distinction between hypothetical constructs and intervening variables. *Psychological Review, 55,* 95–107.

McConaughy, S. H., Achenbach, T. M., & Gent, C. L. (1988). Multiaxial empirically based assessment: Parent, teacher, observational, cognitive, and personality correlates of Child Behavioral Profile types for 6- to 11-year-old boys. *Journal of Abnormal Child Psychology, 16,* 485–509.

McGee, R., & Williams, S. (1988). A longitudinal study of depression in nine-year-old children. *Journal of the American Academy of Child and Adolescent Psychiatry, 27,* 342–348.

Meehl, P. E. (1954). *Clinical versus statistical prediction: A theoretical analysis and a review of the evidence.* Minneapolis: University of Minnesota Press.

Meehl, P. E. (1962). Schizotaxia, schizotypy, schizophrenia. *American Psychologist, 17,* 827–838.

Milich, R., & Loney, J. (1979). The role of hyperactivity and aggressive symptomatology in predicting adolescent outcome among hyperactive children. *Journal of Pediatric Psychology, 4,* 93–112.

Milich, R., Widiger, R. A., & Landau, S. (1987). Differential diagnosis of attention deficit and conduct disorders using conditional probabilities. *Journal of Consulting and Clinical Psychology, 55,* 762–767.

Olweus, D. (1977). Aggression and peer acceptance in adolescent boys: Two short-term longitudinal studies of ratings. *Child Development, 48,* 1301–1313.

Olweus, D. (1979). Stability of aggressive reaction patterns in males: A review. *Psychological Bulletin, 86,* 852–875.

Olweus, D. (1980). The consistency issue in personality psychology revised: With special reference to aggression. *British Journal of Social and Clinical Psychology, 19,* 377–390.

Patterson, G. R. (1977). Naturalistic observation in clinical assessment. *Journal of Abnormal Child Psychology, 5,* 309–322.

Patterson, G. R. (1982). *Coercive family process.* Eugene, OR: Castalia.

Patterson, G. R. (1986). Performance models for antisocial boys. *American Psychologist, 41,* 432–444.

Puig-Antich, J., & Chambers, W. (1978). *The Schedule for Affective Disorders and Schizophrenia for School-Age Children (Kiddie-SADS).* New York: New York State Psychiatric Institute.

Quay, H. C. (1979). Classification. In H. C. Quay & J. S. Werry (Eds.), *Psychopathological disorders of childhood* (2nd ed., pp. 1–42). New York: Wiley.

Quay, H. C. (Ed.) (1987). *Handbook of juvenile delinquency.* New York: Wiley.

Quay, H. C. (1988). The behavioral reward and inhibition system in childhood behavior disorder. In L. M. Bloomingdale (Ed.), *Attention deficit disorder* (Vol. 3., pp. 176–186). Oxford, England: Pergamon Press.

Quay, H. C., & Peterson, D. R. (1983). *Interim manual for the Revised Behavior Problem Checklist.* Coral Gables, FL: University of Miami.

Quay, H. C., Routh, D. K., & Shapiro, S. K. (1987). Psychopathology of childhood: From description to validation. In M. R. Rosenzweig & L. W. Parter (Eds.), *Annual review of psychology* (Vol. 38., pp. 491–532). Palo Alto, CA: Annual Reviews.

Rapoport, J. L., & Benoit, M. (1975). The relation of direct home observations to the clinic evaluation of hyperactive school age boys. *Journal of Child Psychology and Psychiatry, 16,* 141–147.

Reeves, J. C., Werry, J. S., Elkind, G. S., & Zametkin, A. (1987). Attention deficit, conduct, oppositional, and anxiety disorders in children: II. Clinical characteristics. *Journal of the American Academy of Child and Adolescent Psychiatry, 26,* 144–155.

Reich, W., & Earls, F. (1987). Rules for making psychiatric diagnoses in children on the basis of multiple sources of information: Preliminary strategies. *Journal of Abnormal Child Psychology, 15,* 601–616.

Robins, L. N. (1966). *Deviant children grown up.* Baltimore: Williams & Wilkins.

Robinson, E. A., & Eyberg, S. M. (1981). The Dyadic Parent–Child Interaction Coding System: Standardization and validation. *Journal of Consulting and Clinical Psychology, 49,* 245–250.

Routh, D. K. (1989). Validating diagnostic categories. In C. G. Last & M. Hersen (Eds.), *Handbook of child psychiatric diagnosis* (pp. 41–57). New York: Wiley.

Routh, D. K. (1990). Taxonomy in developmental psychopathology: Consider the source. In M. Lewis & S. M. Miller (Eds.), *Handbook of developmental psychopathology* (pp. 53–62). New York: Plenum.

Russell, A. T., Bott, L., & Sammons, C. (1989). The phenomenology of schizophrenia occurring in childhood. *Journal of the American Academy of Child and Adolescent Psychiatry, 28,* 399–407.

Rutter, M., & Graham, P. (1968). The reliability and validity of the psychiatric assessment of the child: I. Interview with the child. *British Journal of Psychiatry, 114,* 563–579.

Rutter, M., Tizard, J., & Whitmore, K. (Eds.) (1970). *Education, health, and behavior.* London: Longman.

Rydelius, P. A. (1988). The development of antisocial behavior and sudden violent death. *Acta Psychiatrica Scandinavica, 77,* 398–403.

Schonfeld, I. S., Shaffer, D., O'Connor, P., & Portnoy, S. (1988). Conduct disorder and cognitive functioning: Testing three causal hypotheses. *Child Development, 59,* 993–1007.

Shapiro, S. K., Quay, H. C., Hogan, A. E., & Schwartz, K. P. (1988). Response perseveration and delayed responding in undersocialized aggressive conduct disorder. *Journal of Abnormal Psychology, 97,* 371–373.

Shekim, W. O., Cantwell, D. P., Kashani, J., Beck, N., Martin, J., & Rosenberg, J. (1986). Dimensional and categorical approaches to the diagnosis of attention deficit disorder in children. *Journal of the American Academy of Child Psychiatry, 25,* 653–658.

Shinn, M. R., Ramsey, E., Walker, H. M., Steiber, S., & O'Neill, R. E. (1987). Antisocial behavior in school settings: Initial differences in an at risk and normal population. *Journal of Special Education, 21,* 69–84.

Snyder, J., & Patterson, G. R. (1987). Family interaction and delinquent behavior. In H. C. Quay (Ed.), *Handbook of juvenile delinquency* (pp. 216–243). New York: Wiley.

Stewart, M. A., & Kelso, J. (1987). A two-year follow-up of boys with aggressive conduct disorder. *Psychopathology, 20,* 296–304.

Taylor, E., Everitt, B., Thorley, G., Schachar, R., Rutter, M., & Wieselberg, M. (1986). Conduct disorder and hyperactivity: II. A cluster analytic approach to the identification of a behavioral syndrome. *British Journal of Psychiatry, 149,* 768–777.

Taylor, E., Schachar, R., Thorley, G., & Wieselberg, M. (1986). Conduct disorder and hyperactivity: I. Separation of hyperactivity and antisocial conduct in British child psychiatric patients. *British Journal of Psychiatry, 149,* 760–767.

Van Voohis, P., Cullen, F. T., Mathers, R. A., & Garner, C. C. (1988). The impact of family structure and quality on delinquency: A comparative assessment of structural and functional factors. *Criminology, 26,* 235–261.

Walder, L. O., Abelson, R. P., Eron, L. D., Banta, T. J., & Laulicht, J. H. (1961). Development of a peer-rating measure of aggression. *Psychological Reports, 9,* 497–556.

Walker, J. L., Lahey, B. B., Hynd, G. W., & Frame, C. L. (1987). Comparison of specific patterns of antisocial behavior in children with conduct disorder with or without coexisting hyperactivity. *Journal of Consulting and Clinical Psychology, 55,* 910–913.

Webster-Stratton, C. (1985). Mother perception and mother–child interactions: Comparison of a clinic-referred and a nonclinic group. *Journal of Clinical Child Psychology, 14,* 334–339.

Welner, Z., Reich, W., Herjanic, B., Jung, K. G., & Amado, H. (1987). Reliability, validity, and parent–child agreement studies of the Diagnostic Interview for Children and

Adolescents (DICA). *Journal of the American Academy of Child and Adolescent Psychiatry, 26*, 649–653.

Werry, J. S., Methven, J. R., Fitzpatrick, T., & Dixon, H. (1983). The interrater reliability of DSM-III in children. *Journal of Abnormal Child Psychology, 11*, 341–354.

West, D. J. (1987). Review of D. L. Olweus, J. Block, & M. Radke-Yarrow (Eds.), Development of antisocial and prosocial behavior. *Journal of Child Psychology and Psychiatry, 28*, 189.

CHAPTER 5

Attention Deficit-Hyperactivity Disorder in Children

David C. Guevremont
Russell A. Barkley
University of Massachusetts Medical Center

Few disorders of childhood have received as much theoretical and empirical scrutiny in child psychiatry and psychology as that which is subsumed under the classification of attention deficit-hyperactivity disorder (ADHD; American Psychiatric Association, 1987). The quantity of scientific papers devoted to this disorder in the past 25 years is probably related to the fact that children displaying symptoms of ADHD represent one of the most common referral complaints to child mental health professionals in the United States (Ross & Ross, 1982). Despite the wealth of research information available, historical shifts in the conceptualization of causes of ADHD, as well as the symptoms believed to constitute the disorder, have contributed to misconceptions and diagnostic ambiguities on the part of the general public and professionals alike.

Currently, ADHD is considered to be a developmental disorder of age-appropriate attention span, impulse control, rule-governed behavior (i.e., response to rules and verbal instructions), and sometimes motor restlessness or overactivity (American Psychiatric Association, 1987; Barkley, 1981). Previously referred to as hyperkinesis, hyperactive child syndrome, minimal brain dysfunction, and attention deficit disorder (ADD; with or without hyperactivity), the disorder has been relabeled and diagnostic criteria changed as recently as 1987. This relabeling no doubt reflects the rapidly increasing research on the etiologies, primacy of symptoms, associated features, and developmental course of the disorder.

HISTORICAL OVERVIEW

One of the earliest and complete descriptions of children displaying symptoms now ascribed to ADHD was presented by George Still (1902) in a series of published lectures to the Royal College of Physicians in England. Still described a group of children in his clinic practice who were highly emotional, defiant, aggressive, and quite resistant to discipline. Many were also described as excessively active and poor at attending to tasks. Still conceptualized these behavior patterns as resulting from serious deficiencies in the "volitional inhibition" of behavior and arising from various types of "defects in moral control" (p. 1008). Hereditary transmission of these characteristics was posited as a possible etiology, whereas in other children these symptoms were believed to have been acquired as a result of central nervous system damage. Still observed that these symptoms were more common in males and appeared to be accompanied by a higher number of minor physical anomalies in their appearance.

The next 35 years saw few papers on children with these characteristics, although motor restlessness was given emphasis in those that did appear (e.g., Childers, 1935; Levin, 1938). After World War 2, Strauss, Lehtinen, and their colleagues (e.g., Strauss & Lehtinen, 1947) posited that motor restlessness and inattentive behavior in children were the direct result of brain damage. They coined the phrase *minimal brain damage* to describe what they believed was the cause of hyperactivity in children, even where evidence or history of brain injury was lacking. Nonetheless, excessive motor activity remained the defining symptom of this disorder throughout the 1950s and 1960s, although new explanatory mechanisms were being posited (e.g., Laufer, Denhoff, & Solomons, 1957).

By the late 1960s, conclusions regarding brain damage as the primary cause of hyperactivity became less certain, resulting in a shift in diagnostic labels to minimal brain dysfunction (Wender, 1971), hyperactive child syndrome (Chess, 1960; American Psychiatric Association, 1968), or hyperkinetic reaction of childhood. By the mid-1970s, however, a growing body of evidence began to accumulate that also questioned whether "hyperactivity" was in fact the primary deficit of the disorder. A series of studies suggested that children labeled *hyperactive* also showed pronounced deficits with sustaining attention to tasks and controlling impulsive responses in comparison to normal children (e.g., Douglas, 1972). A shift away from viewing overactivity as the primary deficit of the disorder to problems in sustaining attention, inhibiting behavior, and regulating actions in the context of situational demands resulted from this research (American Psychiatric Association, 1980; Routh, 1978).

This conceptual shift was so influential that the disorder was relabeled attention deficit disorder (with or without hyperactivity) by the American Psychiatric Association in 1980. By 1987, a re-emergence in the emphasis given earlier to motor restlessness as a defining symptom of the disorder once again resulted in a relabeling of the disorder to ADHD (American Psychiatric Association, 1987; Barkley, Costello, & Spitzer, 1989). The subtyping, "without hyperactivity" was related to a separate and minimally detailed category of undifferentiated attention deficit disorder (see Barkley, Costello, & Spitzer, 1989).

PRIMARY SYMPTOMS AND SITUATIONAL VARIATIONS

Each of the symptoms constituting ADHD is believed to be multidimensional rather than unitary, although research has been conflictual as to precisely which dimensions are the most distinguishing deficits in the disorder. Nonetheless, research to date suggests that ADHD children have their greatest difficulties with sustained attention or vigilance (Douglas, 1983) versus focused or selective attention and alertness. Thus, clinical complaints often concern incomplete work, off-task behavior, or rapid shifting of activities.

Much of the impairment resulting from ADHD is manifested under conditions in which the child is expected to behave in accordance with age-related situational demands. Consequently, both the frequency and severity of problems may fluctuate across settings, activities, and caregivers (e.g., Tarver-Behring, Barkley, & Karlsson, 1985; Zentall, 1984). Difficulties with sustained attention appear to become more pronounced in the context of especially dull tasks, repetitive or effortful activity, or those tasks having little intrinsic appeal (Barkley, 1989; Luk, 1985). Conversely, problems with sustained attention and other primary symptoms of ADHD may dissipate dramatically under conditions of continuous and immediate reinforcement schedules, as opposed to partial and delayed schedules of reinforcement (Douglas & Parry, 1983), and during self-paced tasks, intrinsically interesting activities (e.g., video games), and novel conditions or unfamiliar settings (Barkley, 1977,

1989; Luk, 1985). In settings with little structure or where demands to follow rules are low, ADHD children may be less distinguishable from normal children (Barkley, 1985; Jacob, O'Leary, & Rosenblad, 1978; Routh & Schroeder, 1976). Moreover, in settings or on tasks in which instructions are repeated frequently, problems with sustained attention are less pronounced (Douglas, 1983). These situational fluctuations in symptoms suggest that the deficits ascribed to ADHD children are highly interactive with and influenced by the environmental context (Barkley, 1981, 1989; Zentall, 1984).

A similar statement can be made about impulsivity, which is believed to be multidimensional in nature (Milich & Kramer, 1985). Impulsive behavior may also show variability across different environmental and reinforcement arrangements (e.g., Douglas & Parry, 1983). Impulsivity in ADHD children has been characterized as a pattern of rapid, inaccurate responding (Brown & Quay, 1977), poor ability to delay immediate gratification (Rapport, Tucker, DuPaul, Merlo, & Stoner, 1986), and a function of limited use of cognitive-mediational strategies that assist in the regulation of one's own behavior (Kendall & Braswell, 1982).

The overlap between attention and response inhibition becomes apparent when one considers that factor analytic studies (Milich & Kramer, 1985) have failed to differentiate an impulsive dimension from those measuring activity and attention. Lahey and colleagues (1988), for example, found support for an inattention and excessive motor activity factor but no support for the notion that impulsivity exists as an independent dimension. Items describing impulsive behavior loaded most strongly with motor hyperactivity items. The interdependence of these constructs calls into question whether such symptoms are merely different facets of one or two deficits rather than three as reflected in current clinical and theoretical writings (American Psychiatric Association, 1980, 1987; Douglas, 1983). Nonetheless, frequent complaints on the part of parents and teachers pertaining to excessive talking, problems waiting for a turn, "blurting out answers" prematurely, and limited awareness of potentially dangerous actions suggest that impulsivity is a defining element in the disorder.

Numerous studies have shown ADHD children to be more active, restless, and fidgety than normal children (Barkley & Cunningham, 1979; Porrino et al., 1983). Factor analytic studies suggest further that overactivity represents a distinct symptom cluster from measures of inattention in ADHD children (e.g., Edelbrock, Costello, & Kessler, 1984; Lahey et al., 1988). Thus, children may display inattention but not hyperactivity. Despite these findings, it has not been convincingly shown that hyperactivity distinguishes ADHD from other clinic-referred groups of children (Firestone & Martin, 1979; Sandberg, Rutter, &

Taylor, 1978). Recent studies, however, suggest that it may be the pervasiveness of the hyperactivity across settings that distinguishes ADHD from other diagnostic groups (Taylor, 1986).

Finally, poor compliance to instructions and rules may also represent a primary deficit in ADHD children (American Psychiatric Association, 1987; Barkley, 1981, 1982, 1989), although it is not yet clear what mechanism(s) may account for these deficits. ADHD children demonstrate significant problems with compliance to parental and teacher commands (Barkley, 1985; Whalen, Henker, & Dotemoto, 1980), with experimental instructions in the absence of the experimenter (Draeger, Prior, & Sanson, 1986), and with prohibitions to defer gratification (Rapport et al., 1986).

Although such problems may be a by-product of poor impulse control and attention, researchers have recently speculated that a "motivational deficit" may partly explain these deficits (Barkley, 1989; Haenlein & Caul, 1987; Van der Meere & Sergeant, 1988a, 1988b). In this view, ADHD children show a deficiency in the way they are regulated by environmental consequences. As noted, ADHD children appear to show an impaired sensitivity to reinforcement and possibly punishment (Douglas & Parry, 1983). Consequently, rules and instructions may fail to develop the meaningful properties necessary to control behavior to the degree expected for the child's chronological or mental age. It appears therefore that ADHD children are primarily "contingency-shaped" rather than rule-governed in their behavior. Given this assertion, these children seem to be influenced more by the immediately available contingencies rather than the previously given or implicit rule (Barkley, 1981, 1987, 1989). Not surprisingly, ADHD children are routinely referred for treatment because of problems with compliance to adult directives and rules and as a group they have been described as discipline-resistant (Barkley, 1981). Although the notion of a motivation deficit and its contribution to ADHD symptomology remains speculative, studies are currently underway to define the underlying mechanisms and parameters of poor rule compliance and responsivity to consequences in this group of children.

SECONDARY AND ASSOCIATED CHARACTERISTICS

In addition to the primary or defining symptoms of the disorder, a large literature exists that indicates a higher prevalence of developmental, behavioral, emotional, and academic difficulties of ADHD children. Accidental poisonings, health problems (e.g., upper respiratory illnesses), sleep disturbances, enuresis, and physical injuries are more common in ADHD than in normal children (Hartsough & Lambert, 1985; Ross & Ross, 1982; Stewart, Thack, & Friedin, 1970). Deficits in general intelligence, academic achievement, motor coordination, and a higher prevalence of learning disabilities are also frequently reported (e.g., Cantwell & Satterfield, 1978; Ross & Ross, 1982; Safer & Allen, 1976).

Peer relationship problems and social rejection are found in as many as 60% of ADHD children (Campbell & Paulauskas, 1979; Johnston, Pelham, & Murphy, 1985; Milich & Landau, 1982). Poor self-esteem and mild forms of depression may emerge as problems of later childhood, possibly as a result of chronic failure and conflict in social, academic, and family functioning (Barkley, 1981; Breen & Barkley, 1985; Weiss & Hechtman, 1986). Problematic and negative social interactions with adults may develop early in such children as they often appear to be more coercive, aggressive, and less able to sustain compliance than normal children in interactions with their mothers (e.g., Barkley, Karlsson, & Pollard, 1985; Cunningham & Barkley, 1979; Mash & Johnston, 1982). These negative interaction patterns also exist in the relations of many ADHD children with their fathers (Tallmadge & Barkley, 1983) as well as with teachers (Whalen et al., 1980).

Thus, ADHD children represent a heterogenous group in which variations and combinations of these associated characteristics appear to increase the risk for developing additional problems in adjustment for some of these children more than others. Perhaps the most distinguishing associated feature, with important implications for both assessment and treatment, involves the presence and severity of aggressive behavior and conduct problems, found in up to 70% of clinic samples (Loney & Milich, 1982). ADHD children with aggression are more likely to suffer poor peer relationships, poorer academic outcomes, greater problems with delinquency, and a higher incidence of psychopathology in their parents than children with lesser degrees of hostile-defiant behavior (Paternite & Loney, 1980; Weiss & Hechtman, 1986).

A second subtyping of characteristics with implications for identifying differential etiologies, outcomes, and treatments involves the presence and degree of hyperactivity. Factor analytic studies have identified a distinct group of children who display inattention but not hyperactivity. It is possible for such children to receive a DSM-III-R diagnosis of ADHD despite the absence of hyperactivity. This group appears to correspond to the diagnosis of attention deficit disorder without hyperactivity (American Psychiatric Association, 1980), where a sluggish cognitive tempo, higher prevalence of anxious and depressive features, social withdrawal, and a greater incidence of learning disabilities have been reported (e.g., Carlson, 1986; Lahey, Schaughency, Hynd, Carlson, & Nieves, 1987). Conversely, those with hyperactivity often display higher levels of aggression, poorer peer interactions, and poorer academic performance (Edelbrock et al., 1984; King & Young, 1982). Such findings suggest that these groups may represent different disorders altogether, possibly requiring different treatment approaches. Highly anxious and depressed ADHD children, for example, may be more prone to poor or adverse reactions to stimulant medications than those without these symptoms (Taylor, 1983; Voelker, Lachar, & Gdowski, 1983), although replication and clarification of these findings awaits more rigorous investigations.

PREVALENCE AND ETIOLOGY

Between 3% and 5% of the school-aged population is believed to be diagnosable as ADHD (Ross & Ross, 1982). The disorder is more prevalent in males, with ratios ranging from 6:1 to 10:1 in clinic samples (American Psychiatric Association, 1980), although epidemiological surveys have reported ratios as low as 3:1 (Trites, Dugas, Lynch, & Ferguson, 1979). The prevalence appears to vary slightly across countries (O'Leary, Vivian, & Nisi, 1985) and socioeconomic groups, but ADHD occurs in all cultures and countries (Taylor & Sandberg, 1984).

To date, no single etiology has adequately accounted for this disorder, although the most consistent findings of research suggest familial-hereditary factors, pregnancy (e.g., alcohol, tobacco consumption), and obstetrical complications (e.g., postmaturity) as possible predisposing influences (Cantwell, 1975; Omenn, 1973; Ross & Ross, 1982). Although structural brain damage has long been implicated in the etiology of ADHD, there is evidence that fewer than 5% to 10% of ADHD children have histories suggestive of brain damage (Rutter, 1977). Recent studies using computerized axial tomography (CAT) have also failed to reveal significant differences between ADD children and matched controls (Shaywitz, Shaywitz, Byrne, Cohen, & Rothman, 1983).

Although brain damage may not be the primary cause of ADHD in most children, there is indirect evidence that neurological functioning in circumscribed cortical and subcortical areas of the brain may be impaired in some children. For example, two studies found that ADHD children had decreased blood flow in the central white matter of the frontal lobes, caudate nucleus, and striatum relative to normal children and children with developmental dysphasia (Lou, Henriksen, & Bruhn,

1984; Lou, Henriksen, Bruhn, Borner, & Nielsen, 1989). In line with such findings are the results of a study using computer averaging of electroencephalograph (EEG) wave patterns during cognitive tasks (Satterfield, 1986). Decreased patterns of activation or reactivity were found in the frontal areas of ADHD children relative to controls. Neuropsychological findings of poorer performance on measures of frontal lobe functioning in ADHD children relative to normal or clinical control groups lend further support to the notion of frontal lobe dysfunction in ADHD (Chelune, Ferguson, Koon, & Dickey, 1986; Grodzinsky, 1990; Mariani, 1990).

These results, as well as additional indirect evidence from neuropsychological and psychophysiological studies (Anastopoulos & Barkley, 1988), would seem to indicate a pattern of underactivity in certain frontal cortical and subcortical areas particularly in the orbital-frontal zone and its connections with the striatum (caudate nucleus) of the brain in some ADHD children. Such neuropsychological findings are quite consistent with the findings from behavioral observations of ADHD children in that the primary symptoms of ADHD are acknowledged to be a function of the integrity of the dorsolateral and orbital regions of the frontal cortex (Stuss & Benson, 1986).

Additional attention has been directed toward the possible causal role played by neurochemical imbalances and/or deficiencies in contributing to neurological dysfunction in ADHD children. In particular, some investigators have reported results consistent with a neurochemical explanation of brain dysfunction, primarily involving dopamine (Shaywitz, Cohen, & Bowers, 1977) and norepinephrine mechanisms (Shekim, Dekirmenjian, Chapel, Javoid, & Davis, 1979), although other studies have not supported the neurochemical hypothesis (e.g., Rapoport, Quinn, & Lamprecht, 1974). Despite the methodological shortcomings in many of these studies, recent reviews of this literature (e.g., Zametkin & Rapoport, 1986) have tentatively concluded that dopamine and/or norepinephrine may be involved in the etiology of ADHD. Such conclusions must remain tentative until further and more rigorous investigations are completed.

Finally, although various toxins, such as food additives, refined sugars, and allergens have been proposed as possible etiologies of ADHD (Feingold, 1975; Taylor, 1980), rigorous investigations have not supported these contentions (Conners, 1980; Gross, 1984; Mattes & Gittelman, 1981). Elevated blood lead levels, however, have been linked, albeit weakly, to the development of hyperactivity in some children (e.g., David, Clark, & Hoffman, 1979; Rummo, Routh, Rummo, & Brown, 1979).

DEVELOPMENTAL COURSE

Earlier research suggested that ADHD children tended to outgrow their problems by adolescence. Recent findings, however, indicate that the majority will continue to show problems with inattention, restlessness, and impulsivity well into adolescence and early adulthood (Mannuzza, Gittelman-Klein, Bonagura, Horowitz Konig, & Shenker, 1988; Weiss & Hechtman, 1986). ADHD is believed to arise in early childhood, with most children being identified as deviant prior to age 7 (Barkley, Fischer, Newby, & Breen, 1988; Ross & Ross, 1982). Difficulties in managing their behavior and toilet training are noted in about half of ADHD children by age 3 (Hartsough & Lambert, 1985; Safer & Allen, 1976).

The majority of these children will have displayed the primary ADHD symptoms by 6 years of age, with oppositional, aggressive, and defiant behavior emerging in many (Ross & Ross, 1982). By the middle childhood years, academic difficulties often surface (Cantwell & Satterfield, 1978) and are frequently accompanied by complaints of poor rule compliance, disruptive behavior, and poor peer relations. Those with a greater degree of oppositional-defiant behavior, lying, and stealing are at greater risk for developing adolescent conduct disorders and antisocial personality in young adulthood (Paternite & Loney, 1980; Weiss & Hetchman, 1986).

The degree and severity of primary symptoms (e.g., inattention, hyperactivity) may dissipate during adolescence, but the majority of ADHD children will continue to deviate from normal adolescents with respect to these symptoms (Gittelman, Mannuzza, Shenker, & Bonagura, 1985). Continued difficulties appear to be more common in those who had developed conduct problems, whereas those without such difficulties may show problems limited primarily to academic underachievement (Paternite & Loney, 1980). ADHD children displaying aggression and conduct problems will have more contacts with police, greater incidences of truancy, drug use, and family conflicts at adolescence than those without significant levels of conduct problems (Weiss & Hetchman, 1986). Poor self-esteem, depression, alcoholism, and social and occupational difficulties continue for a number of these children, particularly those with lower levels of intelligence and socioeconomic status, serious conduct problems, poor social relations, parental psychopathology, and the absence or ineffectiveness of treatment (Loney, Whaley-Klahn, Kosier, & Conboy, 1981; Satterfield, Satterfield, & Cantwell, 1981; Thorley, 1984; Weiss & Hetchman, 1986).

Such predisposing factors may relate to the longer term outcomes for this group. During the young adult years, many appear to show improved social adjustment in comparison to the adolescent years. Still, over 60% continue to report restlessness, inattention, impulsivity, depression, and low self-esteem in comparison with non-ADHD young adults (Weiss & Hetchman, 1986). Moreover, between 25% and 45% continue to display aggression, conduct problems, problems with alcohol, and criminal behavior during the young adult years (Gittelman et al., 1985; Loney et al., 1981; Weiss & Hetchman, 1986).

CURRENT DIAGNOSTIC CRITERIA: REVIEW AND CRITIQUE

The most recent guidelines for diagnosing ADHD appear in the revised Diagnostic and Statistical Manual (DSM-III-R; American Psychiatric Association, 1987) presented in Table 5.1. A cutoff score of at least eight symptoms was established through a clinical field trial as the score with the greatest accuracy in correct classification among several different diagnostic groups. Although the revision provides greater specification of behaviors considered a symptom of the disorder, problems inherent in DSM-III-R include the use of a single fixed cutoff score across all age levels, age of onset and duration criteria that are not empirically established, and the unidimensional listing of symptoms that may not adequately reflect different symptom clusters (e.g., inattention versus hyperactivity) among groups of children. Additional guidelines for establishing a diagnosis have been suggested by Barkley (1982) and are presented in Table 5.2.

Little, if any research has yet been done on the interrater reliability of the DSM-III-R criteria for ADHD. What few studies were done on the earlier DSM-III criteria for attention deficit disorder (ADD) suggested low reliability among clinicians, especially across countries (Pendergrast et al., 1988), although somewhat higher agreements were found among research teams (Lahey et al., 1987; Pendergrast et al., 1988).

The validity of the DSM-III-R criteria are somewhat difficult to establish in view of problems inherent in specifying a criterion or standard for ADHD against which newly proposed criteria can be compared. Prior research on DSM-III ADD criteria did show reasonable concordance with parent and teacher ratings of ADD symptoms (Edelbrock & Costello, 1988), and children selected by those criteria were often significantly different from normal or other diagnostic groups on measures of personality, vigilance, impulsivity, activity level, and parent–child

TABLE 5.1
Criteria for Diagnosing Attention Deficit-Hyperactivity Disorder

A. A disturbance of at least six months during which at least eight of the following are present:
 (1) often fidgets with hands or feet or squirms in seat (in adolescents, may be limited to subjective feelings of restlessness)
 (2) has difficulty remaining seated when required to do so
 (3) is easily distracted by extraneous stimuli
 (4) has difficulty awaiting turn in games or group situations
 (5) often blurts out answers to questions before they have been completed
 (6) has difficulty following through on instructions from others (not due to oppositional behavior or failure of comprehension), e.g., fails to finish chores
 (7) has difficulty sustaining attention in tasks or play activities
 (8) often shifts from one uncompleted activity to another
 (9) has difficulty playing quietly
 (10) often talks excessively
 (11) often interrupts or intrudes on others, e.g., butts into other children's games
 (12) often does not seem to listen to what is being said to him or her
 (13) often loses things necessary for tasks or activities at school or at home (e.g., toys, pencils, books, assignments)
 (14) often engages in physically dangerous activities without considering possible consequences (not for the purpose of thrill-seeking), e.g., runs into street without looking
B. Onset before the age of seven
C. Does not meet criteria for Pervasive Developmental Disorder

Note: From the *Diagnostic and Statistical Manual of Mental Disorders* (3rd ed., rev.) by the American Psychiatric Association, 1987, Washington, DC: Author.

relations (Breen & Barkley, 1985; Mash & Johnston, 1982; McGee, Williams, & Silva, 1988a, 1988b). Even so, the manner in which previous studies established their diagnosis and selection criteria often varied considerably across studies, rarely used parent or teacher rating scales to establish developmental deviance, and often used hetero-

TABLE 5.2
Additional Guidelines for Establishing a Diagnosis of ADHD as Suggested by Barkley (1982)

1. The developmental/statistical deviance of ADHD core symptoms should be established by standardized and well-normed child behavior rating scales.
2. Symptoms of ADHD have a duration of at least 12 months.
3. Symptoms of ADHD have an onset by 6 years of age.
4. Symptoms of ADHD should be established as significantly pervasive across settings.
5. Symptoms of ADHD are not accounted for by significant delays in intellectual development.

geneous samples having high comorbidity for other disorders (e.g., oppositional disorder, conduct disorders, and learning disabilities; Barkley, 1982).

Evidence for the validity of the more recent DSM-III-R criteria can be derived from several sources. One is the process by which items were chosen in the DSM-III-R. Reference was made to factor analytic studies of child behavior rating scales completed by parents and teachers from which were taken items that appeared to load highly on dimensions believed to be indicative of ADHD symptoms (for instance inattention and hyperactivity scales from the Child Behavior Checklist). To the extent that these factors and their respective items have some established validity, this could be said to be true of those items chosen from them for inclusion in the DSM-III-R. Another source of support rests in the field trial of the criteria (Spitzer, Davies, & Barkley, in press) in which the sensitivity and specificity of the items and their odds ratios or discriminating power for ADHD compared to non-ADHD childhood disorders were assessed. These data indicate significantly high odds ratios for all items. They are in fact listed in the DSM-III-R in descending order of their odds ratios (discriminating power). A further source of validation comes from research that has factor analyzed the DSM-III-R item list and found the items to cluster into two factors (inattention and hyperactivity), each of which shows a high degree of internal consistency (DuPaul, 1990a). Finally, some evidence now exists to show that parent and teacher ratings of these 14 symptoms, when cast as a rating scale, correlate significantly with direct behavioral observations of children's inattention in their school classrooms, efficiency of performing academic work, and actual achievement test scores on annual group achievement tests (DuPaul, 1990a). The evidence available to date is therefore quite encouraging concerning the validity of these criteria.

The DSM-III-R criteria are a considerable improvement over those provided in both the DSM-II (American Psychiatric Association, 1968) and DSM-III (American Psychiatric Association, 1980) in a number of ways:

1. The items were selected in part by reference to factor analyses of parent and teacher rating scales such that they were known to load together on factors associated with the major symptoms of ADHD (Barkley, Spitzer, & Costello, in press).

2. In contrast to the DSM-III, symptom items are no longer clustered within the separate categories or constructs of inattention, impulsivity, and overactivity with each having a separate cutoff score for determining its diagnostic significance. The polythetic approach taken in DSM-

III-R makes it more consistent with the dimensional view of child psychopathology taken in more empirical approaches to a taxonomy of childhood disorders (Achenbach & Edelbrock, 1983) as well as with other disorders in the DSM.

3. The DSM-III-R avoids clustering particular items underneath a given construct purely on the basis of committee consensus, as was used in DSM-III. Attempts at factor analyzing the older DSM-III items have shown that the items do not cluster the way they are set forth in DSM-III but instead form a two-dimensional solution of inattentive-restless and hyperactive-impulsive.

4. The cutoff point in DSM-III-R was determined in a quasi-experimental field trial (Spitzer, Davies, & Barkley, in press) and so has some empirical basis for its specification, whereas the separate cutoff scores used in DSM-III for each symptom list were established through consensus decree. This indicates that DSM-III-R criteria are more likely to select a group of children who are truly statistically deviant relative to normal children than are the criteria of DSM-III.

5. The specification of guidelines for establishing the severity of the disorder is important and reflects the research noted earlier that the disorder has significant range of expression and situational variation in its symptoms and that the degree of pervasiveness of the symptoms may be particularly important relative to the severity of the disorder and its associated conditions (Taylor, 1986).

6. Removing affective disorders as an exclusionary condition constitutes an added improvement because it allows for the diagnosis of an affective disorder to be made as a co-morbid condition when it is present and recognizes that these disorders are not associated with each other in any sort of causal direction (e.g., major depressive disorder leads to ADHD and so when it is present it should be excluded). Follow-up research clearly shows that ADHD children are not significantly more likely to develop a major affective disorder and so when such a disorder is present with ADHD it is likely to be an equally primary condition and worthy of separate diagnosis (Weiss & Hechtman, 1986).

7. And finally, DSM-III-R removed the subtyping approach to ADD based on the presence or absence of significant hyperactivity. This was necessary because at the time little research existed to show whether ADD without hyperactivity (ADD/−H) was actually a true subtype of ADD having a shared, common attentional problem but differing mainly in the presence of hyperactivity or comprised an entirely different disorder of attention. Moreover, no research was available to indicate that such a distinction would be clinically meaningful. It is possible to sort ADHD children into all sorts of subtypes but this does not automatically make such an approach useful. The DSM-III-R assigned ADD/−H

to a relatively underdefined status labeled undifferentiated ADD and called for more research on its validity as a subtype of ADHD; a prudent gesture given the findings of subsequent research.

These accolades having been noted, it is worth pointing out that several significant problems remain with the structure of DSM-III-R that are deserving of attention in the development of DSM-IV now underway. Possible solutions to these difficulties are summarized in Table 5.3 and discussed more thoroughly later. However, despite the listing of the items in a single dimension format, recent factor analyses again demonstrate that these items constitute two separate but interdependent factors, which are inattentive-restless and hyperactive-impulsive (DuPaul, 1990a). The DSM-IV committee is considering whether two lists of items each having a separate cutoff score would not be more consistent with empirical research on the disorder. This is to be encouraged.

Another difficulty lies in the use of a fixed cutoff score across so wide an age range of children, adolescents, and even adults. It is well known that the prevalence of these symptoms in children is considerably higher in the preschool years and declines significantly throughout childhood and adolescence. By applying a fixed score (8 of 14) to everyone, this criterion runs the likely risk of overidentifying preschool children as ADHD while underidentifying adolescents. Support for such a problem comes from the DSM-III-R field trial itself, which found the sensitivity and specificity of this cutoff score to decline significantly with age, indicating that it was overly restrictive in the older age groups. Recent research suggests that a score of 6 of 14 may be more appropriate for identifying children 12 years and older whereas a score

TABLE 5.3
Suggested Improvements in Criteria for Attention Deficit-Hyperactivity Disorder for DSM-IV

1. Develop two separate item lists reflecting items pertaining to inattention and items pertaining to hyperactivity and impulsivity, respectively.
2. Create age adjusted cutoff scores for three broad age ranges: 3 to 5 years, 6 to 11 years, and 12 to 18 years.
4. Create sex-adjusted cutoff scores separately for boys and girls.
5. Recommend the use of rating scales to further establish the developmental inappropriateness of the ADHD items.
6. Increase the duration of symptoms to 12 months, especially in diagnosing preschool-age children (3 to 5 years).
7. Emphasize the primary role of impulsive-hyperactive symptoms, or behavioral disinhibition, as a distinguishing feature of the disorder.
8. Create a separate new childhood diagnostic category, symptom item list, and diagnostic criteria for children previously called Attention Deficit Disorder with Hyperactivity, or Undifferentiated Attention Deficit Disorder, outside of the Disruptive Behavior Disorders.

of 10 of 14 would be better for children 5 or younger (Barkley, Fischer, Edelbrock, & Smallish, in press; DuPaul, 1990a) if identifying a relatively consistent threshold for deviance across developmental levels is important (i.e., 97th percentile for age).

A related problem with these criteria is their failure to distinguish different cutoff scores for girls compared to boys. Research on rating scales and developmental psychopathology has repeatedly shown that the prevalence of these symptoms is strongly related to sex of the child. Again, applying a fixed cutoff score to both sexes may overidentify ADHD in boys while underidentifying it in girls. Recent epidemiological surveys of the DSM-III-R item list reveal just such a problem (DuPaul, 1990a). It is to be hoped that the DSM-IV committee will develop separate cutoff scores by sex if it desires to make its diagnostic criteria more consistent with the findings from the field of developmental psychopathology.

A further difficulty with the DSM-III-R criteria is their failure to provide guidance to clinical practitioners and scientists as to how to establish whether a symptom occurs to a degree that is inappropriate for a child's mental age. It is time to acknowledge that well-standardized behavior rating scales offer the best means of determining such deviance available to date and to recommend that practitioners and scientists alike incorporate them into their criteria for establishing a diagnosis of ADHD (Barkley, 1988a).

The requirement that the child's symptoms exist for at least 6 months is also in need of refinement in view of the large number of preschool-age children who are likely to have these characteristics yet whose problems remit within 6 months (Campbell, 1990). Adopting a duration of 12 months would be far more conservative and is likely to identify a group of children whose behavioral problems are considerably more stable over development (Barkley, Fischer, et al., in press; Campbell, 1990).

At the time of its drafting, little research was available to indicate the utility of the subtype of ADD known as ADD/−H, as already noted. However, it is abundantly clear from subsequent research (Barkley, DuPaul, & McMurray, in press; Carlson, 1986) that the distinction is quite useful. It is also becoming clear that ADD/−H is probably not a true subtype of ADD in that it does not share a similar type of attentional deficit. ADD/−H children are not as likely to manifest problems with vigilance, sustained attention, or impulsivity but instead seem to have problems with cognitive processing speed and focused attention (Barkley, DuPaul, & McMurray, in press). They are also more likely to be rated as daydreamy, staring, confused or lost in thought, and sluggish or lethargic than are ADD children with hyperactivity (ADD/+H). The comorbid conditions associated with ADD/−H also appear to be different than for ADD/+H as does the prevalence of particular disorders within the extended family psychiatric histories. ADD/−H children are considerably less likely to be aggressive or conduct disordered and to have such problems in their family histories while they are more likely to have anxiety disorders and learning disabilities among their relatives than are children with ADD/+H (Barkley, DuPaul, & McMurray, in press).

All of this implies that ADD/+H is not a Disruptive Behavior Disorder and may be deserving of a separate, distinct childhood diagnosis than ADD/+H, or ADHD. This is unlikely to occur, however, so long as ADD/−H is defined by the absence of significant hyperactivity yet as having the same attention problems using the same item lists for Inattention and Hyperactivity that are employed in ADHD. The DSM-IV would do well to create a separate expanded list of attention items that incorporates those descriptors of inattention that appear more commonly in ADD/−H, such as daydreamy, confused, and so forth, so that it is a diagnosis made by both distinct inclusion criteria as well as exclusion criteria. This would also eliminate the possibility as now exists that ADD/−H children can meet criteria for ADHD as it is currently defined in the DSM-III-R, although the probability of this occurring has recently been shown to be low (about 20%).

Empirical research is also beginning to hint at the possibility that an attentional deficit, in fact, is not the most distinguishing feature of ADHD but that disinhibition, or impulsive-hyperactive behavior, may well be. This is partially evident in the DSM-III-R field trial that found that the items having the greatest discriminating power from other childhood psychiatric disorders are those pertaining to impulsive and hyperactive behavior, whereas difficulties with attention, although significant as discriminating items, contribute considerably less sensitivity and specificity (Spitzer et al., in press). It is also evident in research using a variety of lab tests of attention and impulsivity that utilize discriminant function analyses to evaluate the relative contribution of these test scores to distinguishing ADHD from normal or clinical control groups of children. Such scores as commission errors on vigilance tests and impulsive responding on delay of gratification tasks as well as measures of activity level contribute most to group differentiation, are more highly associated with parent and teacher ratings of ADHD in the natural setting than lab measures of attention, (Barkley, in press; Douglas, 1983; Grodzinsky, 1990; Werry, Elkind, & Reeves, 1987), and are quite useful in achieving high classification rates (Gordon, 1979; Rapport et al., 1986) between ADHD and normal children. If such evidence continues to accrue in this fashion, it suggests that behavioral disinhibition or hyperactive-impulsive behavior may be the most distinguishing feature of ADHD, rather than inattention, and so this should be stressed in the description of the disorder in DSM-IV. Furthermore, this evidence would intimate that hyperactive-impulsive disorder may be a more appropriate term for ADHD if the most discriminating symptoms are to have priority in the naming of the disorder.

CLINICAL DIAGNOSIS AND ASSESSMENT

Children with ADHD represent a heterogenous group, displaying developmentally deviant levels of the primary symptoms and, frequently, a number of associated behavioral, emotional, learning, and social problems. The manifestation of these primary symptoms along with a profiling of the nature and severity of secondary difficulties provide a useful and necessary approach to determining longer term outcomes and likely treatment approaches. Unfortunately, there is no single diagnostic tool available for determining the presence of this inherently complex disorder.

Based on diagnostic criteria appearing in DSM-III and DSM-III-R, Barkley (1981, 1987) outlined parameters that may be used in a comprehensive multimethod assessment of ADHD. First, measurement of primary symptoms (e.g., sustained attention, impulsivity) should allow age-related comparisons via adequate normative data to establish the developmental deviance of symptoms. Second, the possibility of coexisting problems (e.g., oppositional-defiant behavior, learning disabilities) should be thoroughly assessed. Third, the situational variations of problems dictate that multiple sources of information should be obtained from diverse settings. Finally, the persistence of symptoms across childhood and into adolescence necessitates the use of methods that are sensitive to a wide age range. Four general methods of assessment are employed as part of the clinical protocol: interview, standardized child behavior rating scales, laboratory measures, and direct observation.

Interviews

In-depth parent and child interviews are indispensable for establishing that certain diagnostic criteria are met and that conditions other than ADHD are not primarily responsible for the child's current behavior. The examiner must be familiar with the diagnostic features of ADHD as well as other childhood disorders, as some may masquerade as or overlap with ADHD (e.g., schizotypal personality or thought disorders).

The interview with the parent is designed to obtain a detailed history regarding the (a) child's medical and developmental status; (b) family psychiatric, learning, and developmental disorders; (c) current psychosocial conditions (e.g., marital relations); and the (d) child's school history and intellectual/learning status.

The use of structured interviewing formats for diagnosing childhood psychopathology has been a relatively new development in attempts to enhance the objectivity, reliability, and validity of traditional child diagnostic procedures. Most of these interview schedules have been developed for research purposes or for conducting epidemiological studies regarding the prevalence of psychiatric syndromes (Edelbrock & Costello, 1988). A number of these structured interviewing formats exists, each varying with respect to training required by the interviewer, the degree of structure demanded in the interview process and scoring, and the psychometric properties of the instrument. Most of these instruments provide detailed questioning regarding a large number of psychiatric symptoms, their onset, duration, severity, and associated impairments. Although it may be premature to recommend widespread clinical use of any one interviewing instrument, several show promising psychometric properties and clinical utility.

The Kiddie-Schedule for Affective Disorders for School-Age Children (K-SADS; Puig-Antich & Chambers, 1978) is a semistructured diagnostic interview for children between 6 and 17 years of age. The instrument requires the interviewer to have significant interviewing experience as well as a detailed familiarity with DSM-III and Research Diagnostic Criteria for major affective disorders. Parents are generally interviewed first about the child's psychiatric status and the child is subsequently interviewed to resolve any discrepancies between parent and child reports. The K-SADS yields information on the presence and severity of 49 core symptoms, over 35 of which pertain to depression or to clinical features associated with depression (e.g., social withdrawal). This interviewing instrument was originally developed as a means of selecting subjects for research on childhood depression and it may be clinically useful for diagnosing or ruling out depression in children. Although its psychometric properties appear adequate, it is limited to its focus on affective disorders, and may not provide comprehensive or detailed coverage of disruptive behavior disorders desired in the assessment of ADHD. The Interview Schedule for Children (ISC; Kovacs, 1982) also may be used as a clinical assessment device to identify or rule out depression in children. Like the K-SADS, the ISC focuses primarily on symptoms related to depression in children.

Several additional structured psychiatric interviews for children have shown promise and may be more useful in the clinical assessment of ADHD because of their broader coverage of disruptive behavior disorders. The Diagnostic Interview for Children and Adolescents (DICA; Herjanic & Reich, 1982) is a highly structured diagnostic interview that can be administered to parents or children over the age of 6. The DICA can be administered by clinicians as well as lay interviewers trained specifically to use the instrument. Most of the interview is organized around themes (e.g., behavior at home, behavior at school), whereas other parts cover more specific psychiatric diagnostic classifications. The DICA yields information on the presence or absence of 185 symptoms, including information on their onset, duration, severity, and associated impairments. Scoring of the interview also yields six summary scores pertaining to (a) relationship problems, (b) school behavior, (c) school learning, (d) neurotic symptoms, (e) somatic symptoms, and (f) psychotic symptoms.

The DICA has broad diagnostic coverage that may make it more useful in the assessment of ADHD than the K-SADS or ISC. Interrater reliability appears to be adequate, but test–retest reliability are currently lacking and validation of the instrument has been weak at best. Currently, the DICA may be most suitable for research and for conducting large-scale epidemiological studies (Edelbrock & Costello, 1988).

Like the DICA, the Diagnostic Interview Schedule for Children (DISC; Costello, Edelbrock, Kalas, Kessler, & Klaric, 1982) is a highly structured interview that can be administered by both professionals and lay interviewers with 2 or 3 days of specific training. Parallel versions of the interview are available for parents and children. The DISC offers one of the most comprehensive structured interviewing formats, designed specifically to assess diagnostic criteria set forth in DSM-III. The interview covers almost all diagnoses applied to children and adolescents, providing equal coverage to psychotic, affective, and disruptive behavior disorders. The psychometric features of the DISC are sound, including test–retest, discriminant, and concurrent validity studies (Costello, Edelbrock, & Costello, 1985; Edelbrock, 1984). Like the DICA, the DISC may be more suitable to diagnosing ADHD than other formats that emphasize affective disorders in children.

Despite the promise that these structured interviews hold, a recent review by Edelbrock and Costello (1988) suggests that the currently available interviews are in need of more thorough reliability and validity studies. No single interview format has emerged as superior for all clinical purposes. Pending further studies, widespread clinical use of structured psychiatric interviews for diagnosing ADHD should be done with caution and in the context of a multicomponent assessment approach utilizing other assessment instruments and methods.

Behavior Rating Scales

Standardized, well-normed parent and teacher behavior rating scales with adequate psychometric properties have become an indispensable part of the clinical assessment of ADHD. They provide a means of objectifying the occurrence of behaviors across multiple settings and informants, and for establishing the developmental deviance of problem behaviors by comparison of scores with norms. A detailed review of child behavior rating scales is available in Barkley (1987). Several scales with excellent psychometric properties and normative data are available in the evaluation of ADHD.

Parent Rating Scales

The Child Behavior Checklist (CBCL; Achenbach & Edelbrock, 1983) provides a thorough screening of child psychopathology through the 113-item Behavior Problems Scale. Using factor analyses based on 1,300 children, profiles were derived for boys and girls on the basis of three age groups (i.e., 4 to 5, 6 to 11, and 12 to 16). Based on factor scores, common dimensions of childhood disorders (e.g., aggressive, social withdrawal) can be plotted on profiles containing normative data for the age and gender of the child. This allows the examiner to determine on which dimensions, if any, the child is depicted as statistically deviant. The hyperactivity factor provides a score related to ADHD symptomology for 6- to 11-year-olds and correlates highly with the likelihood of a psychiatric diagnoses of ADHD derived via interviewing (Edelbrock & Costello, 1988). A specific hyperactivity factor was not obtained for children under 6 years of age on the CBCL. Scores pertaining to hyperactivity for this age group appear to load most frequently on the Aggressive Scale. A more recent version of the CBCL for 2- to 3-year-olds contains 100 items pertaining to social interaction, depression, sleep problems, somatic problems, aggressiveness, and destructiveness. Items related to hyperactivity on this version also seem to load on the Aggressive Scale.

Social functioning can also be assessed using the Social Competence Scale of the CBCL. The CBCL is one of the few scales available that includes items pertaining to adaptive behavior and social competence. The psychometric properties of the CBCL are excellent (Barkley, 1987), and it has been shown to discriminate ADHD from normal and other clinic-referred groups of children (Breen, 1986; Mash & Johnston, 1983).

A second useful scale for assessing ADHD is the Conners Parent Rating Scale-Revised (CPRS-R; Goyette, Conners, & Ulrich, 1978). It is the most extensively employed scale in research on the disorder. The revised 48-item questionnaire has the most satisfactory normative data among the different versions of this scale and yields five factor scores: conduct problems, learning problems, psychosomatic, impulsive-hyperactive, and anxiety. Although many of the items overlap with the CBCL, the CPRS-R includes a separate Hyperactive Scale for 3- to 5-

year-olds that is not available on the CBCL. The CPRS-R is also considerably briefer and more useful when readministration of the scale is anticipated, such as in evaluating treatments. Normative data on the CPRS-R were obtained from a sample of 750 3- to 17-year-olds. The psychometric properties are satisfactory. The measure also discriminates ADHD from non-ADHD children, and is sensitive to stimulant medication and parent training interventions (Barkley, 1987).

The Home Situations Questionnaire (HSQ; Barkley, 1981) was developed to evaluate the specific home situations in which problem behaviors occur. The scale supplements measures describing the nature of problem behaviors only. The HSQ is useful in assessing the situational variation in behavior as well as the pervasiveness and severity of behavioral difficulties. The HSQ contains 16 items about common situations occurring at home (e.g., while playing alone) and in public (e.g., while in stores). Parents indicate whether problems exist in each situation and their severity using a scale from 1 (mild) to 9 (severe). The scale yields two scores: number of problem situations and mean severity. Normative data on the HSQ are available for 4- to 12-year-olds (Barkley & Edelbrock, 1987). The scale has been found to differentiate ADHD from normal children and is sensitive to parent training and stimulant medication interventions (Barkley, Karlsson, Pollard, & Murphy, 1985; Befera & Barkley, 1985; Pollard, Ward, & Barkley, 1983). This scale has recently been revised such that its directions specify that inattentiveness is to be rated across these situations rather than the more global construct of "behavior problems." Information of the reliability, validity, and normative data on the revised version are reported by DuPaul (1990b).

A rating scale has been constructed using the 14 items from the DSM-III-R criteria for ADHD with the response format being identical to those anchor points used on the Conners' scales. This ADHD Rating Scale has been factor analyzed, resulting in two separate subscales: inattentive-restless and hyperactive-impulsive. Normative data for a large sample of children ages 5 to 12 years along with information on the scales reliability and validity have been reported by DuPaul (1990a).

Teacher Rating Scales

The Child Behavior Checklist-Teacher Report Form (CBCL-TRF; Achenbach & Edelbrock, 1983) includes many of the same items that appear on the parent version. The instrument includes scales measuring adaptive behavior as well as common dimensions of child behavior problems and psychopathology. The Adaptive Functioning Scale produces five scores pertaining to general school performance, effort, behavior, learning, and the child's general happiness. The 118-item Behavior

Problem Scale yields factor scores (e.g., anxious, obsessive-compulsive), which are plotted on profiles containing normative data available for both sexes and for two age groupings (6 to 11 and 12 to 16). Useful in the assessment of ADHD are the inattentive and nervous-overactive factors. The CBCL-TRF discriminates ADHD from other psychiatric problems (Edelbrock et al., 1984).

The Conners Teacher Rating Scale (CTRS; Conners, 1969; Goyette et al., 1978) is a 39-item version that is the counterpart to the parent version. A 28-item revised version overlaps with the longer version and is completed more quickly. The revised CTRS is well-normed and yields factor scores relevant to the assessment of ADHD, including hyperactive, inattentive-passive, and conduct problem factors. The scale appears to load heavily on problems in conduct and may not be as sensitive as the CBCL in assessing other areas of psychopathology. Nonetheless, the scale has adequate test–retest reliability (Edelbrock, Greenbaum, & Conover, 1985), has been shown to discriminate ADHD children from other children, and is sensitive to stimulant drug treatment effects (Barkley, 1987).

The School Situations Questionnaire (SSQ; Barkley, 1981) assesses the types of situations in which problem behaviors occur in the school setting. Like its home counterpart (HSQ), it allows an estimate of how circumscribed or pervasive behavioral difficulties of the child are at school. The scale contains 12 school-related situations (e.g., while teacher is lecturing) sampling across a variety of structured and unstructured situations. The teacher indicates whether the situation is a problem for the child and how severe on a scale from 1 (mild) to 9 (severe). The number of settings in which problems occur and a mean severity rating are obtained. Norms are contained in the chapter by Barkley and Edelbrock (1987). The SSQ discriminates ADHD from normal children and is sensitive to stimulant drug effects (Barkley, Fischer, et al., 1988). This scale has also been recently revised to reflect ratings pertaining specifically to inattentiveness across these 12 situations, with new normative data as well as information on reliability and validity now available (DuPaul, 1990b).

Three teacher-completed behavior rating scales have been developed that have special relevance for assessing ADHD symptomology. One of these is the ADHD Rating Scale developed by DuPaul (1990a) and described earlier under parent rating scales. Normative data are available on this scale for teacher reports as is information on the reliability and validity of this version (DuPaul, 1990a).

The Attention Deficit Disorder Comprehensive Teacher Rating Scale (ACTeRS; Ullmann, Sleator, & Sprague, 1984) was specifically developed for assessment of attention deficit disorders and treatment responses. The four subscales (i.e., oppositional behavior, attention, hyperactivity, and social problems) can be compared to normative data on a large sample of 5- to 12-year-olds. The ACTeRS has been shown to differentiate ADHD from normal and learning-disabled children (Ullmann et al., 1984). Further research on this scale will be needed before it should be considered a valid instrument for assessing ADHD.

Finally, the Edelbrock Child Attention/Activity Profile (CAP), developed by Edelbrock and derived from the lengthier CBCL (see Barkley, 1987) was developed to assess stimulant drug responses of ADHD children. The five items loading highest on the Overactivity Scale but lowest on Inattention, and the seven loading highest on the Inattention Scale but lowest on Overactivity of the CBCL-TRF were selected for this scale. See Fig. 5.1 for this scale. The CAP appears to be useful for classifying ADHD children according to the subtypes with hyperactivity and without hyperactivity. Normative data are available based on

CAP Rating Scale

Child's Name: Today's Date: Filled Out By:	FOR OFFICE USE ONLY

Below is a list of items that describes pupils. For each item that describes the pupil *now* or *within the past week*, check whether the item is Not True, Somewhat or Sometimes True, or Very or Often True. Please check all items as well as you can, even if some do not seem to apply to this pupil.

	Not True	Somewhat or Sometimes True	Very or Often True
1. Fails to finish things he/she starts	[ ]	[ ]	[ ]
2. Can't concentrate, can't pay attention for long	[ ]	[ ]	[ ]
3. Can't sit still, restless, or hyperactive	[ ]	[ ]	[ ]
4. Fidgets	[ ]	[ ]	[ ]
5. Daydreams or gets lost in his/her thoughts	[ ]	[ ]	[ ]
6. Impulsive or acts without thinking	[ ]	[ ]	[ ]
7. Difficulty following directtions	[ ]	[ ]	[ ]
8. Talks out of turn	[ ]	[ ]	[ ]
9. Messy work	[ ]	[ ]	[ ]
10. Inattentive, easily distracted	[ ]	[ ]	[ ]
11. Talks too much	[ ]	[ ]	[ ]
12. Fails to carry out assigned tasks	[ ]	[ ]	[ ]

Please feel free to write any comments about the pupil's work or behavior in the last week.

FIG. 5.1. The CAP Rating Scale.

TABLE 5.4

Normative Cutoff Points for the Inattention, Overactivity, and Total scores for the Edelbrock CAP Scale

Cutoff Points	*Total (1100)*	*Boys (550)*	*Girls (550)*
		Inattention	
Median	1	2	0
69 Percentile	3	4	2
84 Percentile	6	7	5
93 Percentile	8	9	7
98 Percentile	11	12	10
		Overactivity	
Median	0	1	0
69 Percentile	1	2	1
84 Percentile	4	4	2
93 Percentile	6	6	5
98 Percentile	8	8	7
		Total Score	
Median	2	4	1
69 Percentile	6	7	4
84 Percentile	10	11	8
93 Percentile	14	15	11
98 Percentile	19	20	16

scores obtained from 1,100 children, 6 through 16 years of both sexes (Barkley, 1987) and are shown in Table 5.4. Preliminary studies indicate that the CAP is sensitive to stimulant drug effects on ADHD children (Barkley, McMurray, Edelbrock & Robbins, 1989).

Direct Measures of ADHD Symptoms

Thus far only indirect measures (e.g., interview, ratings) of ADHD symptomology have been reviewed. Two sources of direct measurement that are useful components to the assessment process include systematic observations of behavior and laboratory test measures.

Direct Observation

Direct observational procedures have to be judged according to their psychometric properties, adequacy of sampling, degree of training necessary for the reliable use of the system, and the resources required for their implementation before being considered in a protocol for assessing ADHD. These potential constraints may limit their widespread inclusion in clinical assessment protocols. Nonetheless, several observational systems appear promising in the assessment of ADHD.

Abikoff, Gittleman-Klein, and Klein (1977) were among the first to develop a direct observational code, specifically for measuring ADHD symptoms in the classroom. Fourteen categories reflecting ADHD behaviors (e.g., off-task, movement about the classroom) are scored on an interval basis. Twelve of these 14 codes were found to differentiate ADHD and normal children. The Hyperactive Behavior Code (Jacob et al., 1978) was also developed to assess ADHD symptoms in the classroom. Six behavior codes constituting ADHD-like symptoms (e.g., change of position, daydreaming) are recorded on an interval system and collapsed to yield a single summary score. The summary score discriminates ADHD from normal children in structured classroom situations and correlates highly with teacher ratings of ADHD behaviors on the CTRS.

Observational systems measuring behavior in children's classrooms have been limited largely to research because of the obvious practical constraints encountered in most clinical settings. Clinical analogue observational procedures, however, have been developed that address, at least partially, some of the practical and logistical problems inherent in conducting classroom observations. Roberts (1979) developed a clinic observation system using a playroom setting to record ADHD behavior that was validated by Milich and his associates (e.g., Milich, 1984; Milich, Loney, & Landau, 1982). Children are observed in two 15-minute situations: free play and restricted academic periods.

Barkley (Barkley, 1987; Barkley et al., 1988) adapted this system for use in the clinical evaluations of ADHD children and for assessment of stimulant drug responses. Only the restricted academic period is used in which the child is instructed to complete a set number of mathematics problems selected from workbooks for the child's grade level. The child is asked to remain at the table and not to play with any of the toys in the playroom. The behavior of the child is recorded by an observer using a one-way mirror. The initial occurrence of five behaviors are recorded during each 30-second interval. The coding form appears in Fig. 5.2. The following behaviors are measured: off-task, fidgets, vocalizes, out-of-seat, and plays with objects. Definitions for these categories are provided in Table 5.5. The percentage of occurrence of each of the behaviors can be summarized or collapsed to yield a total summary score of ADHD behavior. This system has been found to discriminate ADHD from normal children (Breen, 1986) and to be sensitive to stimulant medication dose effects (Barkley et al., 1988).

Direct observation should only be considered as one component in

		1	2	3	4	5	6	7	8	9	10	11	12	13	14	15	16	17	18
Off Task																			
Fidgeting																			
Vocalizing																			
Plays w/Obj.																			
Out of Seat																			

Interval #:	19	20	21	22	23	24	25	26	27	28	29	30	Total	Scoring	
Off Task														/30 =	≃
Fidgeting														/30 =	≃
Vocalizing														/30 =	≃
Plays w/Obj.														/30 =	%
Out of Seat														/30 =	%
													Total ADD Beh.	/150 =	≃

Child's Name ________________ Coder Initials __________ Date: __________

Session: Init. Wk1 Wk2 Wk3

Is this a reliability check? YES NO

If so, with whom? __________

Comments:

FIG. 5.2. Academic Situation Code Sheet.

TABLE 5.5
Coding Procedures for the Restricted Academic Situations Test

Instructions for Conducting Observations

Place the child in a playroom having a one-way mirror and intercom facilities, a small table and chair at which the child will work, and a number of toys available. Instruct the child to sit at the small table and work on grade-level arithmetic problems presented on worksheets. Instruct the child to work on the math problems, to remain in the seat, and not to touch any objects in the room.

Begin observing the target child using a stop watch or audiotape that cues interval changes. This tape merely contains voice prompts indicating the beginning of each 30-second interval (i.e., Begin 1 . . . Begin 2 . . . Begin 3 . . . Begin 30 . . .). When the tape sounds the interval number, the coder proceeds to that column on the observation form and places a check mark in that block corresponding to each behavior category. Each category is scored only once during a 30-second interval, regardless of how often it may occur. When the tape recorder sounds the next interval number, the coder moves to the next column and begins marking any behavior categories that occur in that interval.

The following behavior categories are recorded: off-task, fidgeting, vocalizations, plays with object, and out of seat. It *is* possible to score a child as showing any or all of these behavior categories within any 30-second interval.

There are 30 intervals to be coded (15 minutes × 2 intervals each minute). The following definitions are used for each behavior category.

Definitions of Behavior Categories

1. *Off-task*: This category is checked if children interrupt their attention to the tasks to engage in some other behavior. Off-task behaviors are: looking around the room, playing with the pencil, talking to another person, or any other behavior where children are not looking at their task. Children can hum or whistle while working, kick their legs, and even stop using the pencil and still remain "on task," as long as they maintain eye contact with the task. It is essentially the breaking of eye contact with the task that constitutes "off-task" behavior.

2. *Fidgeting*: Any repetitive, purposeless motion of the legs, arms, buttocks, or trunk. The movement must occur at least twice in succession to be considered repetitive, *and* it should serve no purpose. Some examples are: swaying back and forth, kicking one's legs back and forth, shuffling feet from side to side, shifting one's buttocks about in the chair, tapping one's pencil on the desk.

3. *Vocalization*: Any vocal noise or verbalization made by the child excluding statements made toward the teacher. Statements made out loud but to no one in particular or talking to oneself are scored in this category. If children respond to verbalizations from another person directed at them it is not scored in this category. Examples: humming, whistling, throat clearing, clicking one's teeth together, singing.

4. *Plays with Objects*: If the child manually touches any other object in the room that is not related to the task (pencil, paper, and desk) or his or her body (including clothing), it is scored in this category. Playing with one's own body parts or clothing is not scored here.

5. *Out of Seat*: Any time the child's buttocks break contact with the flat surface of the seat, it is coded in this category.

Scoring Dependent Measures

The score for each category is derived by counting the number of check marks for that category and dividing by 30 to yield a percent occurrence.

the overall assessment protocol of ADHD because of limited normative data for interpreting the degree of developmental deviance in scores, problems inherent in obtaining representative sampling, and because of the requirement that other conditions be present or ruled-out as part of the diagnosis.

Laboratory Measures

Standardized laboratory tests with adequate normative data are a second strategy for directly measuring core ADHD symptoms (e.g., attention-span, impulsivity, motor activity). Shortcomings of these tests in assessing ADHD have included limited normative data for establishing developmental deviance as well as limited data to support the validity of these laboratory measures. Recent advances in establishing normative and validity data on several measures have proven promising and the inclusion of these measures in an assessment protocol can provide a useful adjunct to other assessment methods.

Attention Span

One of the most widely used measures for direct assessment of attention-span or vigilance is the Continuous Performance Test (CPT). Common among the variety of CPTs is the requirement that a child observe a screen while stimuli (e.g., numbers, letters) are rapidly projected. The child is instructed to press a button when a certain stimulus or pair of stimuli appear in sequence. The task generally lasts between 9 and 15 minutes and requires continuous attention for maximum performance.

Total correct responses, number of stimuli missed (omissions), and the number of stimuli to which the child incorrectly responded (commissions) are recorded. The total number correct and omission scores are believed to represent sustained attention. Commission scores are assumed to measure impulsivity and possibly sustained attention as well. The CPT has been shown to discriminate ADHD from normal children (Douglas, 1983) and correlates with other measures of attention-span (e.g., behavior ratings of ADHD; Klee & Garfinkel, 1983).

Several computer software programs and a commercially available solid-state computerized device for assessing sustained attention and impulsivity have recently become available (Swanson, 1985). The Gordon Diagnostic System (GDS), for example, is a small, solid-state computerized device that has normative data on over 1,000 children ages 3 to 17 years. The GDS has been shown to discriminate ADHD and normal children (Gordon, 1979, 1983, 1985) and to be sensitive to stimulant drug effects on ADHD children (Barkley et al., 1988).

Impulsivity

Laboratory tests have also been developed to directly measure impulse control. The GDS, for example, includes a test of impulsivity called the Delay Task. Here, the child must delay or inhibit responding to earn points. The task yields three measures: number of correct responses, total number of responses, and the ratio of correct responses to the total number. Each measure has been found to discriminate ADHD and non-ADHD clinic-referred children, and to correlate with ADHD ratings (Gordon, 1979). Barkley and associates (1988) recently found, however, that scores on the Delay Task were not sensitive to stimulant drug effects. Further work is needed to clarify reliability and validity characteristics of this instrument, both as a measure of impulsivity and as a treatment outcome measure.

The most widely employed and well-researched test of impulsivity is the Matching Familiar Figures Test (MFFT; Kagan, 1965). The MFFT is a match-to-sample task in which the child is presented with a sample picture and is instructed to select the same picture from an array of highly similar pictures. The amount of time taken to the first response (response latency) and the number of errors are recorded. The average response latency and total number of errors are then interpreted by comparing them to normative data available on 2,846 5- through 12-year-olds. Scores that deviate from age and gender norms are believed to reflect impulsivity or an impulsive cognitive response style on the part of the child. Both response latency and error scores discriminate ADHD and normal children (Campbell, Douglas, & Morganstern, 1971) and correlate with observational measures of ADHD behaviors (activity, attention; Milich, Landau, & Loney, 1981). Both scores have also been found to be sensitive to stimulant drug effects, albeit inconsistently (Barkley, 1977).

Activity Level

Laboratory instrumentation has long been used in the direct measurement of activity level in children. The actometer and pedometer, for example, are attached to the child's body (e.g., wrist, ankle) to mechanically measure movement. These instruments are commonly used in research but have not been widely employed in clinical assessment protocols of ADHD. The limited use of activity level devices is probably due to the absence of normative data, questionable reliability of scores, as well as obvious practical issues when using specialized instrumentation. The relationship of scores obtained using such devices to other well-founded measures of ADHD have not been very convincing (Barkley & Ullmann, 1975; Milich et al., 1982). Thus, their use in a clinical protocol would necessitate cautious interpretation of findings.

In summary, laboratory tests that attempt to provide direct measures of ADHD symptomology appear to hold promise in the clinical assessment of ADHD. The availability of normative data and acceptable psychometric properties are essential to their inclusion in the assessment protocol. Of course, scores obtained under laboratory or clinic settings may not accurately represent typical performance. Data addressing the ecological validity of laboratory measures has been inconsistent. Thus, cautious interpretation of scores in the context of information obtained through other sources and methods is strongly advocated (Barkley, in press).

RECOMMENDATIONS FOR FUTURE RESEARCH

As yet, there exists no gold standard or litmus test for insuring the validity of the diagnosis of ADHD. Nonetheless, prudence dictates that some homage be paid to the following guidelines if consistency across studies is to be achieved:

Stipulation of whether or not DSM-III-R criteria were followed, how they were applied, and what sources of information were used (e.g., parent or teacher reports or both) should be reported routinely. Structured psychiatric interviews are beneficial in this initial stage of selection as they insure that different examiners apply a uniform procedure and guidelines across subjects (Edelbrock & Costello, 1988). Reporting the means for number of symptoms, duration, and onset where DSM-III-R criteria are being used would also permit comparisons of severity of the disorder across studies and provide useful data on these parameters. Descriptions of the total number of subjects screened for a study to achieve the final sample, as well as the demographic features of this sample, would also be useful.

It should be mandatory that the actual developmental deviance of the subjects' ADHD symptoms be established through the use of a well standardized child behavior rating scale (Barkley, 1982). Although the Conners' scales have served this purpose in many studies, better scales having larger and more representative norms, better item coverage, and greater breadth of symptoms exist, such as the Child Behavior Checklist (Achenbach & Edelbrock, 1983) and should be used more frequently. Child behavior rating scales useful in research have been reviewed elsewhere (Barkley, 1987). It should be said that the Conners' Abbreviated Parent and Teacher scales (also called Hyperactivity Index) should no longer be used in selecting subjects given the confounding of hyperactivity with aggressive symptoms on the scale. Subjects so chosen will almost invariantly not be pure cases of ADHD, but likely mixed ADHD/conduct problems (oppositional-defiant disorder), making it difficult to tell which of these disorders accounts for the findings (Ullman et al., 1984).

This leads to an additional suggestion that researchers make a greater effort to select pure cases (i.e., groups of ADHD without clinical conduct problems or the contrasting of pure groups of ADHD children against the more common mixed ADHD/oppositional-defiant disordered group) so as to clarify what morbidity is actually associated with ADHD alone. It also now seems advisable not to collapse ADHD children with those who are ADD without hyperactivity given emerging evidence that these are not subtypes of the same attention disturbance but may be qualitatively different disorders entirely (Carlson, 1986; Lahey et al., 1988). Whereas the former may be a disorder of sustained attention and impulsivity, the later seems to be more a problem of focused attention (Barkley, DuPaul, & McMurray, in press; Mirsky, 1987).

The pervasiveness of the ADHD symptoms should also be established and reported. Research (Schachar, Rutter, & Smith, 1981; Taylor, 1986) suggests that children showing ADHD at home and school are more deviant and perhaps represent a truly unique syndrome of ADHD than do those deviant in only one of these settings. Whether this merely represents a marker of severity for the disorder along a continuum of symptoms or demarcates a unique syndrome is still unclear, but reporting such parameters will help further clarify the issue. Furthermore, Barkley (1982) suggested that situational pervasiveness should be established separately within the domains of caregiver responsibility for parents and teachers. The Home and School Situations Questionnaires were originally developed toward this end (Barkley & Edelbrock, 1987), but they, too, are hampered by the ambiguity of instructions that confound ADHD with behavior problems. This is being rectified in an ongoing study (DuPaul, 1990b) wherein the scales have been rephrased to refer specifically to attention/concentration problems and are being normed on a much larger sample of children.

Ideally, laboratory measures would be useful to document the existence of the ADHD symptoms more extensively and objectively. Vigilance tasks are the most likely candidates (see Swanson, 1985) given their reliable discrimination of ADHD from normal and other disordered populations. As yet, however, no particular version has emerged as a consensus among researchers as the best one. While Gordon's (1983) vigilance task has a large normative sample across ages 3–17 and offers a durable, portable apparatus, its validity as a measure of inattention and as a diagnostic tool remains hotly contested despite its growing popularity among clinicians. If used, it should be combined with other measures of attention and never used as the sole or definitive source for diagnosis as other psychiatric disorders can also show impaired vigilance (e.g., autism, psychosis, learning disorders).

Whether using rating scales alone or combined with laboratory tests to establish deviance, it seems judicious to correct these scores for the mental age of the subject where this varies more than a standard deviation from the mean for chronological age (Barkley, 1982). This is founded on the reasonable assumption that delays in sustained attention and other ADHD symptoms covary significantly with mental age and are likely to be below-average in children of less than average IQ by virtue of delayed mental development alone. This effect can be somewhat crudely adjusted for by comparing these children to the norms using their mental rather than chronological age to establish the relative deviance of ADHD symptoms.

Where parent reports via interviews or scales serve as the sole source for information on ADHD symptoms, it may be useful to collect parent self-report ratings of depression and marital discord and statistically parcel these out when initially comparing subjects to other control groups. They should also be covaried out of dependent measures to avoid confounds based on factors other than the subject's actual ADHD symptomology. This suggestion is founded on emerging evidence that depressed or maritally discordant parents may report, possibly in an exaggerated manner, greater symptom deviance in their children on rating scales than may actually be true (Forehand & McMahon, 1981; Griest, Wells, & Forehand, 1979).

Other disorders must certainly be excluded in selecting children given their likelihood of confounding ADHD with other, unwanted conditions. Seizure disorders, autism, psychosis, deafness, blindness, significant language delays, and frank brain damage may all introduce a host of deficits, symptoms, or other characteristics not believed to occur in pure ADHD, and will undoubtedly contribute unwanted error variance to the dependent measures. All of these disorders may have associated attentional disturbances that may be qualitatively or etiologically different from the common developmental-idiopathic form of ADHD that is of interest, and these types of attentional disruptions may only confound interpretation of the findings. This is not to say that such children cannot receive a clinical codiagnosis of ADHD, but that their inclusion as research subjects seems unwise.

CONCLUSIONS

Attention deficit-hyperactivity disorder is currently viewed as a developmental disorder with primary deficits in the domains of sustained attention, impulse control, and motor restlessness and overactivity with an early onset in childhood. It is usually chronic in nature and pervasive or cross-situational. A fourth domain, a motivational deficit in which the regulation of behavior by its consequences is deficient, has recently been raised as a possible primary problem in ADHD children, resulting in poor rule compliance. In this context, ADHD symptoms appear to be interactive with the environment and show considerable variability and fluctuation across settings, tasks, caregivers, and reinforcement arrangements. Current research strongly suggests that the disorder has a biological predisposition with multiple etiologies (e.g., Cantwell, 1975; Ross & Ross, 1982). In addition to these primary symptoms, ADHD children show a greater prevalence of associated problems in emotional, behavioral, social, and academic domains. Those displaying significant patterns of aggression, defiance, and oppositional behavior appear at greater risk for continued serious adjustment problems in adolescence and young adulthood.

This chapter has described a diagnostic and assessment protocol for evaluating ADHD in children in both research and clinical settings. A multimethod approach was emphasized. Each method possesses strengths as well as shortcomings in the overall assessment process. The current status of the field strongly suggests that an assessment protocol rely on multiple methods, utilizing several different sources of information obtained from different settings and informants (Barkley, 1981, 1988a). The inclusion of parent and teacher interviews, standardized parent and teacher behavior ratings, several laboratory test measures of sustained attention and impulsivity, and direct observation can provide information pertaining to the onset of symptoms, their chronicity, pervasiveness, developmental deviance of primary symptoms, coexisting behavior difficulties, and the requirement that other conditions (e.g., psychiatric, medical) be excluded. The clinical evaluation and assessment of ADHD in children requires knowledge of the relevant research and clinical literature, knowledge of the various forms of childhood psychopathology, sound clinical judgment, and sufficient resources for obtaining multiple measurements using a variety of instruments and methods.

REFERENCES

Abikoff, H., Gittelman-Klein, R., & Klein, D. (1977). Validation of a classroom observation code for hyperactive children. *Journal of Consulting and Clinical Psychology, 45*, 772–783.

Achenbach, T. M., & Edelbrock, C. (1983). *Manual for the Child Behavior Checklist and revised Child Behavior Profile*. Burlington, VT: Thomas Achenbach.

American Psychiatric Association. (1968). *Diagnostic and statistical manual of mental disorders* (2nd ed.). Washington, DC: Author.

American Psychiatric Association. (1980). *Diagnostic and statistical manual of mental disorders* (3rd ed.). Washington, DC: Author.

American Psychiatric Association. (1987). *Diagnostic and statistical manual of mental disorders* (3rd ed., rev.). Washington, DC: Author.

Anastopoulos, A. D., & Barkley, R. A. (1988). Biological factors in attention deficit-hyperactivity disorder, *The Behavior Therapist, 11,* 47–53.

Barkley, R. A. (1977). A review of stimulant drug research with hyperactive children. *Journal of Child Psychology and Psychiatry, 18,* 137–165.

Barkley, R. A. (1981). *Hyperactive children: A handbook for diagnosis and treatment.* New York: Guilford Press.

Barkley, R. A. (1982). Specific guidelines for defining hyperactivity in children (attention deficit disorder with hyperactivity). In B. Lahey & A. Kazdin (Eds.). *Advances in clinical child psychology* (Vol. 5, pp. 137–180).

Barkley, R. A. (1985). The social interactions of hyperactive children: Developmental changes, drug effects, and situational variation. In R. McMahon & R. Peters (Eds.). *Childhood disorders: Behavioral-developmental approaches* (pp. 228–243). New York: Brunner/Mazel.

Barkley, R. A. (1987). The assessment of attention deficit-hyperactivity disorder. *Behavioral Assessment, 9,* 207–233.

Barkley, R. A. (1988a). Attention deficit disorders. In E. Mash & L. Terdal (Eds.), *Behavioral assessment of childhood disorders* (pp. 69–104). New York: Guilford Press.

Barkley, R. A. (1988b). Child behavior rating scales and checklists. In M. Rutter, H. Tuma, & I. S. Lann (Eds.), *Diagnosis and assessment in child and adolescent psychology* (pp. 113–155). New York: Guilford Press.

Barkley, R. A. (1989). The problem of stimulus control and rule-governed behavior in children with attention deficit disorder with hyperactivity. In I. Bloomingdale & J. Swanson (Eds.). *Attention Deficit Disorders* (Vol. 4, pp. 203–228). New York: Plenum.

Barkley, R. A. (in press). The ecological validity of laboratory and field assessment methods for ADHD. *Journal of Abnormal Child Psychology.*

Barkley, R. A., Costello, A., & Spitzer, R. (1989). *The development of the* DSM-III-R *criteria for attention deficit hyperactivity disorder.* Manuscript submitted for publication.

Barkley, R. A., & Cunningham, C. E. (1979). The effects of Ritalin on the mother–child interactions of hyperactive children. *Archives of General Psychiatry, 36,* 201–208.

Barkley, R. A., DuPaul, G. J., & McMurray, M. (in press). A comprehensive evaluation of attention deficit disorder with and without hyperactivity as defined by research criteria. *Journal of Consulting and Clinical Psychology.*

Barkley, R. A., & Edelbrock, C. (1987). Assessing situational variations in children's behavior problems: The home and school situations Questionnaires. In R. Prinz (Ed.), *Advances in behavioral assessment of children and families* (Vol. 3, pp. 157–176). Greenwich, CT: JAI Press.

Barkley, R. A., Fischer, M., Edelbrock, C. S., & Smallish, L. (in press). The adolescent outcome of hyperactive children diagnosed by research criteria, I: An eight year prospective follow-up study. *Journal of the American Academy of Child and Adolescent Psychiatry.*

Barkley, R. A., Fischer, M., Newby, R., & Breen, M. (1988). Development of a multimethod clinical protocol for assessing stimulant drug responses in ADD children. *Journal of Clinical Child Psychology, 17,* 14–24.

Barkley, R. A., Karlsson, J., & Pollard, S. (1985). Effects of age on the mother–child interactions of hyperactive children. *Journal of Abnormal Child Psychology, 13*, 631–638.

Barkley, R., Karlsson, J., Pollard, S., & Murphy, J. (1985). Developmental changes in the mother–child interactions of hyperactive boys: Effects of two dose levels of Ritalin. *Journal of Consulting and Clinical Psychology, 52*, 750–758.

Barkley, R. A., McMurray, M., Edelbrock, C., & Robbins, K. (1989). The response of aggressive and non-aggressive ADHD children to two doses of methylphenidate. *Journal of the American Academy of Child and Adolescent Psychiatry, 28*, 873–881.

Barkley, R. A., Spitzer, R. L., & Costello, A. (in press). The development of the DSM-III-R criteria for the disruptive behavior disorders. *Journal of the American Academy of Child and Adolescent Psychiatry.*

Barkley, R. A., & Ullmann, D. G. (1975). A comparison of objective measures of activity and distractibility in hyperactive and nonhyperactive children. *Journal of Abnormal Child Psychology, 3*, 231–244.

Befera, M., & Barkley, R. A. (1985). Hyperactive and normal boys and girls: Mother–child interaction, parent psychiatric status, and child psychopathology. *Journal of Child Psychology and Psychiatry, 26*, 439–452.

Breen, M. (1986). *ADD-H in girls: An analysis of attentional, emotional, cognitive, and academic behaviors and parental psychiatric status.* Manuscript submitted for publication.

Breen, M., & Barkley, R. A. (1985). Psychological adjustment in learning disabled, hyperactive, and hyperactive/learning disabled children using the Personality Inventory for Children. *Journal of Clinical Child Psychology, 13*, 232–236.

Brown, R. T., & Quay, H. C. (1977). Reflection-impulsivity of normal and behavior-disordered children. *Journal of Abnormal Child Psychology, 5*, 457–462.

Campbell, S. B. (1987). Parent-referred problem three year olds: Developmental changes in symptoms. *Journal of Child Psychology and Psychiatry, 28*, 835–846.

Campbell, S. B. (1990). *Behavior problems in preschool children: Clinical and developmental issues.* New York: Guilford.

Campbell, S. B., Douglas, V. I., & Morganstern, G. (1971). Cognitive styles in hyperactive children and the effect of methylphenidate. *Journal of Child Psychology and Psychiatry, 12*, 55–67.

Campbell, S. B., & Paulauskas, S. (1979). Peer relations in hyperactive children. *Journal of Abnormal Child Psychology, 20*, 233–246.

Cantwell, D. P. (1975). Genetics of hyperactivity. *Journal of Child Psychology and Psychiatry, 16*, 261–264.

Cantwell, D. P., & Satterfield, J. H. (1978). The prevalence of academic underachievement in hyperactive children. *Journal of Pediatric Psychology, 3*, 168–171.

Carlson, C. (1986). Attention deficit disorder without hyperactivity: A review of preliminary experimental evidence. In B. Lahey & A. Kazdin (Eds.), *Advances in clinical child psychology* (Vol. 9, pp. 153–176). New York: Plenum.

Chelune, G. J., Ferguson, W., Koon, R., & Dickey, T. O. (1986). Frontal lobe disinhibition in attention deficit disorder. *Child Psychiatry and Human Development, 16*, 221–234.

Chess, S. (1960). Diagnosis and treatment of the hyperactive child. *New York State Journal of Medicine, 60*, 2379–2385.

Childers, A. T. (1935). Hyper-activity in children having behavior disorders. *American Journal of Orthopsychiatry, 5*, 227–243.

Conners, C. K. (1969). A teacher rating scale for use in drug studies with children. *American Journal of Psychiatry, 126*, 884.

Conners, C. K. (1980). *Food additives and hyperactive children.* New York: Plenum.

Costello, E. J., Edelbrock, C., & Costello, A. J. (1985). The validity of the NIMH Diagnostic

Interview Schedule for Children: A comparison between pediatric and psychiatric referrals. *Journal of Abnormal Child Psychology, 13,* 579–595.

Costello, A. J., Edelbrock, C., Kalas, R., Kessler, M. D., & Klaric, S. H. (1982). *The NIMH Diagnostic Interview Schedule for Children (DISC).* Unpublished interview schedule, Department of Psychiatry, University of Pittsburgh.

Cunningham, C. E., & Barkley, R. A. (1979). The interaction of hyperactive and normal children with their mothers during free play and structured trask. *Child Development, 50,* 217–224.

David, O. J., Clark, J., & Hoffman, S. (1979). Childhood lead poisoning: A reevaluation. *Archives of Environmental Health, 34,* 106–111.

Douglas, V. I. (1972). Stop, look, and listen: The problem of sustained attention and impulse control in hyperactive and normal children. *Canadian Journal of Behavioural Science, 4,* 259–282.

Douglas, V. I. (1980). Higher mental processes in hyperactive children: Implications for training. In R. Knights & D. Bakker (Eds.), *Treatment of hyperactive and learning disordered children* (pp. 65–92). Baltimore, MD: University Park Press.

Douglas, V. I. (1983). Attention and cognitive problems. In M. Rutter (Ed.), *Developmental neuropsychiatry* (pp. 280–329). New York: Guilford Press.

Douglas, V. I., & Parry, P. A. (1983). Effects of reward on delayed reaction time task performance of hyperactive children. *Journal of Abnormal Child Psychology, 11,* 313–326.

Draeger, S. Prior, M., & Sanson, A. (1986). Visual and auditory attention performance in hyperactive children: Competence or compliance. *Journal of Abnormal Child Psychology, 14,* 411–424.

DuPaul, G. J. (1990a). *The ADHD Rating Scale: Normative data, reliability, and validity.* Manuscript submitted for publication.

DuPaul, G. J. (1990b). *The Revised Home and School Situations Questionnaires: Normative data, reliability, and validity.* Submitted for publication.

Edelbrock, C. (1984, October). *Relations between the NIMH Diagnostic Interview Schedule for Children (DISC) and the Child Behavior Checklist and Profile.* Paper presented at the annual meeting of the American Academy of Child Psychiatry.

Edelbrock, C., & Costello, A. J. (1988). Convergence between statistically derived behavior problem syndromes and child psychiatric diagnosis. *Journal of Abnormal Child Psychology, 16,* 219–231.

Edelbrock, C., Costello, A., & Kessler, M. D. (1984). Empirical corroboration of attention deficit disorder. *Journal of the American Academy of Child Psychiatry, 2,* 285–290.

Edelbrock, C., Greenbaum, R., & Conover, N. C. (1985). Reliability and concurrent relations between the teacher version of the Child Behavior Profile and the Conners Revised Teacher Rating Scale. *Journal of Abnormal Child Psychology, 1,* 295–304.

Feingold, B. (1975). *Why your child is hyperactive.* New York: Random House.

Firestone, P., & Martin, J. E. (1979). An analysis of the hyperactive syndrome: A comparison of hyperactive, behavior problem, asthmatic, and normal children. *Journal of Abnormal Child Psychology, 7,* 261–272.

Forehand, R. L., & McMahon, R. J. (1981). *Helping the noncompliant child: A clinicians' guide to parent training.* New York: Guilford Press.

Gittelman, R., Manuzza, S., Shenker, R., & Bonagura, N. (1985). Hyperactive boys almost grown up. I. Psychiatric status. *Archives of General Psychiatry, 42,* 937–947.

Gordon, M. (1979). The assessment of impulsivity and mediating behaviors in hyperactive and non-hyperactive children. *Journal of Abnormal Child Psychology, 7,* 317–326.

Gordon, M. (1983). *The Gordon Diagnostic System.* Boulder, CO: Gordon Systems.

Gordon, M. (1985, August). *Assessment of ADD/hyperactivity: Research on the Gordon Diagnostic System*. Symposium presented at the American Psychological Association, Los Angeles, CA.

Goyette, C. H., Conners, C. K., & Ulrich, R. F. (1978). Normative data for Revised Conners Parent and Teacher Rating Scales. *Journal of Abnormal Child Psychology, 6*, 221–236.

Griest, D., Wells, K. C., & Forehand, R. (1979). An examination of predictors of maternal perceptions of maladjustment in clinic-referred children. *Journal of Abnormal Psychology, 88*, 277–281.

Grodzinsky, G. (1990). *A developmental neuropsychological assessment of frontal lobe functions in children with attention deficit hyperactivity disorder*. Unpublished doctoral dissertation, Boston College.

Gross, M. D. (1984). Effects of sucrose on hyperkinetic children. *Pediatrics, 74*, 876–878.

Haenlein, M., & Caul, W. F. (1987). Attention deficit disorder with hyperactivity: A specific hypothesis of reward dysfunction. *Journal of the American Academy of Child and Adolescent Psychiatry, 26*, 356–362.

Hartsough, C. S., & Lambert, N. M. (1985). Medical factors in hyperactive and normal children: Prenatal, developmental, and health history findings. *American Journal of Orthopsychiatry, 55*, 190–201.

Herjanic, B., & Reich, W. (1982). Development of a structured interview for children: Agreement between child and parent on individual symptoms. *Journal of Abnormal Child Psychology, 10*, 7–24.

Jacob, R. G., O'Leary, K. D., & Rosenblad, C. (1978). Formal and informal classroom settings: Effects on hyperactivity. *Journal of Abnormal Child Psychology, 6*, 451–458.

Johnston, C., Pelham, W. E., & Murphy, H. A. (1985). Peer relationships in ADDH and normal children: A developmental analysis of peer and teacher ratings. *Journal of Abnormal Child Psychology, 13*, 89–100.

Kagan, J. (1965). Reflection-impulsivity: The generality and dynamics of conceptual tempo. *Journal of Abnormal Psychology, 71*, 17–24.

Kendall, P. C., & Braswell, L. (1982). Cognitive-behavioral self-control therapy for children: A component analysis. *Journal of Consulting and Clinical Psychology, 50*, 672–689.

King, C., & Young, D. (1982). Attentional deficits with and without hyperactivity: Teacher and peer perceptions. *Journal of Abnormal Child Psychology, 10*, 483–496.

Klee, S. H., Garfinkel, B. D. (1983). The computerized continuous performance task: A new measure of attention. *Journal of the American Academy of Child Psychiatry, 11*, 487–496.

Kovacs, M. (1982). *The Interview Schedule for Children (ISC)*. Unpublished interview schedule, Department of Psychiatry, University of Pittsburgh.

Lahey, B. B., Pelham, W. E., Schaughency, E. A., Atkins, M. S., Murphy, H. Allen, Hynd, G., Russo, M., Hartdagen, M., & Lorys-Vernon, A. (1988). Dimensions and types of attention deficit disorder. *Journal of the American Academy of Child and Adolescent Psychiatry, 27*, 330–335.

Lahey, B. B., Schaughency, E. A., Hynd, G. W., Carlson, C. L., & Nieves, N. (1987). Attention deficit disorder with and without hyperactivity: Comparison of behavioral characteristics of clinic-referred children. *Journal of the American Academy of Child and Adolescent Psychiatry, 26*, 718–723.

Laufer, M., Denhoff, E., & Solomons, G. (1957). Hyperkinetic impulse disorder in children's behavior problems. *Psychosomatic Medicine, 19*, 38–49.

Levin, P. M. (1938). Restlessness in children. *Archives of Neurology and Psychiatry, 39*, 764–770.

Loney, J., & Milich, R. (1982). Hyperactivity, inattention, and aggression in clinical practice. In M. Wolrich & D. Routh (Eds.), *Advances in behavioral pediatrics*, (Vol. 2, pp. 113–147). Greenwich, CT: JAI Press.

Loney, J., Whaley-Klahn, M. A., Kosier, T., & Conboy, J. (1981, November). *Hyperactive boys and their brothers at 21: Predictors of aggressive and antisocial outcomes.* Paper presented at the meeting of the Society of Life History Research, Monterey, CA.

Lou, H. C., Henriksen, L., & Bruhn, P. (1984). Focal cerebral hypoperfusion in children with dysphasia and/or attention deficit disorder. *Archives of Neurology, 41*, 825–829.

Lou, H. C., Henriksen, L., Bruhn, P., Borner, H., & Nielsen, J. B. (1989). Striatal dysfunction in attention deficit and hyperkinetic disorder. *Archives of Neurology, 46*, 48–52.

Luk, S. (1985). Direct observations studies of hyperactive behaviors. *Journal of the American Academy of Child Psychiatry, 24*, 338–344.

Mannuzza, S., Gittelman-Klein, R., Bonagura, N., Horowitz Konig, P., & Shenker, R. (1988). Hyperactive boys almost grown up: II. Status of subjects without a mental disorder. *Archives of General Psychiatry, 45*, 13–18.

Mariani, M. (1990). *A neuropsychological assessment of preschool children with attention deficit hyperactivity disorder.* Unpublished doctoral dissertation, Boston College.

Mash, E. J., & Johnston, C. (1982). A comparison of mother–child interactions of younger and older hyperactive and normal children. *Child Development, 53*, 1371–1381.

Mash, E. J., & Johnston, C. (1983). Parental perceptions of child behavior problems, parenting self-esteem, and mothers' reported stress in younger and older hyperactive and normal children. *Journal of Consulting and Clinical Psychology, 51*, 68–99.

Mattes, J. A., & Gittelman, R. (1981). Effects of artificial food colorings in children with hyperactive symptoms. *Archives of General Psychiatry, 38*, 714–718.

McGee, R., Williams, S., & Silva, P. A. (1988b). Behavioral and developmental characteristics of aggressive, hyperactive, and aggressive-hyperactive boys. *Journal of the American Academy of Child Psychiatry, 23*, 270–279.

McGee, R., Williams, S., & Silva, P. A. (1988a). Background characteristics of aggressive, hyperactive, and aggressive-hyperactive boys. *Journal of the American Academy of Child Psychiatry, 23*, 280–284.

Milich, R. (1984). Cross-sectional and longitudinal observations of activity level and sustained attention in a normative sample. *Journal of Abnormal Child Psychology, 12*, 261–276.

Milich, R., & Kramer, J. (1985). Reflections on impulsivity: An empirical investigation of impulsivity as a construct. In K. Gadow & I. Bialer (Eds.), *Advances in learning and behavioral disabilities* (Vol. 3, pp. 117–150). Greenwich, CT: JAI Press.

Milich, R. S., & Landau, S. (1982). Socialization and peer relations in hyperactive children. In K. D. Gadow & I. Bialer (Eds.), *Advances in learning and behavior disabilities* (Vol. 1, pp. 283–339). Greenwich, CT: JAI Press.

Milich, R., Landau, S., & Loney, J. (1981, August). *The interrelationships among hyperactivity, aggression, and impulsivity.* Paper presented at the meeting of the American Psychological Association, Los Angeles.

Milich, R. S., & Loney, J. (1979). The role of hyperactive and aggressive symptomology in predicting adolescent outcome among hyperactive children. *Journal of Pediatric Psychology, 4*, 93–112.

Milich, R., Loney, J., & Landau, S. (1982). The independent dimensions of hyperactivity and aggression: A validation with playroom observation data. *Journal of Abnormal Psychology, 91*, 183–198.

Mirskey, A. F. (1987). Behavioral and psychophysiological markers of disordered attention. *Environmental Health Perspectives, 74*, 191–199.

O'Leary, K. D., Vivian, D., & Nisi, A. (1985). Hyperactivity in Italy. *Journal of Abnormal Child Psychology, 13*, 485–500.

Omenn, G. S. (1973). Genetic issues in the syndrome of minimal brain dysfunction. *Seminars in Psychiatry, 5,* 5–17.

Paternite, C., & Loney, J. (1980). Childhood hyperkinesis: Relationship between symptomology and home environment. In C. K. Whalen & B. Henker (Eds.), *Hyperactive children: The social ecology of identification and treatment* (pp. 105–141). New York: Academic Press.

Pendergrast, M., Taylor, E., Rapoport, J. L., Bartko, J., Donnely, M., Zametkin, A., Ahearn, M. B., Dunn, G., & Wieselberg, H. M. (1988). The diagnosis of childhood hyperactivity: A U.S.-U.K. cross-national study of DSM-III and ICD-9. Journal of Child Psychology and Psychiatry, 29, 289–300.

Pollard, S., Ward, F. M., Barkley, R. A. (1983). The effects of parent training and Ritalin on the parent–child interactions of hyperactive boys. *Child and Family Behavior Therapy, 5,* 51–69.

Porrino, L. J., Rapoport, J. L., Behar, D., Sceery, W., Ismona, D. R., & Bunney, W. E. (1983). A naturalistic assessment of the motor activity of hyperactive boys. *Archives of General Psychiatry, 40,* 681–687.

Puig-Antich, J., & Chambers, W. (1978). *The Schedule for Affective Disorders and Schizophrenia for school-aged children.* Unpublished interview schedule, New York State Psychiatric Institute.

Rapoport, J. L., Quinn, P. O., & Lamprecht, F. (1974). Minor physical anomalies and plasma dopamine-beta-hydroxylase activity in hyperactive boys. *American Journal of Psychiatry, 131,* 386–390.

Rapport, M. D., Tucker, S. B., DuPaul, G. J., Merlo, M., & Stoner, G. (1986). Hyperactivity and frustration: The influence of control over and size of rewards in delaying gratification. *Journal of Abnormal Child Psychology, 14,* 191–204.

Roberts, M. (1979). *A manual for the Restricted Academic Playroom Situation.* Iowa City, IA: Author.

Ross, D. M., & Ross, S. A. (1982). *Hyperactivity: Current issues, research, and theory* (2nd ed.). New York: Wiley.

Routh, D. K. (1978). Hyperactivity. In P. Magrab (Ed.), *Psychological management of pediatric problems* (pp. 3–48). Baltimore, MD: University Park Press.

Routh, D. K., & Schroeder, C. S. (1976). Standardized playroom measures as indices of hyperactivity. *Journal of Abnormal Child Psychology, 4,* 199–207.

Rummo, J. H., Routh, D. K., Rummo, N. J., & Brown, J. F. (1979). Behavioral and neurological effects of symptomatic and asymptomatic lead exposure in children. *Archives of Environmental Health, 34,* 120–124.

Rutter, M. L. (1977). Brain damage syndromes in childhood: Concepts and findings. *Journal of Child Psychology and Psychiatry, 19,* 21–33.

Safer, R., & Allen, D. (1976). *Hyperactive children.* Baltimore, MD: University Park Press.

Sandberg, S. T., Rutter, M., & Taylor, E. (1978). Hyperkinetic disorder in psychiatric clinic attenders. *Developmental Medicine and Child Neurology, 20,* 279–299.

Satterfield, J. (1986). *Preliminary results of BEAM studies of ADD children.* Paper presented at the American Academy of Child Psychiatry, Los Angeles, CA.

Satterfield, J. H., Satterfield, B. T., & Cantwell, D. P. (1981). Three year multimodality treatment study of 100 hyperactive boys. *Journal of Pediatrics, 98,* 650–655.

Schacher, R., Rutter, M., & Smith, A. (1981). The characteristics of situationally and pervasively hyperactive children: Implications for syndrome definition. *Journal of Child Psychology and Psychiatry, 22,* 375–392.

Shaywitz, B. A., Cohen, D. J., & Bowers, M. B. (1977). Cerebrospinal fluid monamine metabolites in children with minimal brain dysfunction-Evidence for alteration of brain dopamine. *Journal of Pediatrics, 90,* 978–982.

Shaywitz, B. A., Shaywitz, S. E., Byrne, T., Cohen, D. J., & Rothman, S. (1983). Attention deficit disorder: Quantitative analysis of CT. *Neurology, 33,* 1500–150.

Shekim, W. O., Dekirmenjian, H., Chapel, J. L., Javoid, J., & David, J. M. (1979). Norepinephrine metabolism and clinical response to dextroamphetamine in hyperactive boys. *Journal of Pediatrics, 95,* 389–394.

Sleator, F. K., & Ullmann, R. A. (1981). Can the physician diagnose hyperactivity in the office? *Pediatrics, 67,* 13–17.

Spitzer, R. L., Davies, M., & Barkley, R. A. (in press). The DSM-III-R field trial of the disruptive behavior disorders. *Journal of the American Academy of Child and Adolescent Psychiatry.*

Stewart, M. A., Thach, B. T., & Freidin, M. R. (1970). Accidental poisoning and the hyperactive child syndrome. *Diseases of the Nervous System, 31,* 403–407.

Still, G. F. (1902). Some abnormal psychical conditions in children. *Lancet, 1,* 1008–1012, 1077–1082, 1163–1168.

Strauss, A. A., & Lehtinen, L. E. (1947). *Psychopathology and education of the brain-injured child.* New York: Grune & Stratton.

Stuss, D. T., & Benson, D. F. (1986). *The frontal lobes.* New York: Raven.

Swanson, L. M. (1985). Measures of cognitive functioning appropriate for use in pediatric psychopharmacological research studies. *Psychopharmacology Bulletin, 21,* 887–890.

Tallmadge, J., & Barkley, R. A. (1983). The interactions of hyperactive and normal boys with their mothers and fathers. *Journal of Abnormal Child Psychology, 11,* 565–579.

Tarver-Behring, S., Barkley, R. A., & Karlsson, J. (1985). The mother–child interactions of hyperactive boys and their normal siblings. *American Journal of Orthopsychiatry, 55,* 202–209.

Taylor, E. A. (1986). Childhood hyperactivity. *British Journal of Psychiatry, 149,* 562–573.

Taylor, E., & Sandberg, S. (1984). Hyperactive behavior in English schoolchildren: A questionnaire survey. *Journal of Abnormal Child Psychology, 12,* 143–156.

Taylor, H. G. (1983). MBD: Meanings and misconceptions. *Journal of Clinical Neuropsychology, 5,* 271–287.

Taylor, J. F. (1980). *The hyperactive child and the family.* New York: Random House.

Thorley, G. (1984). Review of follow-up and follow-back studies of childhood hyperactivity. *Psychological Bulletin, 96,* 116–132.

Trites, R. I., Dugas, F., Lynch, G., & Ferguson, R. (1979). Incidence of hyperactivity. *Journal of Pediatric Psychology, 4,* 179–188.

Ullmann, R. K., Sleator, F. K., & Sprague, R. I. (1984). A new rating scale for diagnosis and monitoring of ADD children. *Psychopharmacology Bulletin, 20,* 160–164.

Van der Meere, J., & Sergeant, J. (1988a). Controlled processing and vigilance in hyperactivity: Time will tell. *Journal of Abnormal Child Psychology, 16,* 641–655.

Van der Meere, J., & Sergeant, J. (1988b). Focused attention in pervasively hyperactive children. *Journal of Abnormal Child Psychology, 16,* 627–639.

Voelker, S., Lachar, D., & Gdowski, C. (1983). The Personality Inventory for Children and response to methylphenidate: Preliminary evidence for predictive validity. *Journal of Pediatric Psychology, 8,* 161–169.

Weiss, G., & Hechtman, I. (1986). *Hyperactive children grown-up.* New York: Guilford Press.

Wender, P. (1971). *Minimal brain dysfunction in children.* New York: Wiley.

Werry, J. S., Elkind, G. S., & Reeves, J. C. (1987). Attention deficit, conduct, oppositional, and anxiety disorders in children: III. Laboratory differences. *Journal of Abnormal Child Psychology, 15,* 409–428.

Whalen, C. K., Henker, B., & Dotemoto, S. (1980). Methylphenidate and hyperactivity: Effects on teacher behaviors. *Science, 208*, 1280–1282.

Zametkin, A. J., & Rapoport, J. L. (1986). The pathophysiology of attention deficit disorder with hyperactivity. *Advances in Clinical Child Psychology, 9*, 177–217.

Zentall, S. (1984). Context effects in the behavioral ratings of hyperactivity. *Journal of Abnormal Child Psychology, 12*, 345–352.

CHAPTER 6

Anxiety Disorders

Richard E. Mattison
Washington University School of Medicine

As research in adult anxiety disorders has accelerated, more attention has now been directed toward anxiety disorders in childhood and adolescence. Current knowledge about anxiety psychopathology in children that meets today's scientific standards is limited. Nevertheless, this chapter reviews accruing objective evidence for the three childhood anxiety disorders that have been the focus of psychiatric research for the past two decades: separation anxiety disorder, avoidant disorder, and overanxious disorder. This review concentrates primarily on studies of these three specific disorders, rather than on reports using more general classification terms, such as *anxiety disorders*.

HISTORICAL BACKGROUND

Modern classification of child and adolescent psychiatric disorders began with DSM-II (American Psychiatric Association [APA], 1968). Two child anxiety diagnoses were included in the section Behavior Disorders of Childhood and Adolescence: withdrawing reaction and overanxious reaction of childhood (or adolescence). The brief description of withdrawing reaction listed the characteristic symptoms of seclusiveness, detachment, sensitivity, shyness, timidity, and general inability to form close personal relationships. The primary symptoms of overanxious reaction were stated as chronic anxiety, excessive and unrealistic fears, sleeplessness, nightmares, and exaggerated autonomic responses. In addition, these youth tended to be immature, self-conscious, grossly lacking in self-confidence, conforming, inhibited, dutiful, approval-seeking, and apprehensive in new situations and unfamiliar surroundings. Review of the literature shows little research into these two DSM-II child diagnostic categories, and consequently little progress in our knowledge of child anxiety disorders during the time of DSM-II.

Two major changes in childhood anxiety disorders were made in DSM-III (APA, 1980). First, a separate diagnostic section was established for Anxiety Disorders of Childhood or Adolescence. Second, in addition to the two anxiety diagnoses of DSM-II (withdrawing reaction was re-named avoidant disorder), a third diagnosis was added, separation anxiety disorder. DSM-III-R (APA, 1987) did not change the names of these three child anxiety disorders. However, some changes in diagnostic criteria have occurred, which are discussed in the next section.

Paralleling the development of the DSM categorical classification system has been the growth of an alternative dimensional classification approach (Quay, 1986). This classification system is based on empirical factor analyses of items on checklists and rating scales completed by parents, teachers, clinicians, or children themselves. Over the years anxiety-named scales have emerged, which Quay (1986) designated as a broad anxious-withdrawal-dysphoria category. More narrow anxiety scales have also been identified. For example, in an extensive study of major parent rating instruments in over 8,100 6- to 16-year-old U.S. and Dutch youth referred for mental health services, analyses determined two narrow syndromes with anxiety symptomatology: anxious/ depressed and withdrawn (Achenbach, Conners, Quay, Verhulst, & Howell, 1989). These scales could be related, respectively, to the DSM-III-R diagnoses of overanxious disorder and avoidant disorder. This dimensional classification of child anxiety psychopathology is discussed further later in this chapter, as well as literature demonstrating specific relationships between the anxiety diagnoses of both classification systems.

DEFINITIONAL ISSUES

The diagnostic criteria for the DSM-III-R childhood diagnoses of separation anxiety disorder (SAD), avoidant disorder (AVD), and overanxious disorder (OAD) are presented in Tables 6.1–6.3. This section focuses on changes that have occurred to the earlier DSM-III criteria.

TABLE 6.1

Diagnostic Criteria for Separation Anxiety Disorder

A. Excessive anxiety concerning separation from those to whom the child is attached, as evidenced by at least three of the following:
   1. unrealistic and persistent worry about possible harm befalling major attachment figures or fear that they will leave and not return
   2. unrealistic and persistent worry that an untoward calamitous event will separate the child from a major attchment figure, e.g., the child will be lost, kidnapped, killed, or be the victim of an accident
   3. persistent reluctance or refusal to go to school in order to stay with major attachment figures or at home
   4. persistent reluctance or refusal to go to sleep without being near a major attachment figure or to go to sleep away from home
   5. persistent avoidance of being alone, including "clinging" to and "shadowing" major attachment figures
   6. repeated nightmares involving the theme of separation
   7. complaints of physical symptoms, e.g., headaches, stomachaches, nausea, or vomiting, on many school days or on other occasions when anticipating separation from major attachment figures
   8. recurrent signs or complains of excessive distress in anticipation of separation from home or major attachment figures, e.g., temper tantrums or crying, pleading with parents not to leave
   9. recurrent signs of complaints of excessive distress when separated from home or major attachment figures, e.g., wants to return home, needs to call parents when they are absent or when child is away from home

B. Duration of disturbance of at least two weeks.

C. Onset before the age of 18.

D. Occurrence not exclusively during the course of a Pervasive Developmental Disorder, Schizophrenia, or any other psychotic disorder.

Note: From *Diagnostic and Statistical Manual of Mental Disorders* (3rd ed., rev.) (pp. 60–65) by the American Psychiatric Association, 1987, Washington, DC: Author.

TABLE 6.2
Diagnostic Criteria for Avoidant Disorder of Childhood or Adolescence

A. Excessive shrinking from contact with unfamiliar people, for a period of six months or longer, sufficiently severe to interfere with social functioning in peer relationships.

B. Desire for social involvement with familiar people (family members and peers the person knows well), and generally warm and satisfying relations with family members and other familiar figures.

C. Age at least $2\frac{1}{2}$ years.

D. The disturbance is not sufficiently pervasive and persistent to warrant the diagnosis of Avoidant Personality Disorder.

TABLE 6.3
Diagnostic Criteria for Overanxious Disorder

A. Excessive or unrealistic anxiety or worry, for a period of six months or longer, as indicated by the frequent occurrence of at least four of the following:
   1. excessive or unrealistic worry about future events
   2. excessive or unrealistic concern about the appropriateness of past behavior
   3. excessive or unrealistic concern about competence in one or more areas, e.g., athletic, academic, social
   4. somatic complaints, such as headaches or stomachaches, for which no physical basis can be established
   5. marked self-consciousness
   6. excessive need for reassurance about a variety of concerns
   7. marked feelings of tension or inability to relax
B. If another Axis I disorder is present (e.g., Separation Anxiety Disorder, Phobic Disorder, Obsessive Compulsive Disorder), the focus of the symptoms in A are not limited to it. For example, if Separation Anxiety Disorder is present,the symptoms in A are not exclusively related to anxiety about separation. In addition, the disturbance does not occur only during the course of a Psychotic Disorder or a Mood Disorder.
C. If 18 or older, does not meet the criteria for Generalized Anxiety Disorder.
D. Occurrence not exclusively during the course of a Pervasive Developmental Disorder, Schizophrenia, or any other psychotic disorder.

The major characteristic for SAD remains excessive anxiety concerning separation from a child's major attachment figures, as exemplified by three of nine possible criteria (Table 6.1). The third, fourth, and sixth criteria have not been changed from DSM-III. The "unrealistic and persistent" worries of Criteria 1 and 2 were formerly described only as "unrealistic." "Clinging" and "shadowing" in the fifth criterion are more specific descriptors that replace the more general DSM-III phrase of "emotional upset if unable to follow the major attachment figure around the home." In Criterion 7, the occurrence of the physical symptoms included only school days in DSM-III. "Signs" in the eighth criterion were not described as "recurrent" by DSM-III, and formerly the distress for children under 6 years of age must have been of panic proportions. Criterion 9 was altered the most and formerly read "social withdrawal, apathy, sadness, or difficulty concentrating on work or play when not with a major attachment figure." Thus, the DSM-III-R changes in SAD criteria appear primarily to emphasize recurrence or persistence.

The criteria for AVD show the least change and are primarily the result of rearrangement (Table 6.2). The current Criteria C and D were originally one criterion in DSM-III. In contrast, Criterion A is a combination of three DSM-III criteria. Finally, the first part of Criterion B originally read only as "desire for affection and acceptance," but in DSM-III-R this phrase has been more generalized to "desire for social involvement."

The changes that have occurred to the DSM-III OAD criteria are much like the changes to the SAD criteria, that is, more a matter of emphasis (Table 6.3). The primary criterion focuses on "excessive or unrealistic anxiety or worry" (rather than "generalized and persistent anxiety or worry"), and it now also incorporates the DSM-III separate criterion of persistence for at least 6 months, while still requiring four of seven possible criteria. Criteria 4, 6, and 7 are unchanged from the DSM-III criteria. Criteria 1, 2, and 3 originally did not contain "excessive" or "excessive and unrealistic." Criterion 5 shows the biggest change with the elimination of the DSM-III phrase "or susceptibility to embarrassment or humiliation."

Thus, the diagnostic criteria for the DSM-III-R childhood anxiety disorders have, in general, not changed in required symptomatology compared to DSM-III. Rather, severity or chronicity has been emphasized with new adjectives such as "excessive," "unrealistic," "persistent," and "recurrent."

REVIEW OF THE LITERATURE

Reliability

Few studies of the reliability of childhood anxiety disorders have been conducted. Reports are reviewed that meet the following criteria: final diagnoses determined from both parent and child information gathered in a standardized manner, and presentation of kappa statistics for individual childhood anxiety disorders. Only five studies met these specifications (Table 6.4).

The methodologies of these selected reports indicate that diagnoses were determined by clinicians using parent and child information obtained from structured or semistructured interviews (except for the Werry study, which used case presentations at ward rounds). The numbers of cases for each anxiety diagnosis were limited: SAD (9–28), OAD (7–32), and AVD (4). Ages of the samples were comparable, ranging from approximately 5 to 17 years old. Interrater reliability was examined in three studies, and test–retest reliability in two studies.

Landis and Koch (1977) proposed a kappa above .75 as excellent reliability, and kappas between .59 and .75 as good reliability. Thus, the reliability for both SAD and OAD was excellent (.81–.85) in the two

TABLE 6.4
Reliability Studies of DSM-III Child Anxiety Disorders

				Kappa			
Study	*Subjects*[a]	*N*	*Interview*	*OAD*	*SAD*	*AVD*	*All Dx*
Ambrosini, Metz, Prabucki, & Lee, 1989	Anxiety clinic	25	K-SADS III-R[b]	.85	.85	—	.86
Canino et al., 1987	Community & outpatient	91	DISC[c]	.35	.51	—	(.10–.75)
Last, Hersen, Kazdin, Finkelstein, & Strauss, 1987	Anxiety clinic	91	ISC[c]	.82	.81	—	(.64–1.00)
Silverman & Nelles, 1988	Anxiety clinic & anxiety parents	51	ADIS[b]	.54	—	—	.78
Werry, Methven, Fitzpatrick, & Dixon, 1983	Inpatient	195	Case presentation[b]	.65	.72	.05	.71

[a]General age range = 5–17 years
[b]Interrater reliability
[c]Test–retest reliability

studies (one interrater and one test–retest) of children seen in outpatient clinics specializing in anxiety disorders. In the other settings the reliability was not as strong, with kappas varying from .35 to .72. In general, throughout the five studies the kappas for OAD and SAD appeared similar to the mean kappa for all diagnoses in each investigation. Only one study reported a kappa for AVD (.05 based on four cases), and thus it must be concluded that the reliability for this child anxiety disorder remains unknown.

In summary, studies are still required to establish reliability for the individual childhood anxiety disorders, specifically to include larger numbers of cases and to investigate DSM-III-R criteria. The kappas for OAD and SAD presenting to anxiety clinics are encouraging, possibly indicating good reliability when the cases are severe enough to be taken to such specialty clinics. Thus, future reliability studies of anxiety cases in general child psychiatry outpatient clinics and in general populations of children will be important. Also crucial will be reliability studies utilizing highly structured lay interviews from which anxiety diagnoses are determined by computer algorithms, for example, the DISC (Edelbrock & Costello, 1988).

Validity

There are several properties of diagnostic categories that determine validity. In addition to the specificity of the clinical features, other important features include natural history, biological correlates, familial patterns, and treatment response. Such information is sparse for child anxiety diagnoses, but these limited data are reviewed.

Clinical Features

Thus far, we have little information describing the specific clinical presentation of OAD, SAD, or AVD, except for clinician ratings of OAD diagnostic criteria in OAD children (Strauss, Lease, Last, & Francis, 1988). That is, a general survey of presenting symptoms has not been conducted in any of these disorders, nor even a more specific survey of possible anxiety symptomatology. The disorders have only been described at the more general levels of diagnostic category or instrument scale. Therefore, the value of the individual operational criteria for each anxiety disorder has yet to be determined.

Comorbidity. The pattern of diagnoses presenting to an outpatient child psychiatry clinic specializing in anxiety disorders has been described by Last and her colleagues (Last, Strauss, & Francis, 1987).

Among 73 consecutive children aged 5 to 18 years, the frequencies of primary diagnoses for the three childhood anxiety disorders were 32.9% for SAD, 15.1% for OAD, and 1.4% for AVD. The SAD and OAD children did not differ significantly for age, sex, or race, but the SAD children were significantly lower for socioeconomic class. Comorbid diagnoses were common in both OAD (72.7%) and SAD (79.2%) children, especially concurrent anxiety disorders (OAD 54.6%; SAD 41.7%). The most common additional diagnoses in the OAD children were social phobia (36.4%), oppositional disorder (36.4%), avoidant disorder (27.3%), and attention deficit disorder (18.2%). Within the SAD children, the most frequent comorbid diagnoses were OAD (33.3%), attention deficit disorder (16.7%), and oppositional disorder (16.7%).

Among the children presenting to the anxiety clinic in the previous study, 15.1% received the primary diagnosis of major depression. All of these depressed children had a concurrent anxiety diagnosis; the frequencies of comorbid childhood anxiety disorders were 45.4%, 27.3%, and 27.3% for OAD, SAD, and AVD, respectively. The comorbidity of a depressive disorder with the primary diagnosis of OAD or SAD was much less (0%–12.5%), and somewhat more common in the SAD children.

Comorbidity with a diagnosis of OAD has also been studied according to age. Patterns of concurrent diagnoses were compared in two age groups of OAD children, less than 12 years old (N=23) and 12 or older (N=32) (Strauss et al., 1988). The younger OAD group was significantly more likely than the older group to have a concurrent diagnosis of SAD (69.6% vs. 21.9%) or attention deficit disorder (34.8% vs. 9.4%). The older group had significantly higher rates of simple phobia (40.6% vs. 8.7%) and major depression (46.9% vs. 17.4%).

The comorbidity of anxiety and depressive disorders has been further investigated (Bernstein & Garfinkel, 1986; Hershberg, Carlson, Cantwell, & Strober, 1982; Kovacs, Feinberg, Crouse-Novak, Paulauskas, & Finkelstein, 1984; Strauss, Last, Hersen, & Kazdin, 1988), with some patterns suggested. Children with depressive disorders commonly report anxiety symptoms, much moreso than children with anxiety disorders report depressive symptoms. Youth with both disorders report more severity of anxiety psychopathology than children with anxiety disorders only. Finally, children with both diagnoses tend to be older.

Comparison with Other Classification Systems. Another approach to confirming the validity of the childhood anxiety disorders is comparison of these diagnoses with those established in another classification system, for example, with childhood syndromes empirically determined by factor analyses of checklists. Researchers in dimensional classification agree that one broad-band factor has been established, termed *anxiety-withdrawal-dysphoria* by Quay (1986) and *internalizing* by Achenbach (1985). More specific narrow-band factors also appear established: anxious-depressed and withdrawn (Achenbach et al., 1989). Thus, the broad-band factor could be equated with the general category of childhood anxiety disorder, and the narrow-band anxious-depressed with OAD and withdrawn with AVD. Indeed, items in the anxious-depressed syndrome include fearful or anxious, needs to be perfect, nervous or tense, and self-conscious, while withdrawn contains prefers to be alone, refuses to talk, secretive, shy or timid, and withdrawn. One could postulate that SAD does not correlate with a particular narrow-band factor because of the lack of items in checklists that address the operational criteria for SAD.

Some research has begun to investigate actual relationships between DSM-III childhood anxiety diagnoses and dimensional categories. Werry and his colleagues (Reeves, Werry, Elkind, & Zametkin, 1987) found children with anxiety disorders to be rated by their parents as significantly higher than matched normal controls on the anxiety-withdrawal factor of Quay's Revised Behavior Problem Checklist. Their teachers also scored them higher than both the controls and hyperactive children on the tension-anxiety factor of the Conners Teacher Rating Scale.

In another report, children with OAD showed a relationship with the schizoid or anxious scale of the parent Child Behavior Checklist (Costello, Edelbrock, Dulcan, Kalas, & Klaric, 1984). The higher the *T* score on the scale, the more likely a diagnosis of OAD, and the more severe the OAD, the more likely a higher *T* score on the scale. In another report that also used the Child Behavior Checklist, OAD boys were characterized by internalizing Child Behavior Profile types (or clusters), particularly the schizoid or anxious type (Mattison & Bagnato, 1987). In contrast, attention deficit disorder boys in the same study were primarily identified as hyperactive or delinquent types. No OAD boy was classified as hyperactive or delinquent, and no attention deficit disorder boy as schizoid or anxious.

In addition to classification by dimensions, research has also examined inborn temperament types in children. Possibly related to child anxiety disorders, especially AVD, are the slow-to-warm children identified by Chess and her colleagues (Thomas, Chess, & Birch, 1969), and/or the inhibited children described by Kagan and his colleagues (Garcia-Coll, Kagan, & Reznick, 1984). The slow-to-warm children were described by initial withdrawal in new situations, slow adaptation, mild moods, quietness, and low activity. The inhibited children were characterized by their reactions to unfamiliar people or objects: delayed interaction, retreat from the unfamiliar, discontinuance of play, clinginess to mother, and fretting or crying. Both temperaments have showed persistence in longitudinal studies. Unfortunately, the relationship of such inborn personality styles to DSM-III or DSM-III-R child anxiety diagnoses has not yet been examined. Such a temperament could precede the development of a child anxiety disorder; that is, these temperament characteristics could become more severe, dysfunctional symptomatology.

Summary. Research remains necessary to clarify the clinical features of the specific childhood anxiety disorders. Surveys of symptomatology should be conducted with interviews and checklists completed by multiple observers to help clarify clinical presentation. Such research would also allow correlation studies with empirically derived anxiety factors, to which especially OAD and AVD may be related. Research thus far suggests that children can present as pure OAD or SAD, but multiple anxiety diagnoses and comorbidity with depressive disorders are also common presentations. Thus, future work should clearly identify these different anxiety groups to determine any important differences that may exist.

Biological Correlates

The primary work in differentiating physical, neurological, or laboratory characteristics of children with anxiety disorders has been conducted by Werry and his colleagues (Reeves et al., 1987; Werry, Elkind, & Reeves, 1987). They compared 21 outpatient children aged 5 to 13 years with an anxiety disorder (OAD, SAD, AVD, or phobic disorder) to matched normal controls and also to groups of outpatients with either attention deficit disorder with hyperactivity (ADDH) or ADDH with a conduct or oppositional disorder. The subjects were all tested on a variety of cognitive, academic, laboratory, physical, and neurological measures.

The anxiety subjects did not differ from the other groups on the test of intelligence (Peabody Picture Vocabulary Test), with a mean IQ of 100. In teachers' assessment of reading, writing, and arithmetic, the anxiety disordered children performed significantly better than the two groups of ADDH children, but showed a trend ($p < .10$) toward inferior performance in reading and arithmetic compared to their matched controls. On a specific reading test of word recognition, the anxiety and control groups did not differ significantly.

The groups were compared on laboratory tests of impulsivity, arousal, motor performance, and activity level. The anxiety children did not differ significantly from their control group on any of these parameters. The two ADDH groups did show significantly greater activity than the anxiety group.

Finally, physical and neurological characteristics of the subjects were investigated: pre-, peri-, or postnatal insults, neurodevelopmental abnormalities, minor physical anomalies, articulation, and right-handedness. Noteworthy findings for the anxiety children were limited. They had suffered significantly less pregnancy or delivery insults (24% with more than one insult) than the two groups of ADDH children. Their only difference from their control group was a trend ($p < .10$) for more physical anomalies (24% vs. 5% with greater than five anomalies).

In summary, these anxiety children investigated by Werry and his colleagues showed few differences from their controls, except for specific trends toward underachievement and more physical anomalies. The ADDH groups were different than the anxiety group in predictable areas, that is, poorer academic performance and increased activity. This series of studies is admirable in its comprehensive evaluation designed to determine differences between the diagnostic groups. The logical next step is to build on this work, especially to improve the methodology with adequate numbers of children with specific anxiety disorders and with more rigorous instrumentation.

Natural History

Child psychiatry currently has little understanding of the course of children with anxiety disorders preceding their presentation for evaluation and treatment. Their follow-up after diagnosis has received some attention, primarily as part of the longitudinal study of other child psychiatric disorders. Additional information concerning the natural history of child anxiety disorders is suggested by adult retrospective studies and also prospective follow-up studies of children with more generally defined anxiety diagnoses.

In one follow-up study, Pfeffer, Lipkins, Plutchik, and Mizruchi (1988) followed children with psychiatric disorders for 2 years to identify factors associated with interim suicidal symptomatology. Among the subjects were 28 children with OAD. The presence of the anxiety disorder was not correlated with an increased risk for suicidal behavior. However, in relationship to the stability of the disorder, 70.6% of the original OAD children maintained the diagnosis.

More recently, Cantwell and Baker (1989) completed a 4-year follow-up study of children (originally aged 2 to 11 years) with speech and language disorders as well as psychiatric disorders. Included in the study were children with specific DSM-III anxiety disorders: OAD

(N=8), SAD (N=9), and AVD (N=14). The courses of the OAD children were as follows: 25% maintained their initial diagnosis; 25% recovered with no diagnosis at follow-up; and the remaining OAD children evolved into another diagnosis, especially an affective disorder or another anxiety disorder (38%). Within the SAD group, at follow-up 11% still had their original diagnosis, 44% had recovered, and the rest had changed diagnosis, especially to another anxiety disorder (33%). For the AVD children, the results were same diagnosis (29%), recovered (36%), and new anxiety or affective diagnosis (43%). Thus, the AVD category showed the most continuity of diagnosis (29%), and SAD the highest recovery rate (44%). Overall, at least one third of each category evolved into either another anxiety disorder or an affective disorder.

In their longitudinal study of DSM-III depressive disorders in childhood, Kovacs, Gatsonis, Paulauskas, and Richards (1989) examined the relationship of depressive disorders to anxiety disorders (SAD and OAD). They found that although anxiety disorders can follow the onset of a depressive disorder and can recover as the depressive illness improves, anxiety illness can also predate or postdate the depression. For example, in 30 cases of major depressive disorder, they found that the onset of the anxiety disorder predated the depression in 19 cases. Furthermore, in 12 cases the anxiety illness persisted after recovery from the depressive episode. This independence was found less in cases of dysthymic disorder.

Earlier research in adults with panic disorder and agoraphobia found a common childhood history of separation anxiety (D. Klein, 1964), indicating a possible evolutionary path for children with SAD. This hypothesis has been the focus of a 20-year follow-up project investigating the course of 45 children treated for school phobia, 42 of whom had childhood history of separation anxiety symptoms (Klein & Last, 1989). Compared to a control group, significantly more of the school phobic children developed agoraphobia with panic disorder, although the percentage was small (7% vs. 0%). Also, more of the probands developed a depressive disorder (31% vs. 18%), although the difference was not significant. Thus, although some proof was found for the original hypothesis, the evidence was not robust. One explanation purports that treatment may have improved the final outcome.

In addition to the work of Klein and his colleagues, other retrospective information from adult studies imply possible courses for children and adolescents with anxiety disorders, particularly continued anxiety morbidity. For example, in the epidemiological adult ECA study, anxiety disorders not only emerged as the most common general diagnosis, but also had the earliest age of onset (Christie et al., 1988). More specifically, researchers in adult generalized anxiety disorder

(GAD) have found this disorder to commonly have an age of onset in late childhood or early adolescence (Barlow, Blanchard, Vermilyea, Vermilyea, & DiNardo, 1986; Reich, 1986). Therefore, because of the similarity in symptomatology between GAD and OAD, the transition from OAD to GAD seems a likely occurrence in many cases. Finally, although no studies have been conducted, one speculation for the course of children with AVD is the outcome of avoidant personality disorder in adulthood because of similar symptomatology.

Other prospective studies of children with possible anxiety disorders seem to indicate that long-term morbidity is not uncommon. For example, in a longitudinal study of neurological soft signs, Shaffer and his fellow researchers (1985) found that children at age 7 with soft signs and anxious-dependent behavior commonly showed anxiety and withdrawal psychiatric disorders (especially OAD) at age 17. Outcome studies of school phobia have been conducted (Klein & Last, 1989), although the equation of school phobia with SAD must be made with caution because of several possible diagnoses in the differential diagnosis of school phobia or school refusal (Hersov, 1985; Last, Francis, Hersen, Kazdin, & Strauss, 1987). The most extensive investigation was the 10-year follow-up of 168 school refusers who had received inpatient psychiatric treatment (Berg & Jackson, 1985). During the interim, 30% had received psychiatric care, and at follow-up 30% were judged to still be disturbed. Finally, in a 20-year study of 34 shy and withdrawn outpatient children (possible AVD?), one-third were found at follow-up to be marginally adjusted in their life-functioning (Morris, Soroker, & Burruss, 1954).

Thus, although more definitive follow-up studies are needed for the specific child anxiety disorders, a variety of evidence suggests that children with anxiety disorders are at risk for ongoing morbidity. They appear particularly vulnerable for anxiety disorders (including continuance into adulthood), and also for affective disorders. On the other hand, it appears that many youth with anxiety disorders may recover to the status of no psychiatric illness. Thus, prospective research can help clarify which children and adolescents with anxiety disorders are at the most risk for ongoing psychopathology.

Family Patterns

Determination of patterns of family psychiatric illness in children with anxiety disorders is in its early stages. Previous studies of the offspring of adults with anxiety disorders suggested that their children were at increased risk for anxiety disorders (Weissman, Leckman, Merikangas, Gammon, & Prusoff, 1984; Turner, Beidel, & Costello, 1987).

More definitive research into the types of psychiatric disorders in the families of anxious children has primarily been generated by Last and her colleagues through their child anxiety clinic at the University of Pittsburgh. They have studied both the mothers and the extended families of children with DSM-III anxiety diagnoses.

In their first study, the mothers of outpatient children with OAD (N=22), SAD (N=19), both OAD and SAD (N=17), and controls with other nonanxiety psychiatric disorders (N=15) were evaluated with a structured clinical interview (Last, Hersen, Kazdin, Francis, & Grubb, 1987). Anxiety disorders were very common in the OAD mothers (86.4%), especially GAD (45.5%), and affective disorders were also frequent (50.0%), particularly major depression (31.8%). The percentages in the SAD mothers were similar, that is, 68.4% with an anxiety disorder (47.4% GAD), and 57.9% with an affective disorder (52.6% major depression). The same pattern was found for the mothers of children with both disorders: 94.1% with an anxiety diagnosis (47.1% GAD), and 64.7% with an affective diagnosis (52.9% major depression). Although these percentages for the specific anxiety categories were consistently higher than the findings for the control mothers, no significant differences were found.

In a related study, mothers were investigated for their rates of OAD and SAD in their childhood (Last, Phillips, & Statfield, 1987). The frequency of SAD did not significantly differ in the mothers of OAD, SAD, both, or nonanxiety psychiatric controls. However, the rate of childhood OAD in the mothers of the OAD children (42%) was significantly higher than the rates for the SAD mothers (9.5%) and the control mothers (15%).

Last and her colleagues are now expanding their family research to determine lifetime psychiatric illness in first- and second-degree relatives of child probands with anxiety disorder (Klein & Last, 1989). The DSM-III-R groups of subjects are 52 children with an anxiety disorder, 40 with attention deficit-hyperactivity disorder, and 54 normal controls. The anxious children included a wide range of anxiety disorders, including OAD (N=10), SAD (N=9), and AVD (N=3). The numbers of relatives of the anxiety group who were studied were 151 first-degree and 447 second-degree. They were at a significantly higher risk for anxiety disorders than the relatives of the controls, and showed a positive trend ($p < .10$) for greater risk compared to the relatives of the hyperactive children. More specifically, the male relatives of the anxiety children were at a significantly higher risk for anxiety disorder than either the hyperactive or control male relatives. In the comparison of female relatives, the anxiety mothers were at significantly increased risk compared only to the control mothers. Although the anxiety and hyperactive mothers did not differ significantly for risk, the types of anxiety disorders found for each group were considered noteworthy. The anxiety mothers were most at risk for simple phobia, OAD, and social phobia, whereas the mothers of the hyperactive group were most at risk for posttraumatic stress disorder and social phobia. Overall, and consistent with the more specific results, individual anxiety families showed the most segregation for anxiety disorders.

The relationship of childhood anxiety disorders to other family or environmental factors, for example, stressors, is not clear. Werry and his colleagues (Reeves et al., 1987) compared a group of anxious children with attention deficit disorder groups and a control group on a number of ecological and parent factors. The anxiety group significantly differed from the control group in three ways: lesser education of the fathers, more marital maladjustment, and increased history of anxiety disorder in the mothers (48% vs. 5%). The anxiety group did not differ significantly from the other groups on the Coddington Life Events scale.

In summary, anxiety disorders do appear to occur commonly in the families of children with anxiety disorders, but they also may be frequent in families of children with nonanxiety psychiatric disorders. Affective disorders also often occur in the mothers of children with anxiety disorders. Thus, more research is necessary to clarify family patterns further, especially using specific DSM-III-R child anxiety diagnoses as probands. Simultaneously, the family environment should also be studied for other possible contributing factors, such as marital tension, abuse, and parenting techniques.

Treatment Response

Over the past decade, reviews have repeatedly stated that studies have yet to establish the proper treatment for child anxiety disorders (Klein & Last, 1989; McDermott, Werry, Petti, Cambrinck-Graham, & Char, 1989; Werry & Aman, 1980). The primary reason is the absence of such investigations. Cognitive-behavioral approaches appear to be most promising because of their success with the symptoms of fears, school phobia, and social withdrawal (Mattison, 1989). Pharmacotherapy remains very conservative, for example, the use of imipramine only in severe and/or treatment-resistant cases of SAD with school phobia (Gittelman & Koplewicz, 1986). The indications and efficacy for family and/or individual therapy continue to be unclear. Nevertheless, excellent resources describing various treatment approaches are available for use by both clinicians and researchers (McDermott et al., 1989; Gittelman, 1986).

Proposals

This review of the literature indicates that our basic knowledge of the DSM-III-R childhood anxiety disorders has only begun to accrue, and is based primarily on DSM-III diagnostic criteria. Thus, it appears premature to propose changes in operational criteria because the status of the criteria (past and present DSM-III) requires further elementary investigation. Similarly, it remains too early to alter the current descriptive information provided in the DSM-III-R manual for each child anxiety disorder. However, at the least, that information must be accepted cautiously, recalling that such data are for the most part derived from very few studies of small numbers of children or adolescents with the specific anxiety disorders.

Of all the work that must be undertaken to establish the validity of the DSM-III-R child anxiety diagnoses, perhaps the most crucial is to determine the actual symptomatology that exists in these children, to thereby confirm, refute, or improve the value of the current criteria. What criteria are the most vital, and should they be described in more specific detail? Are there other important, specific anxiety symptoms that are not currently assessed?

In order to accomplish this step, more detailed assessments of anxiety symptomatology in children and adolescents must be developed. Although dimensional classification has produced anxiety syndromes similar to DSM-III-R diagnoses, the anxiety items of most empirical instruments are quite limited and general in description. The development of more comprehensive anxiety instruments would assist clinicians' assessment of current diagnostic criteria. This would allow future diagnostic study and factor analyses of more comprehensive anxiety data that might describe other anxiety syndromes for clinicians to confirm.

DIAGNOSTIC AND ASSESSMENT PROCEDURES

Several instruments are available to study anxiety psychopathology in children and adolescents (Kratochwill, Morris, & Campbell, 1985). Few have been utilized in the investigation of DSM-III or DSM-III-R child anxiety diagnoses. Thus, an effective battery (self-report, parent, teacher, and direct observation measures) remains to be developed. However, potentially useful instruments can be suggested based on their past implementation in studies of childhood anxiety disorders.

Self-Report Instruments

Three self-report instruments have been utilized commonly in child anxiety research: the State-Trait Anxiety Inventory for Children (STAIC) (Spielberger, 1973), the Fear Survey Schedule—Revised (FSSC-R) (Ollendick, 1983), and the Revised Children's Manifest Anxiety Scale (RCMAS) (Reynolds & Richmond, 1978). All have established psychometric properties. However, their ability to distinguish child anxiety disorders remains unclear.

The state and trait scores of the STAIC were found to significantly distinguish a group of children with both an anxiety disorder and major depression from a group of children with only anxiety disorders and from a control group of children with a psychiatric disorder other than anxiety or major depression (Strauss, Last, Hersen, & Kazdin, 1988). The state score also significantly differentiated the pure anxiety group from the control group. Overall, the order of highest STAIC scores was anxiety plus depression group, pure anxiety group, and control group. In another STAIC study, the mean state and trait scores of this measure were significantly higher in an older group of OAD children than in a younger group (Strauss, Lease, Last, & Francis, 1988). Thus, the STAIC has shown some usefulness in identifying some groups of anxiety children, but its accuracy (sensitivity, specificity, etc.) for the identification of individual children with a general or a specific anxiety disorder has not yet been reported.

In the same two studies in which the STAIC was used, the FSSC-R was also part of the battery. The results were less encouraging. The anxiety plus depression children scored significantly higher than the other two groups on the total score of the FSSC-R. However, the pure anxiety group was not significantly different from the control group, and their mean total scores were quite similar. In the study of the two different age groups of OAD children, the older children had a slightly higher mean total score, but not significantly so. Finally, the FSSC-R was used to compare children with OAD and SAD (Last, Francis, & Strauss, 1989). The two anxiety groups did not significantly differ in overall level of self-rated fear, nor on any of the five factor scores that indicate different general categories of fears.

The RCMAS has been the most extensively used self-report measure in the study of children with anxiety disorders. In addition to a total score, it also includes scores for three narrow scales that have been established through factor analysis: physiological, worry/oversensitivity, and concentration. Again, citing the previous two studies conducted by Strauss and her colleagues, all four scores were significantly higher in the comorbid anxiety/depression children compared to the other two groups. The pure anxiety children were not significantly different from the controls on any of the RCMAS scores and, indeed, they had a higher mean score only on worry/ oversensitivity. This same factor was also the only RCMAS factor that significantly distinguished the older (higher score) from the younger OAD children in the second study.

An earlier version of the RCMAS was used in a study of school phobic children with anxiety and/or affective disorders (Bernstein & Garfinkel, 1986). The total score was significantly higher in the children with both anxiety and affective disorders, compared to groups with neither disorder or only an anxiety disorder. The children with only an anxiety disorder were not significantly differentiated from children with an affective disorder or from children with neither disorder. Bernstein, Garfinkel, and Hoberman (1989) used the current RCMAS in a large survey of rural students in grades 9–12. The students classified as high anxiety were differentiated from the low-anxiety students on the following factors: female, somatic complaints, history of physical and sexual abuse, poor grades, drug use, and family history related to depression.

Of the self-report instruments, only the RCMAS has been examined for its accuracy in distinguishing children with anxiety disorders from children with nonanxiety disorders. Worry/oversensitivity appears to be the most useful RCMAS factor. A *T* score greater than 60 on worry/oversensitivity differentiated children with a DSM-III anxiety diagnosis from children with a nonanxiety diagnosis with 40.9% sensitivity and 80.0% specificity (Mattison, Bagnato, & Brubaker, 1988). In a study of boys with OAD compared to boys with dysthymic disorder or attention deficit disorder with hyperactivity, sensitivity was 31.0% and specificity 80.0% with the same cutoff procedure (Mattison & Bagnato, 1987). Thus, the RCMAS has shown some value in correctly identifying children without an anxiety disorder (true negatives). The latter study demonstrated improved accuracy when the RCMAS was used with a parent checklist.

Parent Instruments

As discussed in the earlier comparison of DSM-III anxiety disorders with dimensional classification, empirically derived anxiety scales have emerged, and some relationships between the two systems have been demonstrated. However, only one study has investigated the accuracy of a parent instrument in differentiating childhood anxiety disorders. The Child Behavior Checklist (CBCL) (Achenbach & Edelbrock, 1983) was examined with OAD boys 8 to 12 years old (Mattison & Bagnato, 1987). Within the small group of 16 OAD boys, the narrow-band internalizing scales showed the highest percentages of pathological elevations, as did the broad-band Internalizing scale in comparison to the Externalizing scale (50% vs. 31%). The most common Child Behavior Profile type within the OAD boys was schizoid-anxious (38%). When this specific type was used to classify the OAD boys in comparison to boys with dysthymic or attention deficit disorders, the sensitivity was 37% and specificity 95%. When combined with an either/or cutoff procedure with the worry/oversensitivity factor of the RCMAS, sensitivity improved to 56% while specificity decreased to 76%. This modest study suggested that the most accurate identification of OAD would most likely be produced by a multimethod assessment procedure.

Other Procedures

The usefulness of teacher checklists and direct observation procedures has not yet been studied for the identification of childhood anxiety disorders. However, specific interviews that are administered to children and their parents have been developed. These include sections to elicit anxiety symptomatology of the DSM-III-R child anxiety diagnoses. The most current forms of the semistructured Kiddie-SADS for clinicians and the structured DISC for trained lay interviewers are examples of such general interviews, reviewed recently by Edelbrock and Costello (1988). Another semistructured interview, the Anxiety Disorders Interview Schedule (ADIS), has been developed for use with children and their parents as a comprehensive survey specifically for anxiety symptomatology (Silverman & Nelles, 1988). At this point, a single interview has not emerged as the most useful for diagnosis of anxiety disorders in children.

Finally, psychobiological measures would be desirable in a battery to evaluate children for a possible anxiety disorder. No such measure has emerged for anxiety disorders because such studies are lacking. Moreover, Ferguson and Bawden (1988) reviewed studies of electrophysiological, biochemical, physical and motor, and perceptual and cognitive measures in the identification of specific child psychiatric disorders and found only weak associations and an overall lack of specificity. Although they suggested further research to uncover possible associations, they also advocated defining psychobiological groups and then determining their distinguishing psychopathology.

In summary, several instruments are promising components for a diagnostic battery to determine anxiety diagnoses in children and adolescents. However, few have been used, either alone or in combination, in studies of the individual anxiety disorders. Accuracy also has not been the focus of much attention. Thus, clinicians may look for the future development of empirically sound instruments that comprehensively address in more detail the potentially rich variety of anxiety symptomatology in children and adolescents.

SUMMARY AND DIRECTIONS

The summaries at the end of each section within this chapter indicate that our overall knowledge of childhood anxiety psychopathology is, for the most part, in its infancy. However, the new attention to child anxiety disorders by modern science should replace discouragement with anticipation. What will evolve from more detailed, comprehensive investigations into this basic mood state in children and adolescents? Speculation should at this time be cautious, but yet is tantalizing.

More specific and intensive examination of anxiety psychopathology will expand our appreciation of children's anxiety states and traits. Such research will increase our understanding of normal or age-appropriate and deviant types of anxiety in children. The development of instruments to drive such research will additionally provide clinicians with improved measures to better identify and understand anxious children. These studies will lead to the refinement of DSM-III-R classification of child anxiety disorders, if not the reconceptualization. Evidence for a wider range of childhood anxiety psychopathology has recently begun to emerge from initial studies of other DSM-III-R anxiety disorders in children, such as the seminal work by Rapoport and her colleagues in obsessive compulsive disorder (Rapoport, 1986).

Pure and comorbid anxiety diagnoses appear to exist, indicating the need for careful distinction by researchers. Natural courses most likely are multiple, including disappearance, continuance of the same symptomatology, or evolution into another type of anxiety or psychiatric disorder, especially depressive illness. Early identifying characteristics may gradually emerge through the study of such varied diagnostic possibilities, with subsequent etiology and treatment implications.

The biology of children with anxiety symptoms is rudimentary, but it will evolve. Its determination may partially be aided by genetic research into families with histories of specific anxiety disorders. Animal research as well as advances in adult psychopharmacology and neurophysiology should also provide contributions. Medications may then serve more important specific treatment roles.

The research necessary to address these speculations is on the horizon. Childhood anxiety has always been a key concept in psychiatry, but its scientific advancement has lagged behind its conceptual pace. A more complete understanding of anxiety psychopathology in children and adolescents may have important ramifications for all of psychiatry that cannot yet be appreciated, including nosological considerations.

REFERENCES

Achenbach, T. M. (1985). *Assessment and taxonomy of child and adolescent psychopathology.* Beverly Hills, CA: Sage Publications.

Achenbach, T. M., Conners, C. K., Quay, H. C., Verhulst, F. C., & Howell, C. T. (1989). Replication of empirically derived syndromes as a basis for taxonomy of child/adolescent psychopathology. *Journal of Abnormal Child Psychology, 17,* 299–323.

Achenbach, T. M., & Edelbrock, C. (1983). *Manual for the Child Behavior Checklist and the Revised Child Behavior Profile.* Burlington, VT: University of Vermont, Department of Psychiatry.

Ambrosini, P. J., Metz, C., Prabucki, K., & Lee, J. (1989). Videotape reliability of the third revised edition of the K-SADS. *Journal of the American Academy of Child and Adolescent Psychiatry, 28,* 723–728.

American Psychiatric Association. (1968). *Diagnostic and statistical manual of mental disorders* (2nd ed.). Washington, DC: Author.

American Psychiatric Association. (1980). *Diagnostic and statistical manual of mental disorders* (3rd ed.). Washington, DC: Author.

American Psychiatric Association. (1987). *Diagnostic and statistical manual of mental disorders* (3rd ed., rev.). Washington, DC: Author.

Barlow, D. H., Blanchard, E. B., Vermilyea, J. A., Vermilyea, B. B., & DiNardo, P. A. (1986). Generalized anxiety and generalized anxiety disorder: Description and reconceptualization. *American Journal of Psychiatry, 143,* 40–44.

Berg, I., & Jackson, A. (1985). Teenage school refusers grow up: A follow-up study of 168 subjects, ten years on average after in-patient treatment. *British Journal of Psychiatry, 147,* 366–370.

Bernstein, G. A., & Garfinkel, B. D. (1986). School phobia: The overlap of affective and anxiety disorders. *Journal of the American Academy of Child Psychiatry, 25,* 235–241.

Bernstein, G. A., Garfinkel, B. D., & Hoberman, H. M. (1989). Self-reported anxiety in adolescents. *American Journal of Psychiatry, 146,* 384–386.

Canino, G. J., Bird, H. R., Rubio-Stipec, M., Woodbury, M. A., Ribera, J. C., Huertas, S. E., & Sesman, M. J. (1987). Reliability of child diagnosis in a Hispanic sample. *Journal of the American Academy of Child and Adolescent Psychiatry, 26,* 560–565.

Cantwell, D. P., & Baker, L. (1989). Stability and natural history of DSM-III childhood diagnoses. *Journal of the American Academy of Child and Adolescent Psychiatry, 28,* 691–700.

Christie, K. A., Burke, J. D., Regier, D. A., Rae, D. S., Boyd, J. H., & Locke,

B. Z. (1988). Epidemiologic evidence for early onset of mental disorders and higher risk of drug abuse in young adults. *American Journal of Psychiatry, 145*, 971–975.

Costello, A. J., Edelbrock, C. S., Dulcan, M. K., Kalas, R., & Klaric, S. H. (1984). *Report to NIMH on the NIMH Diagnostic Interview Schedule for Children (DISC)*. Washington, DC: National Institute of Mental Health.

Edelbrock, C., & Costello, A. J. (1988). Structured psychiatric interviews for children. In M. Rutter, A. H. Tuma, & I. S. Lann (Eds.), *Assessment and diagnosis in child psychopathology* (pp. 87–112). New York: Guilford Press.

Ferguson, H. B., & Bawden, H. N. (1988). Psychobiological measures. In M. Rutter, A. H. Tuma, & I. S. Lann (Eds.), *Assessment and diagnosis in child psychopathology* (pp. 232–263). New York: Guilford Press.

Garcia-Coll, C., Kagan, J., & Reznick, J. S. (1984). Behavioral inhibition in young children, *Child Development, 55*, 1005–1019.

Gittelman, R. (1986). *Anxiety disorders of childhood*. New York: Guilford Press.

Gittelman, R., & Koplewicz, H. S. (1986). Pharmacotherapy of childhood anxiety disorders. In R. Gittelman (Ed.), *Anxiety disorders of childhood* (pp. 188–203). New York: Guilford Press.

Hershberg, S. G., Carlson, G. A., Cantwell, D. P., & Strober, M. (1982). Anxiety and depressive disorders in psychiatrically disturbed children. *Journal of Clinical Psychiatry, 43*, 358–361.

Hersov, L. (1985). School refusal. In M. Rutter & L. Hersov (Eds.), *Child and adolescent psychiatry: Modern approaches* (pp. 382–389). Boston: Blackwell Scientific Publications.

Klein, D. F. (1964). Delineation of two drug-responsive anxiety syndromes. *Psychopharmacologica, 3*, 397–408.

Klein, R. G., & Last, C. G. (1989). *Anxiety disorders in children*. Newbury Park, CA: Sage Publications.

Kovacs, M., Feinberg, T. L., Crouse-Novak, M., Paulauskas, S. L., & Finkelstein, R. (1984). Depression disorders in childhood: I. A longitudinal prospective study of characteristics and recovery. *Archives of General Psychiatry, 41*, 229–237.

Kovacs, M., Gatsonis, C., Paulauskas, S. L., & Richards, C. (1989). Depressive disorders in childhood: IV. A longitudinal study of comorbidity with and risk for anxiety disorders. *Archives of General Psychiatry, 46*, 776–782.

Kratochwill, T., Morris, R., & Campbell, K. (1985). Assessment of children's anxiety-related disorders. In J. Berg (Ed.), *School psychology in contemporary society: An introduction* (pp. 163–206). Columbus, OH: Merrill.

Landis, J. R., & Koch, G. G. (1977). The measurement of observer agreement for categorical data. *Biometrics, 33*, 159–174.

Last, C. G., Francis, G., Hersen, M., Kazdin, A. E., & Strauss, C. C. (1987). Separation anxiety and school phobia: A comparison using DSM-III criteria. *American Journal of Psychiatry, 144*, 653–657.

Last, C. G., Francis, G., & Strauss, C. C. (1989). Assessing fears in anxiety-disordered children with the revised Fear Survey Schedule for Children (FSSC-R). *Journal of Clinical Child Psychology, 18*, 137–141.

Last, C. G., Hersen, M., Kazdin, A. E., Finkelstein, R., & Strauss, C. C. (1987). Comparison of DSM-III separation anxiety and overanxious disorders: Demographic characteristics and patterns of comorbidity. *Journal of the American Academy of Child and Adolescent Psychiatry, 26*, 527–531.

Last, C. G., Hersen, M., Kazdin, A. E., Francis, G., & Grubb, H. J. (1987). Psychiatric illness in the mothers of anxious children. *American Journal of Psychiatry, 144*, 1580–1583.

Last, C. G., Phillips, J. E., & Statfield, A. (1987). Childhood anxiety disorders in mothers and their children. *Child Psychiatry and Human Development, 18,* 103–112.

Last, C. G., Strauss, C. C., & Francis, G. (1987). Comorbidity among childhood anxiety disorders. *Journal of Nervous and Mental Disease, 175,* 726–730.

Mattison, R. E. (1989). Pediatric management of anxiety disorders. *Pediatric Annals, 18,* 114–121.

Mattison, R. E., & Bagnato, S. J. (1987). Empirical measurement of overanxious disorder in boys 8 to 12 years old. *Journal of the American Academy of Child and Adolescent Psychiatry, 26,* 536–540.

Mattison, R. E., Bagnato, S. J., & Brubaker, B. A. (1988). Diagnostic utility of the Revised Children's Manifest Anxiety Scale in children with DSM-III anxiety disorders. *Journal of Anxiety Disorders, 2,* 147–155.

McDermott, J. F., Werry, J., Petti, T., Combrinck-Graham, L., & Char, W. F. (1989). Anxiety disorders of childhood or adolescence. In American Psychiatric Association, *Treatments of psychiatric disorders* (Vol. 1, pp. 401–446). Washington, DC: American Psychiatric Association.

Morris, D. P., Soroker, E., & Burruss, G. (1954). Follow-up studies of shy, withdrawn children: I. Evaluation of later adjustment. *American Journal of Orthopsychiatry, 54,* 743–754.

Ollendick, T. H. (1983). Reliability and validity of the Revised Fear Survey Schedule for Children (FSSC-R). *Behavior Research and Therapy, 21,* 685–692.

Pfeffer, C. R., Lipkins, R., Plutchik, R., & Mizruchi, M. (1988). Normal children at risk for suicidal behavior: A two-year follow-up study. *Journal of the American Academy of Child and Adolescent Psychiatry, 27,* 34–41.

Quay, H. C. (1986). Classification. In H. C. Quay & J. S. Werry (Eds.), *Psychopathological disorders of childhood* (3rd ed., pp. 1–34). New York: Wiley.

Rapoport, J. (1986). Annotation: Childhood obsessive compulsive disorder. *Journal of Child Psychology and Psychiatry, 27,* 289–295.

Reeves, J. C., Werry, J. S., Elkind, G. S., & Zametkin, A. (1987). Attention deficit, conduct, oppositional, and anxiety disorders in children: II. Clinical characteristics. *Journal of the American Academy of Child and Adolescent Psychiatry, 26,* 144–155.

Reich, J. (1986). The epidemiology of anxiety. *Journal of Nervous and Mental Disease, 174,* 129–136.

Reynolds, C. R., & Richmond, B. O. (1978). What I Think and Feel: A revised measure of children's manifest anxiety. *Journal of Abnormal Child Psychology, 6,* 271–280.

Shaffer, D., Schonfeld, I., O'Connor, P. A., Stokman, C., Trautman, P., Shafer, S. D., & Ng, S. (1985). Neurological soft signs: Their relationship to psychiatric disorder and intelligence in childhood and adolescence. *Archives of General Psychiatry, 42,* 342–351.

Silverman, W. K., & Nelles, W. B. (1988). The Anxiety Disorders Interview Schedule for Children. *Journal of the American Academy of Child and Adolescent Psychiatry, 27,* 772–778.

Spielberger, C. D. (1973). *State-Trait Anxiety Inventory for Children.* Palo Alto, CA: Consulting Psychologists Press.

Strauss, C. C., Last, C. G., Hersen, M., & Kazdin, A. E. (1988). Association between anxiety and depression in children and adolescents with anxiety disorders. *Journal of Abnormal Child Psychology, 16,* 57–68.

Strauss, C. C., Lease, C. A., Last, C. G., & Francis, G. (1988). Overanxious disorder: An examination of developmental differences. *Journal of Abnormal Child Psychology, 16,* 433–443.

Thomas, A., Chess, S., & Birch, H. G. (1969). *Temperament and behavior disorders in children.* New York: New York University Press.

Turner, S. M., Beidel, D. C., & Costello, A. (1987). Psychopathology in the offspring of anxiety disorder patients. *Journal of Consulting and Clinical Psychology, 55,* 229–235.

Weissman, M. M., Leckman, J. F., Merikangas, K. R., Gammon, G. D., & Prusoff, B. A. (1984). Depression and anxiety disorders in parents and children: Results from the Yale Family Study. *Archives of General Psychiatry, 41,* 845–852.

Werry, J. S., & Aman, M. G. (1980). Anxiety in children. In G. D. Burrows & B. Davies (Eds.), *Handbook of studies on anxiety* (pp. 165–192). Amsterdam: Elsevier/North-Holland.

Werry, J. S., Elkind, G. S., & Reeves, J. C. (1987). Attention deficit, conduct, oppositional, and anxiety disorders in children: III. Laboratory differences. *Journal of Abnormal Child Psychology, 15,* 409–428.

Werry, J. S., Methven, R. J., Fitzpatrick, J., & Dixon, H. (1983). The interrater reliability of DSM III in children. *Journal of Abnormal Child Psychology, 11,* 341–354.

CHAPTER 7

Eating Disorders of Infancy and Early Childhood

Susan Dickerson Mayes
Pennsylvania State University College of Medicine

This chapter focuses on childhood eating disorders, excluding anorexia nervosa and bulimia nervosa (which are covered in *Developmental Disorders*, chap. 8). Along with anorexia and bulimia nervosa, the DSM-III-R (American Psychiatric Association, 1987) lists only two other childhood and adolescent diagnostic categories under the heading of Eating Disorders: rumination disorder of infancy and pica. Obesity is not considered an eating disorder because "it is not generally associated with any distinctly psychological or behavioral syndrome" (p. 65). If, however, "psychological factors are of importance in the etiology or course of a particular case of obesity, this can be indicated by noting Psychological Factors Affecting Physical Condition" (p. 65).

This chapter is divided into three major sections. The first two sections, Rumination and Pica, are organized in a similar manner. Both disorders reflect discrete behavioral symptoms, and research to date is less extensive than that for other DSM-III-R childhood disorders, so a thorough review of the literature is provided for each disorder. This is followed by a comparison of existing knowledge with the DSM-III-R information. All of the DSM-III-R headings for rumination and pica are addressed, including the description of the disorder, associated features, age at onset, course, impairment, complications, predisposing factors, familial pattern, prevalence, sex ratio, differential diagnosis, and diagnostic criteria. Modifications in the DSM-III-R descriptions consistent with published research are suggested.

The third and final section briefly summarizes three diagnostic categories that share many features and etiological variables. These are reactive attachment disorder (RAD), nonorganic failure to thrive (NFTT), and psychosocial dwarfism (PSD). Only RAD is a DSM-III-R diagnosis, found under the heading "Other Disorders of Infancy, Childhood, or Adolescence." All three disorders may present with a similar symptom constellation including: growth retardation; impaired social relatedness; disturbance in the caretaker–child relationship; mood, behavioral, and developmental correlates; and reversal of symptoms with removal from the environment and appropriate care. The use of three different diagnostic labels for similar, if not the same, disorders leads to confusion and interferes with the integration of knowledge across disciplines. To assist in achieving diagnostic clarification and integration of research, a single category incorporating RAD, NFTT, and PSD is proposed for the Eating Disorders section of the *Diagnostic and Statistical Manual.*

RUMINATION

Overview

A computerized literature search using *Medline* and *Psychological Abstracts* was conducted for the years 1972 through 1988 to locate published reports on rumination. The reference lists from these articles were reviewed to identify pertinent publications that may have been missed in the search or that were published prior to 1972. Sixty-three articles representing 123 cases of rumination were analyzed.

Rumination is a voluntary and pleasurable act involving the repeated regurgitation of stomach contents. Foods or fluids are brought up into the mouth and either spit out or reswallowed. For many ruminators, this process occurs almost effortlessly, without observable straining or insertion of fingers into the mouth (Mayes, 1988; Mayes, Humphrey, Handford, & Mitchell, 1988).

Based on the literature review, it is evident that there are two distinct types of rumination: rumination in infants, the majority of whom are developmentally normal, and rumination in mentally retarded individuals of any age. The prevailing theory regarding rumination in infants suggests that it is secondary to a disturbance in the caretaker–child relationship. In contrast, rumination in retarded individuals may occur in the presence of warm and nurturing parents. The process underlying rumination in mentally retarded persons, 93% of whom are severely or profoundly retarded, is felt to be the same as that for other forms of self-stimulation commonly present in this population.

The two types of rumination share some commonalities. In both, rumination is self-induced, purposeful, and pleasurable, and the individual turns inward for gratification, versus deriving satisfaction externally from the environment and others. Also, the incidence for both types is greater in males than in females. The two subtypes of rumination are described in the following sections.

Rumination in Infants

Infant Characteristics. Across the 47 cases of infant rumination reported in the literature (Table 7.1), rumination is 3.7 times greater in males than in females (male to female ration 37:10), and the disorder occurs in both Whites and non-Whites. Mean age at onset was 5.7 months, with the disorder beginning as early as the neonatal period and as late as 17 months. At treatment, the infants had a mean age of 9 months with a range of 1 to 20 months. Developmental functioning for the majority was within normal limits. A developmental delay was specified in only eight cases (17%). In 26 cases (55%) the infants were reported to be progressing normally in development, and in 13 cases (28%) developmental status was not mentioned. Sauvage, Leddet, Hameury, and Barthelemy (1985) followed 20 infant ruminators up to 5 years after diagnosis. The four subjects who did not earn a developmental quotient $\geq$ 80 at follow-up had diagnoses of trisomy 13, congenital hyperammonemia with severe neonatal complications, autism, and atypical pervasive developmental disorder. These diagnoses suggest an organic basis for the presence of mental retardation.

For the majority of the 47 cases reviewed in the literature (87%), the infant ruminators had not achieved expected weight or were losing weight. However, for six infants, weight was within normal limits. These articles did not investigate mortality rates in infant ruminators; however, a review by Sajwaj, Libet, and Agras (1974) suggested that the risk of mortality may be decreasing with time. They reported a mortality rate of 12.5%, in contrast to 17% in a 1959 publication and 21% in 1957.

The literature suggests that infants with rumination do not present with homogeneous social and emotional features. Some authors described the infants as lethargic (e.g., Sajwaj et al., 1974; Sheagren, Mangurten, Brea, & Lutostanski, 1980), whereas others portrayed the infants as alert and responsive (e.g., Richmond, Eddy, & Green, 1958; Sheinbein, 1975). In a review of 20 infant ruminators conducted by Sauvage

TABLE 7.1
Rumination References

Infant Cases	*Mentally Retarded Cases*
Arensberg, 1956	Azrin & Wesolowski, 1975
Chatoor, Dickson, & Einhorn, 1984	Ball, Hendricksen, & Clayton, 1974
Cunningham & Linscheid, 1976	Barmann, 1980
Ferholt & Provence, 1976	Barton & Barton, 1985
Flanagan, 1977	Becker, Turner, & Sajwaj, 1978
Fleisher, 1979	Borreson & Anderson, 1982
Fullerton, 1963	Bright & Whaley, 1968
Hollowell & Gardner, 1965	Conrin, Pennypacker, Johnston, & Rast, 1982
Lang & Melamed, 1969	Daniel, 1982
Linscheid & Cunningham, 1977	Davis, Wieseler, & Hanzel, 1980
Madison & Adubato, 1984	Duker & Seys, 1977
Menking, Wagnitz, Burton, Coddington, & Sotos, 1969	Foxx, Snyder, & Schroeder, 1979
Mestre, Resnick, & Berman, 1983	Galbraith, Byrick, & Rutledge, 1970
Murray, Keele, & McCarver, 1976	Hogg, 1982
Richmond, Eddy, & Green, 1958	Humphrey, Mayes, Bixler, & Good, 1989
Sajwaj, Libet, & Agras, 1974	Jackson, Johnson, Ackron, & Crowley, 1975
Sauvage, Leddet, Hameury, & Barthelemy, 1985	Kohlenberg, 1970
Sheagren, Mangurten, Brea, & Lutostanski,1980	Libby & Phillips, 1979
Sheinbein, 1975	Lobato, Carlson, & Barrera, 1986
Stein, Rausen, & Blau, 1959	Luckey, Watson, & Musick, 1968
Toister, Condron, Worley, & Arthur, 1975	Marholin, Luiselli, Robinson, & Lott, 1980
Wright, Brown, & Andrews, 1978	Mayes, 1988
	Mayes & Humphrey, 1989
	Mayes, Humphrey, Handford, & Mitchell, 1988
	McKeegan, Estill, & Campbell, 1987
	Minness, 1980
	Mulick, Schroeder, & Rojahn, 1980
	O'Neil, White, King, & Carek, 1979
	Rast, Ellinger-Allen, & Johnston, 1985
	Rast & Johnston, 1986
	Rast, Johnston, Allen, & Drum, 1985
	Rast, Johnston, & Drum, 1984
	Rast, Johnston, Drum, & Conrin, 1981
	Rast, Johnston, Lubin, & Ellinger-Allen, 1988
	Simpson & Sasso, 1978
	Singh, Manning, & Angell, 1982
	Smith & Lyon, 1976
	Watkins, 1972
	White & Taylor,1967
	Whitehead, Drescher, Morrill-Corbin, & Cataldo, 1985
	Wright & Menolascino, 1970
	Wright & Thalassinos, 1973

and associates (1985), 10 of the 14 ruminators whose developmental quotients (DQs) at diagnosis were > 80 were considered to be normal in terms of behavior, temperament, and communication, and 4 appeared unhappy and apathetic. For the three ruminators with DQs ranging from 70 through 80, one was described as depressed and withdrawn and two as irritable. Other self-stimulating behaviors were also present for some ruminators. Six of the 20 engaged in head- or body-rocking and 12 in excessive mouthing. Finally, in the majority of studies in the literature that addressed treatment effects, significant improvements in mood, social responsiveness, and development were reported, suggesting that prior to intervention, infant ruminators may have exhibited deficits in these areas.

Environmental and Familial Characteristics. In all of the 45 published case reports in which caretaker or environmental variables were discussed, pathology was suggested. In 41 cases, familial or caretaker–infant disturbances were apparent, including psychosocial stress, marital problems, a separation from the mother that disrupted the mother–infant relationship, physical neglect, emotional deprivation, and maternal psychiatric disorders. With respect to maternal psychiatric disorders, the most frequent diagnosis was depression, followed by anxiety disorder, and then by a variety of diagnoses including personality disturbance, antisocial disorder, substance abuse, schizophrenia, and traumatic brain injury. Sauvage and associates (1985) reported that for the 20 ruminators in their study, rumination "occurred in the context of disturbed relationships (chronic tensions and/or deprivation)" (p. 202). In three cases reported by Sheagren and associates (1980), rumination began while the infants were in the neonatal intensive care unit. These infants had significant medical problems (two had necrotizing enterocolitis and one had bronchopulmonary dysplasia), and they were deprived of a normal parent–child nurturing relationship and home environment while residing in the hospital.

Etiology. Historically, most authors who have speculated on the etiology of infant rumination postulate that it is secondary to a disturbance in the mother–infant relationship, with the mother being incapable of fulfilling a warm, loving, and nurturing role (Bakwin & Bakwin, 1972; Chatoor, Dickson, & Einhorn, 1984; Flanagan, 1977; Fleisher, 1979; Fullerton, 1963; Menking, Wagnitz, Burton, Coddington, & Sotos, 1969; Richmond, Eddy, & Green, 1958; Sheinbein, 1975; Stein, Rausen, & Blau, 1959; Wright, Brown, & Andrews, 1978). The majority of authors conceptualize infant rumination from a psychodynamic perspective and view it as a form of self-stimulation with the infant resorting to internal gratification through the regurgitation of food as a substitute for the absent external gratification normally provided through a nurturing relationship with the caretaker. Some authors further speculate that infant rumination is a means of relieving stress-related tension, while others postulate that rumination reflects depression or anxiety on the part of the infant.

Holvoet (1982) found that familial stress was present in all 19 cases of infant rumination examined in her review. Although inadequate mothering and stress were associated with rumination, she cautioned that these factors were primarily identified by therapists who were searching for psychopathology. Controlled studies are necessary, therefore, in order to empirically establish the determinants of rumination in infants. Additionally, research is needed to investigate the possible role of the infant in contributing to the impaired caretaker–infant relationship and subsequent development of rumination (e.g., pre-existing pathology and temperament variables).

Complications and Treatment Response. Rumination may lead to weight loss, growth retardation, and, in some cases, death. Mortality is a relatively rare consequence today because of such advances as parenteral hyperalimentation. Additional complications may include malnutrition, dehydration, gastric disorders, aspiration, pneumonia, esophagitis, tooth decay and tooth erosion, electrolyte imbalance, anemia, and lowered resistance to disease. Rumination also interferes with the development of functional behaviors and social relationships (Mayes, 1988). It is a very unpleasant and noxious disorder that has a negative impact on others, which may lead to avoidance of the ruminator.

The case studies reported in the literature include data on intervention designed to treat infant rumination. The treatment used most frequently (i.e., in 39 cases) was providing the hospitalized infant with noncontingent attention, nurturance, and care. This approach was used alone in 14 cases and combined with psychotherapy for the natural mother or parents in 23 cases. In one instance, special attention was used in conjunction with both time-out from reinforcement and a verbal reprimand whenever the infant ruminated; in another case, it was combined with surgical intervention (i.e., a Nissen fundoplication to tighten the lower esophageal sphincter). In the remaining eight cases, behavioral techniques were used. Five infants were treated using punishment procedures contingent on rumination. These included electric shock in three cases, oral administration of a taste-aversive substances (i.e. either lemon juice or Tabasco sauce) in two cases, and time-out paired with a verbal reprimand in one case. The last case was also the only infant not hospitalized for treatment. In the remaining cases, contingent social reinforcement when not ruminating was paired with the administration of a taste-aversive substance (one case) or hand restraints (one case) in response to rumination. In all reported cases, treatment resulted in a significant decrease in rumination or its elimination and increased weight gain, regardless of treatment strategy. In 59% of the cases, the authors also reported improvements in the infant's mood, responsiveness to the environment and others, and developmental functioning.

The case study literature also reports treatments that were ineffective in reducing rumination. Such interventions included thickened feedings, reduced amounts at meals, dietary changes, hand restraints, parent therapy, taste-aversive conditioning using lemon juice, and hospitalization with special attention. As previously noted, the latter two modes of intervention were employed successfully in other cases. Therefore, effective treatment with one ruminator may be ineffective with another. Critical analyses of the treatment literature are found in publications by Davis and Cuvo (1980), Tierney and Jackson (1984), and Winton and Singh (1983a).

Rumination in Mentally Retarded Individuals

Individual Characteristics. Seventy-six cases of rumination in mentally retarded individuals are reported in the literature (Table 7.1). The male-to-female ratio in these cases is three to one (57 : 19), similar to that found for rumination in infants. As with infant rumination, rumination in mentally retarded persons is found in both White and non-White populations.

The mean age of onset for the 76 cases reviewed was 5.7 years, although this varied extensively, ranging from 3 months to 21 years. This reflects a significantly later age of onset than that for rumination in infants. The mean age at treatment for the mentally retarded ruminators was 14.9 years, but this also ranged widely from 11 months to 36 years. The mean difference of 9.2 years between mean age at onset and mean age at treatment suggests that rumination is a potentially chronic condition in mentally retarded individuals.

The incidence of rumination appears to increase with severity of retardation. Seventy-three percent of the cases reviewed were profoundly retarded, 20% severely retarded, and 7% moderately retarded. An attempt was made to estimate the mental age at onset of rumination. This entailed multiplying the individual's chronological age at onset by the IQ divided by 100. For cases in which IQ was not reported, the IQ was approximated using the mean IQ for the individual's particular level of retardation, as defined by the American Association on Mental Retardation. Using this procedure, the estimated mean mental age at onset of rumination was 9.5 months, with a range of 7.0 days to 4.3 years. Although this is close to the mean age of onset for psychogenic rumination in infants, rumination in mentally retarded individuals still occurs significantly later in the developmental sequence than does rumination in presumably nondelayed infants.

As with infant rumination, failure to gain expected weight or loss of weight is common in mentally retarded ruminators, but not always present. Weight was not mentioned in 24% of the cases reviewed. For 62%, weight problems were evident (i.e., less than ideal body weight for age or height, failure to thrive, or weight loss). The remaining 14% were not underweight, with two ruminators described as obese. Of the 58 cases reporting weight data, 81% were below weight expectations or losing weight. In a review of adult ruminators at a large institution for mentally retarded individuals, 96% were greater than 10% below their estimated ideal body weight (Rast, Ellinger-Allen, & Johnston, 1985). However, there is a positive association between growth failure and mental retardation independent of rumination (Crump, 1987). Therefore, impaired growth in some mentally retarded ruminators may precede rumination. Like rumination in infants, rumination in mentally retarded individuals is potentially fatal, with mortality rates ranging from 12% to 30% for retarded individuals in residential care (Rast, Ellinger-Allen, & Johnston, 1985).

Environmental Variables and Etiology. Unlike rumination in infants, rumination in mentally retarded persons is not typically considered to be a consequence of poor parenting or lack of fulfillment of emotional needs, as it may occur in the presence of warm and nurturing parents. It is speculated that the individual's neurological-cognitive impairment interferes with the normal utilization of external sources of gratification and predisposes the individual to atypical, self-stimulating behaviors as a source of pleasure.

Rumination is also considered to be a self-injurious behavior (Demchak & Halle, 1985). As is typical of self-stimulating and self-injurious behaviors, the frequency of rumination appears to be affected by the opportunity to engage in appropriate activities as an alternative to rumination, such as interaction with others or the environment. Favell, McGimsey, and Schell (1982) found that self-injurious behaviors were more frequent when the subjects in their study were alone and unoccupied and less frequent when opportunities for play with toys were available. Low levels of self-injurious behaviors associated with availability of toys was also found in a study by Iwata, Dorsey, Slifer,

Bauman, and Richman (1982). In a study of a profoundly retarded 12-year-old ruminator (Humphrey, Mayes, Bixler, & Good, 1989), rumination was lowest during school versus nonschool hours, whereas within the school program, rumination rates varied with the amount of individual attention. Frequency was lowest in school when the child was receiving one-to-one instruction, higher during group activities, and highest during independent play. Furthermore, rumination frequency was significantly associated with the degree to which individual caretakers liked the child (i.e., the child ruminated less with caretakers who liked him more, and vice versa). Although rumination in mentally retarded individuals is not felt to be a consequence of the individual's social and physical environment, these factors may influence the degree of rumination. This is not surprising, because one would expect most behaviors to be influenced by social and environmental variables.

Rumination is fairly common in residential care settings for mentally retarded individuals, with incidence rates ranging from 6% to 10% (Rast, Ellinger-Allen, & Johnston, 1985; Rast, Johnston, Drum, & Conrin, 1981; Rojahn, 1984; Singh, Manning, & Angell, 1982). Of the total 76 cases of rumination in mentally retarded persons reported in the literature, 69% of the individuals were in residential care, and 31% were living at home. The extent to which the occurrence of rumination is disproportionately higher in institutionalized versus noninstitutionalized retarded persons however, remains to be determined.

Complications and Treatment Response. The possible complications of rumination in mentally retarded persons are the same as for infant ruminators. However, treatment for the two types of rumination may differ in several respects. According to the literature, for mentally retarded ruminators, intervention occurred in residential, school, home, and hospital settings, whereas 98% of infant ruminators were hospitalized for treatment.

Of the case studies providing treatment data, the most frequently employed intervention technique for mentally retarded ruminators was aversive conditioning (24 cases). The oral administration of a taste-aversive substance (i.e., lemon juice, Tabasco sauce, or vanilla extract), contingent on rumination, was used in nine cases and electric shock in seven cases. Two ruminators were treated using overcorrection and five by combining overcorrection and taste-aversive procedures. In another case, the child was pinched each time she ruminated.

The second commonly used technique was food satiation (21 cases). The ruminators were allowed to eat to satiation, usually three to six times the normal meal quantity, so that rumination lost its reinforcing value and the individuals were no longer motivated to ruminate.

Intervention for nine other cases involved either the presentation or withdrawal of reinforcement contingent on rumination. Differential reinforcement of other behaviors (DRO) and reinforcement of incompatible behaviors (RIB) were used in four of these cases, time-out from reinforcement in two cases, and a combination of time-out and DRO or RIB in three cases.

Treatment for the remaining ruminators (17 cases) involved a variety of different strategies. Four received noncontingent increased attention and stimulation, and four were treated with peanut butter therapy (i.e., administering three tablespoons of creamy peanut butter every 2 to 3 hours and restricting fluids during meals). For three ruminators, the feeding process was modified to decrease the rate of feeding and increase the degree of participation on the part of the ruminator. For three others, medication was prescribed (metoclopramide hydrochloride or bethanechol chloride) to quicken gastric emptying and improve lower esophageal sphincter tone. Two ruminators were simply held before, during, and after meals. Finally, the remaining ruminator was required to walk around a 5-foot square each time he ruminated. As with rumination in infants, all reported treatment modalities resulted in a significant decrease in rumination or its elimination. Positive nutritional, developmental, social, and emotional gains were also reported across many of these studies.

Although there is some overlap in the treatment strategies used to intervene with both rumination in infants and rumination in mentally retarded individuals, there is a marked difference. Noncontingent special attention in a hospital setting, alone or with psychotherapy for the parents, was used to treat 79% of the infants with rumination. In contrast, the combination of noncontingent attention, stimulation, and care was employed with only 5% of the mentally retarded ruminators. This discrepancy most likely reflects the perceived etiological distinction between the two subtypes of rumination.

As with infant rumination, the literature contains reports of unsuccessful treatment regimens used with rumination in mentally retarded persons. These included thickened feedings, dietary changes, hand restraints, noncontingent special attention, food satiation, and reinforcement or punishment procedures (i.e., DRO, RIB, time-out, verbal reprimand, and presentation of an aversive smell contingent on rumination). As is true for rumination in infants, some of these ineffective strategies proved to be successful with other cases, again suggesting individual differences in response to treatment. Several publications provide critical reviews of this treatment literature (Davis & Cuvo, 1980; Starin & Fuqua, 1987; Tierney & Jackson, 1984; Winton & Singh, 1983a).

Assessment and Differential Diagnosis

Organic Conditions

Rumination is a nonorganic disorder that must be distinguished from physiological or medical conditions that have regurgitation as a symptom. The first step in diagnosis is usually to obtain appropriate medical studies, such as an upper gastrointestinal (GI) study, to rule out anatomical-medical problems. Organic conditions reported in the literature that may cause regurgitation include hiatal hernia, pyloric stenosis, lower esophageal stenosis, diaphragmatic hernia, intestinal obstruction, and gastrointestinal infection. A common type of physiologically based regurgitation is an involuntary gastroesophageal reflux secondary to lower esophageal sphincter pathology (Mayes, 1988). However, the differential diagnosis between this and rumination cannot always be made on the basis of an upper GI study alone, because the two may appear identical radiographically. The radiologist can diagnose reflux but may be unable to determine whether it is voluntary or involuntary. Therefore, clinical observations and a careful history must be the basis for a differential diagnosis in such cases. If the regurgitation does not appear to be voluntary and pleasurable (e.g., the individual shows surprise or distress), the regurgitation is likely to be an involuntary gastroesophageal reflux. If the act seems to be intentional, the individual appears content while regurgitating, and associated features are present (e.g., severe to profound mental retardation and other self-stimulating behaviors or, in an infant, a disturbance in the parent–child relationship), the regurgitation is probably rumination.

Treatment varies considerably for organic and nonorganic regurgitation, thus making the differential diagnosis important. For example, intervention for an involuntary gastroesophageal reflux could involve surgery (e.g., Nissen fundoplication), medication (e.g., metoclopramide or bethanechol), or anti-reflux positioning following meals. In contrast, the behavioral and social treatments most frequently employed to treat rumination are based on the assumption that the rumination is voluntary and under the individual's control.

Vomiting Versus Regurgitation

Rumination involves the *regurgitation* of stomach contents, which is distinct from vomiting. Regurgitation is the reflux or backward flowing of undigested foods or fluids into the esophagus or mouth. In contrast, vomiting is the forcible expulsion of stomach contents through the mouth. Therefore, conditions with vomiting as a symptom should not be confused with rumination. Medical problems that may cause vomiting include food allergies, GI infections, or a sensitive GI system. Vomiting may occur during the feeding process as a result of motor dysfunction or hyperreactive oral-esophageal-gastric mechanisms. Vomiting also may follow feeding in children who have eating disorders (e.g., food aversion).

Furthermore, vomiting may be a symptom of psychiatric disorders. In addition to vomiting associated with anorexia or bulimia nervosa, the literature contains several case descriptions of individuals with other types of psychogenic vomiting. According to Leibovich (1973), "Every variety of personality and every psychiatric disorder may show functional vomiting as a manifestation" (p. 264). Eight cases of psychogenic vomiting were reviewed (Alford, Blanchard, & Buckley, 1972; Leibovich, 1973; Spergel, 1975; Wright & Thalassinos, 1973). The most common diagnosis in these cases was anxiety disorder (three individuals), followed by depression (two persons). One received a diagnosis of hysterical neurosis, one of childhood schizophrenia, and one was undetermined. Within this subsample, psychogenic vomiting was three times greater in females than males (ratio = 6 : 2), and the age at onset ranged from 5.5 to 34 years (mean = 20 years). Thus, psychogenic vomiting differs in many respects from rumination disorder.

Anxiety-Related Regurgitation

Lastly, a case study reported in the literature (Griffin, 1977) suggests that the symptom of regurgitation (versus vomiting) may occur under conditions of stress and in association with anxiety. However, the regurgitation does not have the self-stimulating and pleasurable features of rumination. Griffin (1977) described a 7-year-old male referred for treatment because of regurgitation, which the parents felt was associated with "emotional stress." At 2 years of age, the child's appetite decreased and regurgitation began. At the time of treatment, the child also presented with enuresis and bruxism. Griffin (1977) reported that when the child "was worried about something, his stomach would begin to hurt, and he would then bring up food, thereby relieving the discomfort" (p. 243).

A similar case involved a 4-year-old male referred for evaluation and treatment of regurgitation that had begun at age 2, coinciding with the onset of his parents' marital problems (Mayes, 1989a). The child also presented with enuresis, psychosomatic leg pain, and severe nail-biting. The regurgitation appeared to be stress-related, with an increase in frequency during periods of stress. The child did not experience the regurgitation as pleasurable, and he complained of gastric discomfort. Additionally, the process of regurgitation appeared to be involuntary and the child actively tried to suppress it. Thus, these two cases are not consistent with the definition of rumination as a purposeful, pleasurable, self-stimulatory act.

Diagnostic and Statistical Manual of Mental Disorders

The DSM-III-R provides only one diagnostic category for rumination, Rumination Disorder of Infancy. The DSM-III-R description for rumination is the same as that found in the DSM-III (1980), with the exception of a few changes involving syntax and one small content modification (i.e., adding "laboratory tests" to the measures undertaken in making a differential diagnosis). In the DSM-II (1968), "feeding disturbance" was a diagnostic category, but this was not defined, and rumination was not specifically mentioned. The *International Classification of Diseases-Ninth Revision-Clinical Modification* (ICD-9-CM) (National Center for Health Statistics, 1978) provides a description of rumination that is almost identical to that found in the DSM-III-R. The reference citation for this definition is the American Psychiatric Association Task Force, thus accounting for the similarity between the DSM-III-R and ICD-9-CM descriptions.

Only four cases of eating disorders were included in the original DSM-III field trials. The diagnoses for these were unspecified, and it cannot be determined whether any had diagnoses of rumination disorder. No new field studies in the eating disorders category were conducted for the DSM-III-R. This comprehensive review of the literature did not reveal any concordance studies investigating the reliability of diagnosing rumination disorder. The act of rumination or regurgitation is an objectively defined and observable behavior. However, the determination of whether the regurgitation is voluntary or involuntary may be complex. Sometimes organic etiologies are readily apparent through appropriate medical examinations and laboratory studies. Even so, misdiagnoses occur. For example, Sauvage and colleagues (1985) reported cases of rumination that were initially diagnosed incorrectly as pyloric stenosis or chronic indigestion. Conversely, Herbst, Friedland, and Zboralske (1971) reviewed three cases of "rumination" that were actually organically based with regurgitation secondary to hiatal herniae. Additionally, individuals may present with involuntary gastroesophageal reflux in the absence of obvious organic pathology (e.g., an upper GI study may show reflux, but otherwise appear normal). In these cases, the differential diagnosis involves a clinical judgment as to whether the regurgitation is a purposeful, pleasurable, and self-stimulating act (i.e., rumination) versus an involuntary gastroesophageal reflux. Lastly, the distinction between vomiting (i.e., the forcible expulsion of stomach contents through the mouth) and regurgitation (i.e., the backward flowing of stomach contents into the esophagus or mouth) is not always made in the literature. Many investigators use the terms synonymously, and they sometimes inaccurately refer to valid cases of rumination as vomiting.

The following excerpts are verbatim quotes covering the entire DSM-III-R section on rumination disorder. Each excerpt is followed by a discussion and suggested modifications in light of published research reports.

> The essential feature of this disorder is repeated regurgitation of food, with weight loss or failure to gain expected weight, developing after a period of normal functioning. Partially digested food is brought up into the mouth without nausea, retching, disgust, or associated gastrointestinal disorder. The food is then ejected from the mouth or chewed and reswallowed. A characteristic position of straining and arching the back, with the head held back, is observed. The infant makes sucking movements with his or her tongue and gives the impression of gaining considerable satisfaction from the activity. (American Psychiatric Association, 1987, p. 70)

A review of the literature reveals two distinct subtypes of rumination disorder. Therefore, it is recommended that the diagnostic category be subdivided into rumination in infants and rumination in mentally retarded individuals. The essential feature of the disorder is indeed repeated regurgitation of food. However, it is advised that the voluntary and self-stimulatory aspects of this disorder be emphasized at the outset. This could be accomplished by modifying the phrasing to "purposeful and pleasurable repeated regurgitation of stomach contents in the absence of an organic cause."

Weight loss or failure to gain expected weight is associated with rumination in approximately 85% of cases. However, decreased weight does not always accompany rumination, especially if the degree of rumination is mild or the regurgitated food is reswallowed. It is evident from the cases in the literature that diagnoses of rumination were based solely on the presence of rumination, without considering weight as a criterion. In fact, in 24% of the reported cases of rumination in mentally retarded individuals, weight was not mentioned. Therefore, the possible condition of failure to gain expected weight or weight loss may more appropriately be considered a complication of rumination rather than a criterion for diagnosis.

The literature also does not support the notion that rumination must occur "after a period of normal functioning." Rumination disorder has been reported as early as the neonatal period, and Sauvage and colleagues (1985) stated that "rumination rarely started suddenly; other symptoms usually appeared earlier, such as regurgitations before the second month" (p. 198). Additionally, rumination in mentally retarded individuals is preceded by retarded development and often other forms of self-stimulation. Thus, these individuals were not functioning normally prior to the onset of rumination.

The DSM-III-R description of the process of rumination is consistent with that found in the literature; that is, "partially digested food is brought up into the mouth without nausea, retching, disgust, or associated gastrointestinal disorder" and the ruminator "gives the impression of gaining considerable satisfaction from the activity" (American Psychiatric Association, 1987, p. 70). The DSM-III-R description also states that "the food is then ejected from the mouth or chewed and reswallowed." This is again consistent with the literature except that stomach contents are not necessarily "chewed" before being reconsumed or spit out (especially if the regurgitated material is liquified). Lastly, the DSM-III-R descriptions of "straining and arching" and "sucking movements" are not necessarily true for all ruminators. For many, rumination is accomplished in an almost effortless manner.

> Associated features. The infant is generally irritable and hungry between episodes of regurgitation. (American Psychiatric Association, 1987, p. 70)

This description may be true for some infant ruminators, but the literature indicates that infant ruminators present with heterogenous features in terms of mood and behavior. Sauvage and colleagues (1985) studied 20 infant ruminators and, of the 14 whose development was within normal limits at diagnosis, 10 were described as normal in terms of temperament, behavior, and communication, and 4 were considered to be unhappy. Of the three with developmental quotients from 70 to 80, one was described as depressed and two as irritable. The remaining three children had developmental quotients ≤ 50. An associated feature that does emerge in the literature for both rumination in infants and mentally retarded persons is the presence of other self-stimulating behaviors. For example, 30% of the ruminators in the Sauvage and associates (1985) study engaged in head- or body-rocking, and 60% exhibited excessive sucking or mouthing.

> Age at onset. The disorder usually appears between 3 and 12 months of age. In children with Mental Retardation, it occasionally begins later. (American Psychiatric Association, 1987, p. 70)

Based on the 123 cases of rumination reported in the literature, rumination in infants can begin as early as the neonatal period and as late as 17 months, with a mean age of onset of 5.7 months. In contrast, rumination in mentally retarded individuals begins significantly later, with a mean age of onset of 5.7 years and a range of 3 months to 21 years. Even when mental age is taken into consideration, rumination in mentally retarded persons occurs significantly later in the developmental sequence than does rumination in infants. The estimated mean mental age at onset for mentally retarded ruminators is 9.5 months, with a range of 7 days to 4.3 years.

> Course. The disorder is potentially fatal. A mortality rate from malnutrition as high as 25% has been reported. In severe cases, although the infant is apparently hungry and ingests large amounts of food, progressive malnutrition occurs because regurgitation immediately follows the feedings. Spontaneous remissions are thought to be common. (American Psychiatric Association, 1987, p. 70)

Although rumination disorder is potentially fatal, Sauvage and colleagues (1985) stated that their longitudinal study of 20 infant ruminators does not support the high mortality rate reported in the DSM-III-R. Furthermore, mortality rates in the literature suggest that deaths secondary to rumination are declining with time. According to Sajwaj and colleagues (1974), a 1957 publication indicated a 21% mortality rate, in contrast to the 12.5% rate in their 1974 publication. Mortality rates for institutionalized mentally retarded ruminators may be higher, with estimates ranging from 12% to 30% (Rast, Ellinger-Allen, & Johnston, 1985).

A comprehensive review of the literature did not reveal any studies investigating the frequency of spontaneous remissions. The literature reports treated rumination cases and describes treatment outcomes versus spontaneous remissions. However, some indirect evidence exists that rumination in infants may be a time-limited disorder, because the oldest case reported in the literature was 20 months of age. In contrast, rumination in mentally retarded individuals appears to be a more chronic disorder. For mentally retarded ruminators described in the literature, the difference between mean age at onset versus mean age at treatment was 9.2 years.

> Impairment. If failure to gain expected weight or severe malnutrition develops, developmental delays in all spheres often occur, and impairment can be severe. (American Psychiatric Association, 1987, p. 70)

Developmental functioning for the majority of infant ruminators is within normal limits and a developmental delay was specified in only 17% of the 47 cases reported in the literature. Additionally, it cannot be assumed that if a developmental delay is present, it is secondary to either rumination or weight/nutritional factors. For example, in the follow-up study of 20 infant ruminators by Sauvage and colleagues (1985), 16 had developmental quotients (DQs) within normal limits, and 4 had DQs less than 80. These four had diagnoses of Trisomy 13, congenital hyperammonemia with severe neonatal complications, autism, and atypical pervasive developmental disorder, suggesting an organic etiology for their developmental delays, independent of rumination or problems with weight and nutrition. Furthermore, the onset of rumination in mentally retarded individuals is preceded by their mental retardation and not vice versa.

The extent of social, emotional, and behavioral impairment secondary to rumination has not been definitively established, and individual differences are apparent. Sauvage and associates (1985) reported that half of the 20 infant ruminators in their study were normal in terms of development, behavior, temperament, and communication. In contrast, the majority of treatment outcome studies report a decrease in or elimination of rumination along with improved mood, social responsiveness, and overall developmental functioning, thereby implying deficits in the latter areas prior to intervention. However, this does not prove a causal relationship. It may be that rumination, problems with mood, and decreased responsivity to the environment and others together reflect the underlying problem of the individual turning inward for gratification, as opposed to seeking external satisfaction.

Certainly, severe malnutrition can affect functioning in many developmental areas, but degree of impairment secondary to failure to gain expected weight is less clear. To date, no studies are available in the literature that examine the relationship between varying degrees of weight problems and developmental, social, emotional, and behavioral functioning in ruminators. Furthermore, a variety of other factors are likely to have an impact on extent of impairment: frequency and severity of rumination, environmental variables that may have precipitated or exacerbated rumination, and individual characteristics of the ruminator (e.g., other associated handicaps, the presence of additional self-stimulating or self-injurious behaviors, and temperament).

> Complications. A frequent complication of this disorder is that the caretaker becomes discouraged by failure to feed the infant successfully, and then becomes alienated from the child. The noxious odor of the regurgitated material may cause the caretaker to avoid the infant, which results in understimulation. (American Psychiatric Association, 1987, p. 70)

In addition to possible detachment from and avoidance of the ruminator, a variety of other complications are reported in the literature: malnutrition, dehydration, gastric disorders, aspiration, aspiration pneumonia, esophagitis, tooth decay, electrolyte imbalance, anemia, and lowered resistance to disease. It is also recommended that failure to gain expected weight or weight loss be included in the list of potential complications and excluded as a criterion for diagnosis, because this is a problem for the majority of ruminators, but not necessarily for all.

> Predisposing factors and familial pattern. No information. (American Psychiatric Association, 1987, p. 70)

Rumination in infants is associated with familial or caretaker–infant disturbances, including psychosocial stress, marital problems, separation from the mother disrupting the mother–infant relationship, physical neglect, emotional deprivation, and caretaker psychiatric disorders. Rumination also has been reported in infants hospitalized in a neonatal intensive care unit. Thus these infants resided in an atypical environment and were deprived of normal parent–child nuturing relationships. The predisposing factors for rumination in mentally retarded individuals are severe to profound mental retardation (i.e., 93% of ruminators are functioning at these levels of retardation) and a tendency to engage in self-stimulating behaviors.

> Prevalence. The disorder is apparently very rare. (American Psychiatric Association, 1987, p. 70)

Data on the incidence of rumination in infants are not available. However, prevalence rates of 6% to 10% have been reported for rumination among mentally retarded individuals in residential care (Rast, Ellinger-Allen, & Johnston, 1985; Rast et al., 1981; Rojahn, 1984; Singh et al., 1982). Incidence rates for rumination among noninstitutionalized mentally retarded individuals are not known.

> Sex ratio. The disorder is equally common in males and in females. (American Psychiatric Association, 1987, p. 70)

Based on a review of the 123 cases of rumination disorder reported in the literature, the disorder is 3.24 times more common in males than in females. The ratio of males to females is similar for both rumination in infants (3.7 : 1) and rumination in mentally retarded individuals (3 : 1).

> Differential diagnosis. Congenital anomalies, such as pyloric stenosis, or infections of the gastrointestinal system, can cause regurgitation of food, and need to be ruled out by appropriate physical examinations and laboratory tests. (American Psychiatric Association, 1987, p. 70)

Organic conditions with regurgitation as a symptom must indeed be differentiated from rumination through appropriate medical examinations and laboratory tests. In addition to pyloric stenosis and gastrointestinal infections, other conditions reported in the literature that may cause regurgitation include lower esophageal stenosis, hiatal and diaphragmatic herniae, and intestinal obstruction. An involuntary gastroesophageal reflux secondary to lower esophageal sphincter pathology must also be ruled out. This may not be readily apparent based on radiographic studies alone, and clinical observations and a careful interview covering features associated with rumination may be needed to determine if the regurgitation is rumination (i.e., a voluntary and pleasurable act) or an involuntary reflux.

Rumination (i.e., the regurgitation or backward flowing of stomach contents into the esophagus or mouth) must also be distinguished from disorders with the symptom of vomiting (i.e., the forcible expulsion of stomach contents through the mouth). Vomiting may be caused by medical problems (e.g., food allergies or GI infections) or feeding disorders (e.g., in children with motor impairments or food aversion), or it may be a symptom of a variety of psychiatric disorders. Lastly, rumination must be distinguished from anxiety- and stress-related regurgitation, which does not have the voluntary, pleasurable, and self-stimulatory characteristics of rumination.

The DSM-III-R lists two diagnostic criteria for rumination disorder of infancy: "repeated regurgitation, without nausea or associated gastrointestinal illness, for at least one month following a period of normal functioning" and "weight loss or failure to make expected weight gain" (American Psychiatric Association, 1987, p. 70). As noted previously, the literature does not support the position that rumination occurs only after a "period of normal functioning" or that failure to maintain or gain weight always accompanies rumination. Therefore, it is advised that

TABLE 7.2
Rumination

Proposed Diagnostic Criteria for Rumination

A. Purposeful and pleasurable repeated regurgitation of stomach contents in the absence of organic cause.

Types

A. Rumination in Infants: This subtype of rumination occurs in infants (mean age of onset 5.7 months), and the majority are developmentally within normal limits. The disorder is felt to be secondary to a disturbance in the caretaker–child relationship, occurring in association with, for example, physical neglect, emotional deprivation, separation from the parent, psychosocial stress, and parent psychiatric disorders.

B. Rumination in Mentally Retarded Individuals: This subtype of rumination occurs in mentally retarded persons of any age, the vast majority of whom are functioning in the severely or profoundly retarded range. The etiology of rumination is thought to be the same as that for other forms of self-stimulatory behavior commonly present in this population.

these two stipulations be eliminated as diagnostic criteria. Additionally, the criterion of rumination "for at least one month" appears arbitrary and may have negative ramifications if it deters prompt diagnosis and treatment of this potentially life-threatening disorder. Rumination disorder as described in the literature has four essential features: (a) regurgitation (vs. vomiting), (b) nonorganic etiology, (c) purposeful, pleasurable, and self-stimulatory behavior, and (d) repetitive act. Therefore, it is advised that the diagnostic criteria for rumination disorder be rephrased as follows: purposeful and pleasurable repeated regurgitation of stomach contents in the absence of an organic cause. It is also recommended that rumination disorder be subdivided into two types (rumination in infants and rumination in mentally retarded individuals), similar to the division of conduct disorder into multiple types in the DSM-III-R. In conclusion, the proposed diagnostic criteria and subtypes for rumination are presented in Table 7.2.

Directions for Future Research

Research is needed to confirm the diagnostic validity of the two rumination disorder subgroups, rumination in infants and rumination in mentally retarded individuals. The reliability of diagnosing these subgroups needs to be established, as well as the reliability of differentiating rumination from regurgitation secondary to organic causes, psychogenic vomiting, and anxiety-related regurgitation.

Prospective studies using comparison groups are essential in order to empirically substantiate the etiological hypothesis that rumination in infants is secondary to a disturbance in the caretaker–infant relationship. Case studies reported in the literature imply that family pathology (e.g., psychosocial stress, marital problems, separation from the parent, physical neglect, emotional deprivation, and parent psychiatric disorders) precedes the onset of rumination, but this needs to be empirically confirmed. Characteristics of the infant before the onset of rumination also need to be investigated to determine whether or not pathological features are evident before the emergence of rumination and to investigate the role of the infant in contributing to the impaired caretaker–child relationship. For example, it will be important to examine the degree to which specific infant congenital and temperamental characteristics interfere with the attachment process and the subsequent development of a nurturing and mutually fulfilling relationship with the caretaker.

Based on descriptions in the literature, infant ruminators appear to represent a heterogenous group in terms of developmental, social, emotional, and behavioral functioning. This needs to be studied further, as well as investigating the range of impairment associated with rumination and factors affecting degree of impairment. The issue of spontaneous recovery in the absence of treatment has not yet been addressed, and all case studies reported in the literature are of treated ruminators. Additionally, current mortality data need to replace the older mortality rates quoted in the literature that predate medical advances that are likely to affect the lethality of rumination in infants. Prevalence rates for rumination disorder in infants and among noninstitutionalized mentally retarded individuals also need to be established.

PICA

Overview

Using *Medline* and *Psychological Abstracts*, a computer literature search was conducted for the years 1972 through 1988 to obtain publications on pica. The reference lists for these articles were also reviewed to locate additional pertinent research and articles prior to 1972. According to the majority of authors, pica is an eating disorder characterized by the persistent and repeated ingestion of inedible, nonfood substances. However, definitional discrepancies are apparent. Of the 34 articles that define pica, 82% limit pica to the consumption of nonfood materials. However, even within this subgroup, semantic differences in definition are present. The term *inedible* is used in 32% of the research publications defining nonfood pica (Ausman, Ball, & Alexander, 1974; Barltrop, 1966; Finney, Russo, & Cataldo, 1982; Hawass, Alnozha, & Kolawole, 1987; Kaplan & Sadock, 1985; Madden, Russo, & Cataldo, 1980; Millican, Layman, Lourie, Takahashi, & Dublin, 1962; Mulick, Barbour, Schroeder, & Rojahn, 1980; Singh & Winton, 1984). *Nonfood* is the descriptor in 29% of the articles (Bruhn & Pangborn, 1971; Gallacher, Elwood, Phillips, Davies, & Jones, 1984; Glickman et al., 1981; Kinnell, 1985; Lourie, Layman, & Millican, 1963; Posner, McCottry, & Posner, 1957; Sayers et al., 1974; Singhi & Singhi, 1983). *Nonnutritive* is the criterion in 14% of the publications (Albin, 1977; Foxx & Martin, 1975; Matson, Stephens, & Smith, 1978; Woolston, 1983) and *unnatural* or *foreign* in 14% of the articles (Bronstein & Dollar, 1974; Cavdar, Arcasoy, Cin, Babacan, & Gozdasoglu, 1983; Halsted, 1968; Kolandaivelu & Balan, 1979). An additional 11% of the publications specify that pica involves the eating of *nonnutritive* or *inedible* substances (McAlpine & Singh, 1986; Singh & Bakker, 1984; Winton & Singh, 1983b). Overall, 72% of these definitions include the terms *inedible* or *nonfood*.

However, in 18% of the 34 publications defining pica, the disorder is described as the repeated and compulsive ingestion of any substance, including normal foods (Bucher, Reykdal, & Albin, 1976; Danford, 1982; Danford & Huber, 1982; Feldman, 1986; Mokhobo, 1986; Sayetta, 1986). According to these definitions, pica is characterized by the compulsive, pathological, and excessive consumption of food items, as well as the repeated ingestion of nonfood substances.

There is no proof, though, that nonfood and food pica are manifestations of the same disorder. Certainly, it could be argued that the ingestion of nonfood substances is a more aberrant practice than the compulsive consumption of food items, and the point at which ingestion of specific food items becomes "pathological" may be difficult to determine. Research comparing nonfood and food pica is exceedingly limited, and the study of mentally retarded adults in residential care by Danford and Huber (1982) suggests that the two types of pica differ on important dimensions. Nonfood pica was significantly more common than food pica, accounting for approximately two thirds of the cases. Food pica was most prevalent among individuals functioning in the borderline range of mental retardation. In contrast, the highest incidence of nonfood pica was found among profoundly retarded residents, with a zero incidence rate for individuals in the borderline and mild ranges of mental retardation. Thus, for the purposes of this review, pica will be limited to the ingestion of nonfood substances, as opposed to abnormal food cravings, to be consistent with the prevailing definitions of pica (82%). This will insure definitional clarity and enhance the comparability of findings across studies on pica.

In addition to problems of definition, it is sometimes difficult to distinguish the abnormal practice of pica from cases in which the ingestion of nonfood substances may not be pathological. As aptly stated by Danford (1982), "the diagnosis of pica depends upon cultural attitudes as well as amounts ingested and degrees of craving. No sharp demarcation exists between pathological states and normality, nor between the ages at which some form of pica is considered normal" (p. 304). The literature reviewed here discloses three types of pica, two of which are considered by all investigators to be abnormal (i.e., pica in children over the age of 18 months and pica in developmentally disabled individuals of any age). The third type, cultural pica, is considered by only a minority to be pathological. This type reflects a historical custom or tradition of certain ethnic subgroups and is not considered to be aberrant by those practicing it. Cultural pica differs from pica in children and developmentally disabled individuals in the narrow and specific range of substances consumed and in its prevalence among distinct population subgroups. The three subtypes of pica are described in the following sections.

Pica in Children

Definition. There is almost unanimous agreement among investigators addressing the age at which pica becomes pathological that it must be distinguished from the normal developmental stage of indiscriminant oral exploration. As stated by Sayers and colleagues (1974), "only when a child who is old enough to have learnt what is expected of him persists in the infantile behavior pattern may the term pica be applied" (p. 1659). Most investigators agree that the ingestion of substances should not be considered pathological unless the behavior persists beyond 18 months of age (Barltrop, 1966; Kaplan & Sadock, 1985; Lourie et al., 1963; McAlpine & Singh, 1986; Singh & Bakker, 1984).

Prevalence. Across studies investigating the prevalence of pica among children in the United States, the median incidence rate is 22%. With the exception of one study (Glickman et al., 1981), prevalence data are generally consistent. Wortis and colleagues (1962) studied 272 thirty- to thirty-three-month-old children who were born premature and reported that 22% engaged in pica. In a group of 108 nonepileptic 1- to 3-year-olds, Glickman, Cypess, Crumrine, and Gitlin (1979) found a 19% incidence of pica. Barltrop (1966) studied two groups of 1- to 6-year-olds, one using a parent interview format ($N = 439$) and the other a mail survey ($N = 277$). The obtained prevalence rates for pica were 18.5% and 32.1%, respectively. Two investigations compared incidence rates for Black and White children. Among 386 Black children 7 months of age and older, Cooper (1957) found an incidence rate of 27.2% for pica, versus 16.8% among 398 White children in Baltimore. Millican and associates (1962) reported prevalence rates of 32.3% in 486 Black 1- to 6-year-olds and 10.0% in 294 White children of the same age.

In contrast to these comparable prevalence data for children overall, Glickman and associates (1981) reported a 71% incidence of pica among 100 one- to six-year-old children of low socioeconomic status (SES) participating in a county health department program in Allegheny County, Pennsylvania. The reasons for discrepancies among studies are unclear, although they may be attributed in part to demographic differences and the manner in which pica is defined and measured. Furthermore, prevalence rates may be spuriously high because of the inclusion of children less than 18 months of age in many studies (and thus failure to exclude normal instances of oral exploration) and because of the loose definitions of pica (e.g., in some studies, the act of mouthing or chewing inedible substances was included with ingestion in determining incidence rates).

Gender. Data on gender suggest that pica is relatively equally common among girls and boys in the United States. In a survey of 784 children by Cooper (1957), 44% of the total sample was female and 43% of the pica cases were females. Similarly, Millican and associates (1962) reported nonsignificant differences as a function of gender for both Black and White children in their study of pica. In an investigation of 272 premature children by Wortis and colleagues (1962), incidence was approximately equal, with 25% of the females and 17% of the males exhibiting pica.

Substances Ingested. Across the studies reviewed, the most common material ingested by children is dirt, followed by chips or pieces of paint and plaster, paper, string, cloth, vegetation (e.g., grass, leaves, or sticks), hair, household products (e.g., soap), feces, and a variety of small objects (e.g., stones, crayons, buttons, and insects). Based on a survey by Singhi and Singhi (1982b) of 180 children in India with pica, the average number of nonfood materials ingested was three per child.

Associated Variables. Pica is most common in children up to 6 years of age (Barltrop, 1966; Cooper, 1957; Feldman, 1986; Glickman et al., 1981; Kaplan & Sadock, 1985; Lourie et al., 1963), and the range of materials ingested and prevalence of pica decrease with age from 1 to 6 years (Baltrop, 1966; Danford, 1982; Halsted, 1968; Kaplan & Sadock, 1985). In a survey of 859 children conducted at Children's Hospital in Washington, DC (Lourie et al., 1963), the greatest incidence of pica was among 1½- to 2-year-olds. Pica decreased in prevalence after age 2 and was rare in children beyond the age of 6. Similarly, Cooper (1957) reported on a study of 172 children with pica and found that, "in a very small number of cases the habit persisted until the age of six or seven" (p. 66).

The significant relationship with age is logical given the increases in judgment and adherence to behavioral expectations and limits and the decrease in oral, infantile behavior between the ages of 1 and 6. However, a few instances of pica in older children have been reported, including published cases of a 9-year-old female (Kolandaivelu & Balan, 1979) and a 10-year-old male (Garcia, Schulbe, Markowitz, & Young, 1987), both of whom consumed stones. Cooper (1957) also reported a single case involving a 10-year-old female who ate clay. In this instance, the child's mother and grandmother also ate clay, so familial or cultural influences may have contributed to the girl's continuation of pica.

A number of authors have linked pica with behavioral and emotional disturbances (Danford, 1982; Feldman, 1986; Glickman et al., 1981; Wortis et al., 1962). In the study of 180 children in India who exhibited pica (Singhi & Singhi, 1982a), 57% had additional behavior problems, the most common of which were tantrums, bruxism, breath-holding, and thumb-sucking. A comparison between 50 of these children and 50 nonpica controls revealed a significantly higher incidence of aggressive behavior in the children with pica. In contrast, the study by Cooper (1957) did not show a significant relationship between pica and other behavior problems.

An association between pica and mental retardation and pica and organic impairment also has been reported (Danford, 1982; Glickman et al., 1979, 1981; Wortis et al., 1962). Glickman and colleagues (1979) found that 64% of the 84 epileptic children studied (25% of whom were hyperactive and 38% mentally retarded) had a history of pica at 1 to 3 years of age versus only 19% of the 108 comparison children without seizure disorders. Wortis and colleagues (1962) studied 272 premature children at 30 to 33 months of age. The subset of the sample with pica (22%) had a greater incidence of neonatal insults, neurological defects, deviant behavior, and developmental delays, and they experienced poorer living conditions than the children without pica. Similarly, across two studies involving a total of seven children hospitalized in Baltimore with lead poisoning secondary to pica, 43% were functioning in the mentally retarded range (Finney et al., 1982; Madden et al., 1980). However, the survey by Cooper (1957) failed to disclose a significant relationship between pica and intelligence or the age at acquisition of major developmental milestones.

Research suggests that pica is associated with a host of interrelated variables including ethnicity, cultural factors, socioeconomic status (SES), and psychosocial stress. Epidemiological data for the United States indicate that pica is more prevalent among Black than White children. Reported prevalence rates for Blacks versus Whites are 23% and 15% (Barltrop, 1966), 27% and 17% (Cooper, 1957), and 32% and 10% (Millican et al., 1962), respectively. At all year levels from 1 to 6 years, Millican and associates (1962) found a significantly higher incidence of pica in 486 Black children than in 294 White children. The authors hypothesized that "cultural and economic factors contributed to this difference" (p. 213). They noted that pica was often an acceptable behavior within the Black sample and that many mothers of these children practiced pica. Lourie and colleagues (1963) also found an association between pica and familial and cultural patterns. The investigators stated that pica in children "is especially prevalent among children whose mothers have pica themselves and among children whose mothers have come from communities where clay eating and starch eating are a part of the cultural pattern" (p. 145).

In the United States, the incidence of pica also appears to be most common among children from low versus higher SES families (Danford, 1982; Feldman, 1986; Glickman et al., 1981; Sayetta, 1986). Lourie and associates (1963) reported an incidence of 50% to 60% for pica among lower SES $1\frac{1}{2}$- to 2-year-olds, versus 30% for the same age children at higher SES levels. Pica in older children was also found to be disproportionately greater in the lower versus higher SES groups. The only exception to this pattern is again the work of Cooper (1957), which did not reveal an association between pica and per capita family income in a sample of children residing in Baltimore.

Pica also has been linked with psychosocial stress and family pathology (Danford, 1982; Feldman, 1986; Sayetta, 1986). Bithoney, Snyder, Michalek, and Newberger (1985) studied 23 one- to four-year-old ingestion victims hospitalized in Boston and compared the findings with those of 23 children hospitalized with an acute illness. Family stress and maternal depression were significantly higher among the ingestion versus acute illness patients. The authors reviewed three other studies showing that accessibility of poisons did not differ between the ingestion and noningestion subgroups, but that families of poison victims had greater stress, marital conflict, mental illness, and personal loss. A study conducted in India by Singhi, Singhi, and Adwani (1981) compared 50 children with iron deficiency anemia and pica with 50 anemic children without pica matched on age, sex, SES, and degree of anemia. The pica group earned significantly higher stress scores than the nonpica group, reflecting maternal depression, parental separation, joint family, caretaker other than mother, neglect, physical abuse, and decreased parent–child interaction. A later study by Singhi and Singhi (1983) compared 180 children with pica with 180 without pica. SES was not significantly related to pica but, again, a substantial association was found between pica and psychosocial stress ("mainly in the form of inadequate mothering," p. 349). Additionally, in approximately one third of the cases, the onset of pica coincided with acute stress.

Several hypotheses may be generated to explain the association between psychosocial stress and family variables and pica: inadequate supervision; absence of sanctions against pica; the influence of family pathology on the development of maladaptive behaviors in the child; regression under stress to infantile, oral behavior; and psychodynamic interpretations, such as unmet oral needs secondary to the unavailability of the mother. Additional research is needed to partial out the relationship between pica and the host of interrelated variables, individually and in combination. All, some, or only a few may have a causal relationship with pica.

Complications and Treatment Response. One of the most frequently reported consequences of pica in children is lead poisoning. More than 30% of children with pica have significantly elevated blood lead levels, and 70% to 90% of children with severe lead poisoning have pica (Danford, 1982; Feldman, 1986). Other complications reported in the literature include accidental poisoning, choking, gastric ulcer, constipation, bowel obstruction or perforation, gastrointestinal (GI) infections, tetanus, parasitic infections, bezoars (e.g., hair balls), achlorhydria, and nutritional complications, particularly iron deficiency anemia. Previously it was thought that an iron-deficient state might trigger pica, and some studies suggested that mineral repletion therapy decreased or eliminated pica. However, in studies reported by Lourie and associates (1963), placebos were equally as effective in reducing pica as both intramuscular iron injections and a multivitamin-mineral preparation. Thus, placebo effects and possibly implied sanctions against pica may have been responsible for decreases in pica following mineral therapy. The majority of evidence seems to indicate that pica may lead to nutritional deficiencies, and not vice versa.

Psychosocial and environmental approaches to treatment have included family counseling, education regarding supervision and child safety, and improvements in living conditions. Behavioral techniques have been used successfully to intervene directly with children, including discrimination training (i.e., teaching children to distinguish between inedible and edible substances), differential reinforcement of other behavior (i.e., reinforcing children for intervals during which they did not engage in pica), and overcorrection procedures (e.g., requiring children to brush their teeth and mouth with Listerine for 1 minute in response to each instance of pica) (Finney et al., 1982; Madden et al., 1980).

Pica in Developmentally Disabled Individuals

Prevalence. Pica is reported to be common among psychotic mentally retarded persons (Danford, 1982) and autistic individuals (Cohen, Johnson, & Caparulo, 1976). In a study of 70 autistic patients (mean age = 31 years), Kinnell (1985) reported a prevalence rate of 60% for pica. Several studies have investigated the prevalence of pica among institutionalized mentally retarded individuals, involving primarily adult populations. These studies yielded incidence rates of 8% (Singh & Bakker, 1984), 8.4% (Winton & Singh, 1983b), 9.2% (McAlpine & Singh, 1986, who also included mouthing in their definition of pica), and 21% for nonfood pica (Danford & Huber, 1982).

Gender. Data on the prevalence of pica as a function of gender suggest that pica is equally common in males and females. In a study of 607 mentally retarded individuals aged 5 to 73 years, in institutional care, males accounted for 63% of the residential population and 57% of the pica cases (McAlpine & Singh, 1986). Conversely, females comprised 37% of the total population and 43% of the pica cases. Twenty-seven case studies of pica in mentally retarded persons (mean age = 19 years, range 4 to 57 years) reveals a ratio of 14 females to 13 males (Ausman et al., 1974; Bucher et al., 1976; Foxx & Martin, 1975; Kinnell, 1985; Lobato, Carlson, & Barrera, 1986; Matson et al., 1978; Mayes, 1989b; Mulick, Barbour, Schroeder, & Rojahn, 1980; Mulick, Schroeder, & Rojahn, 1980; Paniagua, Braverman, & Capriotti, 1986; Singh & Bakker, 1984; Singh & Winton, 1984; Winton & Singh, 1983b).

Substances Ingested. Across the 27 case reports and the large-scale institutional studies conducted by Danford and Huber (1982) and McAlpine and Singh (1986), the following substances are the most frequently consumed by mentally retarded individuals and are listed in descending order of preference: string and cloth, any objects or materials small enough to consume, feces, dirt, cigarettes, paper, stones, and pills. Together, the first two categories listed accounted for almost half of the substances consumed.

Etiology and Associated Variables. Pica in developmentally disabled individuals appears to be attributable, in large part, to organic damage resulting in impaired judgment and a predisposition to engage in atypical behaviors. In all of the individual case studies of pica in mentally retarded individuals, other self-stimulating, self-injurious, maladaptive, or atypical behaviors are present. Similarly, McAlpine and Singh (1986) reported that the 56 pica patients studied in their investigation engaged in self-stimulating behaviors an average of 57.2% of the time. Further support for a neurological etiology for pica is demonstrated by the existence of specific central nervous system (CNS) disorders (e.g., Kleine–Levin and Kluver–Bucy syndromes) that have morbid hunger or bizarre oral behavior as symptoms. Research by Danford and her colleagues (Danford & Huber, 1982; Danford, Smith, & Huber, 1982) led to the conclusion that pica is not secondary to the inability of mentally retarded individuals to discriminate food from nonfood substances. In a study of pica among mentally retarded adults in a residential setting, 83% with pica preferred a single nonfood item and many tenaciously searched for their substance of choice (Danford & Huber, 1982).

Consistent with the neurological etiological hypothesis, the prevalence of pica increases with increasing retardation. In the large-scale institutional survey conducted by Danford and Huber (1982), nonfood pica was not found among any of the borderline or mildly retarded individuals. Although 8% of the institution population was moderately retarded, only 1% of the pica individuals came from this subgroup. Similarly, 26% of the total resident population was functioning in the severely retarded range, but only 14% of these individuals exhibited pica. In contrast, the incidence of pica was disproportionately high among the profoundly retarded residents, who accounted for 60% of the institution population and 85% of the pica cases. Similar proportions are found in other reviews. According to McAlpine and Singh (1986), 76% of the individuals with pica in their study were profoundly retarded, 12% severely retarded, 12% moderately retarded, and 0% mildly retarded. Across the 27 individual clinical and published case reports of pica in mentally retarded individuals, 93% are profoundly retarded and 7% severely retarded.

In general, the incidence of pica decreases with age. McAlpine and Singh (1986) found this to be true after the age of 10 in their study of

607 institutionalized retarded individuals, 5 to 73 years of age. Similarly, Danford and Huber (1982) reported declining prevalence of pica with age in their study of 991 eleven- to eighty-eight-year-old retarded persons in residential care. The only exception was an elevation in the oldest age group, 71 years and above. This suggests that increasing mental age may play a role in the reduction of pica, which is consistent with the pattern for pica in children, which generally disappears by age 6.

Complications and Treatment Response. The complications of pica in mentally retarded individuals are similar to those for pica in children: choking, gastric or bowel perforations, constipation, intestinal obstruction (in some cases necessitating surgery), tetanus and parasitic infections (particularly for individuals who consume dirt or feces), GI infections, accidental poisoning, bezoars, achlorhydria, and nutritional abnormalities. Regarding this latter complication, Danford found that certain types of pica, especially the ingestion of dirt, were associated with low iron and zinc levels—even though dietary intake of these minerals was within the recommended range—and elevated copper levels (Danford, 1983; Danford et al., 1982). Furthermore, the degree of iron and zinc deficiency was related to the amount of soil consumed. Danford and colleagues (1982) also found a nonsignificant difference in nutrient intake between mentally retarded individuals with and without pica. Thus, as with pica in children, research suggests that pica in mentally retarded individuals may result in mineral deficiency, and not vice versa.

Many cases of pica in mentally retarded individuals are treated through the use of noncontingent restraints to prohibit the behavior (e.g., employing elbow splints, fencing masks, and mesh jackets). In other cases, behavioral strategies have been utilized to eliminate pica so that physical restraints are not necessary. Of the individual case studies described in the literature, the results of intervention were reported for 23 subjects. Overcorrection procedures were effectively implemented in 10 cases. The procedure most frequently used was that described by Foxx and Martin (1975), which involved 10 minutes of oral hygiene (i.e., cleansing the mouth), 10 minutes of personal hygiene (i.e., washing hands), and 10 minutes of positive practice (e.g., sweeping the floor, picking up debris, and emptying trash) contingent on pica. In eight cases, contingent physical restraint, which the individuals experienced as aversive, was used in response to pica. The remaining five cases were treated using a variety of techniques, including contingent restraint plus differential reinforcement of other behavior (two cases), overcorrection plus the taste-aversive consequence of brushing teeth with hot sauce (one case), contingent blindfold (one case), and antipsychotic medication (one case). Two studies were conducted to determine the relative effectiveness of overcorrection versus contingent physical restraint. In one study, overcorrection was more successful and in the other study, physical restraint had a greater impact on pica. Intervention techniques reported to be ineffective in some studies included medication, time-out, differential reinforcement of other behavior, contingent reprimand, and physical restraint. Thus, what is effective with one individual may not be with another.

Cultural Pica

Definition. For some ethnic or geographic subgroups, pica appears to represent a long-standing cultural custom or tradition that is not considered aberrant by those who practice it. Cultural pica differs from pica in children and mentally retarded individuals in the restricted range of substances consumed, the most common of which is clay or soil (i.e., *geophagia*). Pica, particularly geophagia, is most common among Africans, Aboriginals in Australia, and Blacks in the United States, especially women living in the southeastern portion of the country. However, the literature also contains reports of cultural pica among people in South America, India, Saudia Arabia, Iran, Morocco, Turkey, Portugal, and Puerto Rico, as well as among migrant workers in California. According to Eastwell (1979), geophagia has a "wide distribution among the world's poorer or more tribally oriented people" (p. 264). Similarly, other authors state that the practice is most common among poverty populations (Bronstein & Dollar, 1974; Halsted, 1968; Hawass, Alnozha, & Kolawole, 1987) and in underdeveloped or third world countries (Morgan, 1984; Sayetta, 1986). Cultural pica is primarily practiced by women and is rare in men.

According to Danford (1982), pica is a "world-wide" phenomenon that is often "a consequence of cultural patterns ingrained in the food habits of a region" (p. 303). Similarly, Vermeer and Frate (1979) stated that geophagia "represents a common custom stemming from deeply imbedded cultural traditions and attitudes" (pp. 2134–2135). The practice of geophagia is often quite refined. For example, among southeastern Blacks in the United States, specific types of clay are preferred, the clay is often prepared for consumption by baking, it is commercially available in some areas, and it is sometimes sent to relatives who live in the north where the clay is unavailable. Morgan (1984) stated that such forms of pica represent a "normal, usually harmless, cultural activity" and must be differentiated from the "pathological variety" (p. 1054).

Historical Etiology. Several etiological hypotheses have been offered for cultural pica, all of which may have contributed to its origin. Danford (1982) traced pica back to a Greek practice in 40 B.C. involving the eating of earth to treat a variety of medical conditions. Danford (1982) speculated that the development of pica may be related to ancestral shortages of food, and some authors state that geophagia has a satiating effect, allaying hunger (Bateson & Lebroy, 1978; Halsted, 1968). Historically, earth has religious and magical properties as well as ceremonial applications in some subcultures (Bateson & Lebroy, 1978; Danford, 1982). Eastwell (1979) described the practice among Australian Aboriginals of painting white clay on their bodies during ceremonies and applying the clay to women's nipples after childbirth to increase the flow of milk. Traditionally, earth and clay have been used medicinally (Danford, 1982), particularly for the treatment of gastrointestinal problems (Bateson & Lebroy, 1978; Eastwell, 1979).

The adult outpatients studied by Sayers and associates (1974) in Johannesburg, South Africa were asked to explain why they consumed earth or ash. Although many could not specify reasons, some offered medicinal or religious reasons, and others simply stated that they liked the taste. Therefore, although pica may have originated for a variety of reasons (e.g., hunger, medicinal, religious, or magical), some individuals may continue the practice today for the sake of tradition or because it has become a pleasurable oral habit.

Substances Ingested. The most common form of cultural pica is geophagia, or the eating of earth (i.e., clay or soil), and the second most common form is *amylophagia,* the consumption of laundry starch. Prevalence data across studies suggest that more than 90% of the cases of cultural pica involve the consumption of earth or starch. Historically, amylophagia is a more recent practice than geophagia and many speculate that the consumption of starch has developed as a substitute for geophagia (e.g., ingested by southern Black women who have moved to the north where the clay normally consumed is unavailable) (Halsted, 1968; Vermeer & Frate, 1979). Lourie and associates (1963) found that "several mothers took up starch eating after moving to the District of Columbia, where their favorite clay was not available" (p. 146). Related to, but far less common than the ingestion of earth and starch, are reports of the consumption of ash, plaster, cement, and food items such as powdered milk, baking soda, baking powder, and flour—all similar in texture to clay and starch.

Prevalence by Ethnicity, Gender, and Age. Current estimates of the incidence of cultural pica are lacking in the literature and existing data suggest that the practice may be declining with time. According to

Danford's (1982) review of published reports of pica, approximately 50% of southern Black women ingest clay or starch. Vermeer and Frate (1979) reported data for Holmes County, Mississippi. In a survey of 229 Black individuals, prevalence rates for geophagia (i.e., clay-eating) were 57% for women, 16% for children (all but two of whom were 1 to 4 years of age), and 0% for adolescent and adult males. According to Halsted (1968), a survey of 302 general medical adult outpatients in Columbus, Ohio revealed a 25% rate of geophagia. Of the individuals who practiced geophagia, 76% were female, and 89% were Black, even though Blacks accounted for only 58% of the sample. Bruhn and Pangborn (1971) conducted a study of 65 adult female migrant workers in California. Thirty-eight percent of the women of Mexican descent knew pregnant women who ate dirt or starch, 15% knew nonpregnant women who did so, and none knew of any men who engaged in pica. For the women of Anglo descent, 19% knew pregnant women, 7% knew nonpregnant women, and 0% knew men who consumed dirt or starch.

Prevalence rates for subcultures in other parts of the world also demonstrate that pica is more common in women than in men or children. A survey of 348 adult outpatients in Johannesburg, South Africa revealed that 33% of the women versus 11% of men ate earth or ash. Additionally, women consumed greater quantities than men (Sayers et al., 1974). In a study of 293 Black 4- to 6-year-olds in South Africa, Deveaux, Kibel, Dempster, Pocock, and Formenti (1986) found pica to be present in only 3.4% of the children. According to Eastwell (1979), pica among Australian Aboriginals occurs primarily in adult females. In a study of 11 Aboriginals who consumed clay (Bateson & Lebroy, 1978), 7 were women (16 to 45 years of age), 3 were children (2 to 5 years of age), and only 1 was a man (46 years of age).

Pica During Pregnancy. Among some subgroups, the practice of pica is greatest during pregnancy (Lourie et al., 1963; Sayers et al., 1974), or even limited to pregnancy (Feldman, 1986). Again, geophagia and amylophagia are the most common types, although *pagophagia* (i.e., the excessive consumption of ice or ingestion of freezer frost) is also reported. According to *Williams Obstetrics* (Pritchard, MacDonald, & Gant, 1985), pica during pregnancy is "in large part a social custom" (p. 262).

In a survey of pregnant and postpartum Black women in Mississippi, Vermeer and Frate (1979) found that 47% practiced pica. Twenty-eight percent engaged in geophagia, and 19% ingested other substances, mostly laundry starch, powdered milk, and baking soda. The women who practiced geophagia were older than the women ingesting other substances. A study of 410 pregnant women in Georgia, most of whom were Black and of low SES, (Bronstein & Dollar, 1974) disclosed a 16%

prevalence rate for pica. Of the women practicing pica, 46% consumed laundry starch, 35% "chalk" (white clay), 9% clay, and 10% other substances. O'Rourke, Quinn, Nicholson, and Gibson (1967) conducted a study of 200 non-White, low-SES obstetric patients in Augusta, Georgia, which has one of the world's largest deposits of kaolin, a white clay consumed by many during pregnancy. Fifty-five percent of the women practiced pica during pregnancy, with 32.5% ingesting clay, 11.5% starch, 7.5% both, and 3.5% other substances. For the vast majority, pica was practiced only during pregnancy. A survey of 600 predominantly Black, low-SES prenatal patients at Harlem Hospital (Posner et al., 1957) disclosed that 18% practiced amylophagia, 5% pagophagia, and 1.5% geophagia.

As with cultural pica among nonpregnant individuals, pica during pregnancy is considerably less common among Whites than non-Whites (Halsted, 1968). In a review of studies by Bruhn and Pangborn (1971), 41% of a sample of pregnant Black women in Mississippi consumed starch, versus 10% for Whites, and 27% ingested clay, versus 7% for Whites. Keith, Rosenberg, Brown, and Webster (1969) surveyed 500 patients in labor in a hospital in Chicago and found that 120 of the 425 Black women (28%) practiced amylophagia, whereas none of the 75 White women did so. Thus, similar to cultural pica in nonpregnant women, the practice also appears to be less common among northern than southern Blacks. As previously mentioned, in the study of migrant workers in California by Bruhn and Pangborn (1971), more women of Mexican descent knew pregnant women who practiced pica than did women of Anglo heritage.

The practice of pica during pregnancy appears to be declining with time. A decreasing rate is shown in the review of studies from 1937 through 1979 conducted by Danford (1982). Similarly, Bronstein and Dollar (1974) found an 18% rate of pica during pregnancy among primarily Black, low-SES women in rural Georgia. This was in contrast to a rate of 55% in the same geographic area in a 1966 study. According to Keith and colleagues (1969), the incidence of amylophagia in their study represented a lower rate in comparison to data collected at the same hospital on obstetric patients in 1964.

Complications and Treatment Response. The effects of cultural pica vary considerably from one study to another, with degree and type of pica in large part accounting for the discrepant complications. Severe side effects have been reported by several authors. For example, Cavdar and associates (1983) described a syndrome in Turkey comprised of prolonged geophagia (consumption of Turkish clay), iron deficiency anemia, growth retardation, hypogonadism, and zinc deficiency.

Severance, Holt, Patrone, and Chapman (1988) reported a case study of a 43-year-old Black woman in North Carolina with a 25-year history of geophagia involving the ingestion of more than a cup of clay per day. Six months before hospital admission, the patient was consuming more clay than food. The authors reported that geophagia resulted in muscle weakness, hypokalemia, myositis, and anemia. The patient's symptoms disappeared following discontinuation of geophagia and potassium replacement therapy. The authors noted two other cases with similar symptoms associated with geophagia published in the literature. In a study of Aboriginals by Bateson and Lebroy (1978), a high incidence of complications was reported, including perforated colon, bowel obstruction, and GI infection. Other complications reported in the literature included constipation, parasitic infections, and tetanus.

Nutritional deficiencies have long been associated with pica, varying as a function of the amount and type of material ingested. Geophagia may lead to the malabsorption of iron and zinc (Cavdar et al. 1983; Danford, 1983; Danford, Smith, & Huber, 1982) and potassium (Severance et al., 1988). Bronstein and Dollar (1974) reported a higher incidence of iron deficiency anemia and significantly lower serum albumin and urea/creatine ratios among pregnant women who practice pica in comparison to those without pica. Keith and colleagues (1969) found a borderline significant relationship between amylophagia and anemia in their study of 500 obstetric patients. Others have reported a nonsignificant relationship between geophagia and iron deficiency anemia (Bateson & Lebroy, 1978; Vermeer & Frate, 1979). Again, quantity and type of clay or soil ingested appear to be the major factors determining the presence or degree of complications. As noted by Sayers and associates (1974), the iron-binding properties of different clays vary. Based on a study of 200 pregnant women, O'Rourke and colleagues (1967) found a nonsignificant difference in anemia between individuals who did versus those who did not practice pica. However, 31% of the pica patients developed toxemia, whereas only 13% of the nonpica patients did so. This finding was in contrast to a previously published study showing no apparent association between pica and toxemia.

In the past, it was speculated that individuals with iron or zinc deficiency engaged in pica because of a craving for these depleted minerals. However, existing data do not generally support this speculation. Of individuals with anemia, only a few exhibit pica (Danford, 1982), and substances ingested do not characteristically contain the depleted nutrients (Feldman, 1986; Mokhobo, 1986; Singhi & Singhi, 1982b).

In a study by Vermeer and Frate (1979) of geophagia among Blacks in Mississippi, the authors concluded that the practice had little negative impact on health. Similarly, Pritchard and colleagues (1985) state that the custom of consuming clay or starch during pregnancy is not harmful if the substances are consumed in moderation, if parasites are not present, and if diet is adequate.

In the cases reported in the literature in which treatment of cultural pica was deemed necessary, intervention usually entailed education and counseling regarding appropriate dietary intake, discouragement of pica, and, when indicated, repletion therapy to treat nutrient deficient states.

Diagnostic and Statistical Manual of Mental Disorders

In the DSM-III-R, all types of pica are subsumed under the single category of *pica*. Pica as delineated in the DSM-III-R is almost identical to that described in the DSM-III (1980), with only four changes. Toxoplasm was added as a possible complication of the ingestion of dirt or feces, mineral deficiency was deleted as a predisposing factor, and the differential diagnosis section was reworded, although the content is basically the same. A major change is found in the section on prevalence and sex ratio. In the DSM-III, pica was simply described as, "a rare disorder" (p. 71). In the DSM-III-R, the description has been expanded; "pica is rare in normal adults, but is occasionally seen in young children, in persons with mental retardation, and in pregnant females" (p. 69). Thus, this description is consistent with the three subtypes of pica identified in the literature. Pica was not specifically noted as a diagnosis in the DSM-II (1968). The DSM-II had a Feeding Disturbance category, but this was not defined beyond its label.

The definition of pica provided by the *International Classification of Diseases-Ninth Revision-Clinical Modification* (ICD-9-CM) is, in most respects, the same as that provided by the DSM-III-R, and the ICD-9-CM lists as its source the American Psychiatric Association Task Force on Nomenclature and Statistics. According to the ICD-9-CM glossary of mental disorders, pica is defined as, "perverted appetite of nonorganic origin in which there is persistent eating of nonnutritive substances. Typically, infants ingest paint, plaster, string, hair, or cloth. Older children may have access to animal droppings, sand, bugs, leaves, or pebbles. In the adult, the eating of starch or clay-earth has been observed" (p. 1110). This definition differs from that provided in the DSM-III-R in its omission of pica associated with mental retardation and in its inclusion of the consumption of starch or clay by adults.

Only four cases of eating disorders were included in the field trials for the DSM-III. Diagnoses were not specified, thus it is not known whether any of the cases were pica. No new eating disorder field studies were conducted for the DSM-III-R. A comprehensive literature search did not disclose concordance studies on the reliability of diagnosing pica. Pica is an objectively defined and observable behavior that, according to the majority of researchers and clinicians, is the persistent ingestion of inedible, nonfood substances beyond the age of 18 months. However, unanimous agreement on the definition of pica has not been established, which may negatively affect reliability of diagnosis and comparability of findings across research studies.

The following are verbatim excerpts from the complete DSM-III-R section on pica. Each section quoted from the DSM-III-R is followed by a discussion and suggested modifications based on published research reports.

> The essential feature is the persistent eating of a nonnutritive substance. Infants with the disorder typically eat paint, plaster, string, hair, or cloth. Older children may eat animal droppings, sand, insects, leaves, or pebbles. There is no aversion to food. (American Psychiatric Association, 1987, p. 69)

In 82% of the definitions of pica reported in the literature, the disorder is limited to the ingestion of nonfood substances and does not include the pathological consumption of food items. Among the definitions excluding food from the pica category, 72% use the terms *inedible* or *nonfood* or both. Only 14% defined pica as the ingestion of *nonnutritive* materials. The majority of authors further specified that pica should be distinguished from the normal infant stage of oral exploration persisting up to 18 months of age. Therefore, it is advised that the term *infants* be deleted from the DSM-III-R description and that pica be defined as "repeated ingestion of an inedible, nonfood substance persisting beyond the age of 18 months." The exclusion of the term *nonnutritive* is advised not only for consistency with the literature, but also because some of the materials listed as examples by the DSM-III-R actually have nutritive value (e.g., insects and leaves). Findings in the literature corroborate the DSM-III-R statement that pica is not associated with food aversion. It is recommended that the three subtypes of pica (i.e., pica in children, pica in developmentally disabled individuals, and cultural pica) be delineated at the outset and that examples of substances ingested be provided separately for each subtype because of the differences between types. These criteria are summarized in Table 7.3.

> Associated Features. There are no regularly associated features. (American Psychiatric Association, 1987, p. 69)

TABLE 7.3
Pica

Proposed Diagnostic Criteria for Pica

A. Repeated ingestion of an inedible, nonfood substance persisting beyond the age of 18 months.

B. Does not meet the criteria for Kleine–Levin or Kluver–Bucy Syndromes.

Types

A. Pica in Children: Pica in children occurs beyond the age of 18 months, thus differentiating it from normal infant oral exploration. Pica usually subsides by age 6, although occasional cases in older children have been reported. Substances commonly consumed include dirt, paint, plaster, paper, string, cloth, vegetation (e.g., grass, leaves, and sticks), hair, household products (e.g., soap), feces, and a variety of small objects (e.g., stones, crayons, buttons, and insects).

B. Pica in Developmentally Disabled Individuals: Pica in mentally retarded, autistic, and psychotic individuals may occur at any age. The vast majority are functioning in the profoundly retarded range. Commonly ingested materials include string, cloth, small objects, feces, dirt, and paper.

C. Cultural Pica: Cultural pica differs from pica in children and developmentally disabled individuals in terms of the distinct subgroups that practice it and the narrow and specific range of substances ingested. Cultural pica reflects a historical custom or tradition and is not considered to be aberrant by those who engage in it. The consumption of clay or soil (geophagia) and laundry starch (amylophagia) account for more than 90% of the cases of cultural pica. Cultural pica is a world-wide phenomenon. In the United States, it is most common among, although not limited to, Black women living in the southeastern portion of the country.

D. Pica Not Otherwise Specified: Pica that does not meet the criteria for one of the preceding types of pica.

Based on published research reports, pica in children is associated with other types of behavioral and emotional disturbances. In virtually all cases of pica in mentally retarded individuals, other forms of self-injurious, self-stimulating, and maladaptive behavior are evident.

> Age at onset. Age at onset is usually from 12 to 24 months, but may be earlier. (American Psychiatric Association, 1987, p. 69)

Little research has been conducted investigating the age at onset of pica in children, although prevalence increases with decreasing age. By definition, the behavior is not considered pathological until 18 months of age. The onset of pica in developmentally disabled individuals may be later than that in normally developing children. The practice of cultural pica typically begins in females at puberty or during pregnancy.

> Course. Pica usually remits in early childhood, but may persist into ado-

> lescence or, rarely, continue through adulthood. (American Psychiatric Association, 1987, p. 69)

In children, the practice of pica declines with age and usually ends by age 6, although occasional cases of pica beyond this age are found in the literature. Pica among developmentally disabled individuals is often a chronic disorder persisting indefinitely if not treated. However, in large-scale surveys of mentally retarded adults in institutional care, the prevalence of pica decreases with age. Cultural pica does not typically begin until puberty, and, although not related to age per se, the custom itself appears to be declining with time.

> Impairment. None. (American Psychiatric Association, 1987, p. 69)

As with other maladaptive behaviors, pica may interfere with more functional behavior. This is particularly a problem for developmentally disabled individuals who may devote much time and effort to securing and ingesting inedible substances.

> Complications. Lead poisoning may result from the ingestion of paint or paint-soaked plaster; hairball tumors may cause intestinal obstruction. Toxoplasma or toxocara infections may follow ingestion of feces or dirt. (American Psychiatric Association, 1987, p. 69)

The complications of pica vary considerably with the nature and quantity of the materials ingested. According to the literature, possible complications of pica include choking, gastric ulcer or perforation, constipation, intestinal obstruction or perforation, GI infections, tetanus, parasitic infections, achlorhydria, and nutritional complications. Depending on the substances ingested, accidental poisoning may be a risk for children and developmentally disabled individuals. As noted by the DSM-III-R, the ingestion of paint or plaster may cause lead poisoning, and bezoars may develop from the consumption of hair. Additionally, geophagia has been implicated in the malabsorption of iron, zinc, and potassium, depending on the quantity and type of clay or soil consumed. According to the literature, cultural pica is often a benign habit, but it can produce severe complications, again varying as a function of the type and degree of substances ingested.

> Predisposing factors. Mental retardation, neglect, and poor supervision may be predisposing factors. (American Psychiatric Association, 1987, p. 69)

The majority of research evidence suggests that pica in children is associated with neurological, developmental, and behavior deficits and a variety of interrelated factors reflecting psychosocial stress (e.g., family pathology, impaired parent–child relationships, neglect, abuse, and low SES). The prevalence of pica is apparently greater among Black than White children and among children whose mothers or ethnic subgroup practice cultural pica. Pica among developmentally disabled individuals is clearly associated with degree of mental retardation. Across studies investigating pica in mentally retarded persons, 85% are profoundly retarded, 11% severely retarded, 4% moderately retarded, and 0% mildly retarded. The emergence of cultural pica is directly linked to the customs of the subgroup to which the individual belongs.

> Prevalence and sex ratio. Pica is rare in normal adults, but is occasionally seen in young children, and persons with Mental Retardation, and in pregnant females. (American Psychiatric Association, 1987, p. 69)

Across seven studies published from 1957 through 1981, the median prevalence rate for pica in children is 22%. This rate may be inflated because some studies included infants in the surveys, used loose definitions of pica (e.g., including mouthing or chewing with the actual ingestion of substances), or failed to exclude normal instances of oral exploration and experimentation. The prevalence of pica in children appears to be fairly evenly distributed between males and females. Four studies investigating the incidence of pica among mentally retarded adults in institutional care yielded prevalence rates of 8.0%, 8.4%, 9.2%, and 21.0%. Prevalence of pica among autistic individuals is less well studied, and the only published investigation reported an incidence rate of 60%. Existing data indicate that pica is equally prevalent among developmentally disabled males and females. Recent data on the prevalence of cultural pica are lacking. Across surveys conducted prior to 1980, geophagia or amylophagia were practiced by approximately 50% of Black women residing in the southeastern portion of the United States. Across studies, the prevalence of geophagia or amylophagia during pregnancy was approximately 32% for Black women living in the south and 21% for those residing in the north. Existing data suggest that the practice of cultural pica is declining with time.

> Familial pattern. No information. (American Psychiatric Association, 1987, p. 69)

A study by Barltrop (1966) indicated that siblings of children with pica were significantly more likely to exhibit pica than siblings of children who did not evidence pica. Lourie and colleagues (1963) found that pica was more common among children whose mothers or subculture members consumed clay or starch. Cultural pica is strongly related to familial and cultural patterns and is passed on from one generation to the next.

> Differential Diagnosis. In Autistic Disorder, Schizophrenia, and certain physical disorders, such as Kleine–Levin syndrome, nonnutritive substances may be eaten. In such instances, pica should not be noted as an additional diagnosis. (American Psychiatric Association, 1987, p. 69)

In agreement with the DSM-III-R, it is advised that pica not be an additional diagnosis for individuals with Kleine–Levin Syndrome (as well as Kluver–Bucy Syndrome), because morbid hunger and bizarre oral behavior are essential features of these disorders. However, although pica is associated with autistic disorder and schizophrenia, it is not a symptom of these disorders, and many autistic or schizophrenic individuals do not exhibit pica. Therefore, if pica is present, it is advised that it be noted as an additional diagnosis. By doing so, this will serve to enhance the clinical understanding of pica and further research in this area.

The DSM-III-R lists two diagnostic criteria for pica: "repeated eating of a nonnutritive substance for at least one month" and "does not meet the criteria for either Autistic Disorder, Schizophrenia, or Kleine–Levin syndrome" (American Psychiatric Association, 1987, p. 69). It is recommended that the DSM-III-R diagnostic criteria be revised as suggested in Table 7.3.

Directions for Future Research

In order to better understand pica, it is essential that diagnostic criteria be firmly established and that future research studies conform to these criteria. According to the majority of publications, pica is the repeated ingestion of inedible, nonfood substances beyond the age of 18 months. However, research on pica is not always based on samples consistent with this definition. In some studies, infants are included and either mouthing or chewing or the compulsive, pathological consumption of normally ingested food items is included as a form of pica. The pathological consumption of food items has not been as extensively studied as nonfood pica. This is necessary so that its features can be understood and a determination made as to whether or not this should constitute a separate type of eating disorder.

The diagnostic validity of the three proposed subtypes of pica (i.e., pica in children, pica in developmentally disabled individuals, and cultural pica) needs to be empirically determined and reliability of these diagnoses established. Furthermore, an agreement needs to be reached on whether or not cultural pica is indeed a pathological practice and, subsequently, whether or not it should be included as an eating disorder. Cultural pica is not considered to be aberrant by individuals who engage in it, and many researchers consider it to be a usually benign cultural custom, possibly akin to other oral habits, such as smoking, chewing tobacco, or chewing gum.

There is a critical need to update epidemiological data on pica. Recent research on pica in children and cultural pica is meager, and much of our knowledge is based on older studies that may now be outdated. Current prevalence rates should be established, and research needs to confirm the apparent decline in cultural pica and the apparent equal prevalence by gender for both pica in children and in developmentally disabled individuals.

Research on pica in children suggests that the disorder is associated with a host of variables including neurological or developmental deficits, behavior problems, psychosocial stress, family pathology, SES, ethnicity, and cultural factors. Many of these variables are interrelated, so future empirical endeavors need to partial out these relationships and isolate the essential factors related to and possibly predisposing children to pica.

Lastly, the relationship between pica and nutrition needs to be investigated further. Existing research indicates that pica may lead to nutritional deficiencies (e.g., geophagia interfering with the absorption of iron, zinc, or potassium). Continued research in this area is necessary to gain a better understanding of the relationship between nutrition and the various forms and degrees of pica.

REACTIVE ATTACHMENT DISORDER, NONORGANIC FAILURE TO THRIVE, AND PSYCHOSOCIAL DWARFISM

This final section briefly summarizes three diagnostic categories that share similar, if not the same, symptoms and etiological factors. These diagnoses are reactive attachment disorder in infancy or early childhood (RAD), nonorganic failure to thrive (NFTT), and psychosocial dwarfism (PSD). The latter is also referred to as deprivation, psychosomatic, or abuse dwarfism. The features common to the three disorders include growth retardation; impaired social relatedness; a disturbance in the caretaker–child relationship; mood, behavioral, and developmental correlates; and reversal of symptoms with appropriate care. It is argued that the use of three different labels for what may be the same disorder causes confusion and impedes the synthesis of knowledge and research across disciplines. Therefore, diagnostic criteria integrating RAD, NFTT, and PSD into one category are proposed. Growth retardation is a major feature, thus the diagnostic category may best be included with the other eating and feeding disorders in the *Diagnostic and Statistical Manual*. Currently, only RAD is an Axis I diagnosis in the DSM-III-R. However, in the literature, RAD is a little recognized and researched entity in comparison to NFTT and PSD. Furthermore, the establishment of a diagnostic category integrating RAD, NFTT, and PSD would help to rectify an apparent discrepancy in the DSM-III-R nosology regarding the way in which rumination disorder and RAD are conceptualized. For rumination disorder, the symptom and diagnosis is rumination and, according to the literature, the hypothesized etiology for infants is an impaired caretaker–child relationship. In contrast, the DSM-III-R diagnosis for RAD focuses on the apparent etiology (i.e., a disturbance in the caretaker–child relationship). This apparent inconsistency is discussed further in the following sections along with a presentation of the commonalities and differences among RAD, NFTT, and PSD.

Symptoms and Associated Features

Growth Retardation/Failure to Gain Weight

In the DSM-III, a criterion for RAD was "weight loss or failure to gain appropriate amount of weight for age unexplainable by any physical disorder" (p. 60). Tibbits-Kleber and Howell (1985) and Kaplan and Sadock (1985) also considered failure to thrive to be a component of RAD. However, in the DSM-III-R, failure to thrive is now noted as an associated symptom and, if present, is coded on Axis III (p. 93).

For NFTT, failure to thrive in the absence of an organic cause is the essential feature. Some authors define this as both weight and height below the third percentile for age (Bell & Woolston, 1985; Fischhoff, Whitten, & Petit, 1971; Pollitt, Eichler, & Chan, 1975; Tibbits-Kleber & Howell, 1985). However, for the majority of authors, weight is the primary criterion, usually specified as falling below the third percentile (Altemeier, O'Connor, Sherrod, & Vietze, 1985; Bithoney, 1986; Cupoli, Hallock, & Barness, 1980; Gagan, Cupoli, & Watkins, 1984; Holmes, 1979; Mitchell, Gorrell, & Greenberg, 1980; Oates, 1984a; Rosenn, Loeb, & Jura, 1980; Sills, 1978).

In PSD, growth retardation is also present, but Oates (1984a) contended that height, as opposed to weight, is the primary consideration. According to Oates (1984a), PSD is characterized by "short stature" and "weight in proportion to height or mild loss" (p. 443). In contrast, the major feature in NFTT is "weight loss" with "short stature . . . less marked than weight loss" (p. 443). However, this distinction is not universally accepted, and Bowden and Hopwood (1982) specified that height and weight are both below the third percentile in PSD.

Impaired Social Relatedness

According to the DSM-III-R, one of the diagnostic criteria for RAD is "markedly disturbed social relatedness" (p. 93), such as significantly reduced initiation of and responsiveness to social interaction and indiscriminate social behavior. This essential feature is corroborated by other authors (Call, 1984; Kaplan & Sadock, 1985; Tibbits-Kleber & Howell, 1985). In the syndrome of NFTT, impaired social relatedness is also found (Altemeier et al., 1985; Goldbloom, 1982; Rosenn et al., 1980; Woolston, 1983). Similarly, children with PSD are described as socially withdrawn and unresponsive with impaired interpersonal relationships (Bowden & Hopwood, 1982; Green, Campbell, & David, 1984; Money, 1977; Tibbits-Kleber & Howell, 1985).

Disturbance in the Caretaker–Child Relationship

According to the DSM-III-R, another diagnostic criterion for RAD is "grossly pathogenic care" (p. 93), which precedes and is assumed to be the cause of the attachment disorder. Kaplan and Sadock (1985) also contended that parental pathology and neglect are components of RAD. Furthermore, the DSM-III-R states that pathogenic care may be accompanied by failure to adequately feed the child. Similarly, Tibbits-Kleber and Howell (1985) reported that emotional deprivation in RAD cases may be associated with inadequate nutrition.

For NFTT, the vast majority of authors cite the presence of a disturbance in the caretaker–child relationship, including parental pathology, neglect, deprivation, and decreased interaction (Altemeier et al., 1985; Berkowitz & Senter, 1987; Casey, 1983; Cupoli et al., 1980; Evans, Reinhart, & Succop, 1972; Fischhoff et al., 1971; Gagan et al., 1984; Pollitt et al., 1975; Shaheen, Alexander, Truskowsky, & Barbero, 1968; Sills, 1978). Some authors more specifically relate NFTT to a disturbance in the attachment process (Bell & Woolston, 1985; Gordon & Jameson, 1979; Singer, 1987). Other authors contend that NFTT is a consequence of a disturbed parent–child relationship as well as inadequate nutrition (Casey, Bradley, & Wortham, 1984; Oates, 1977, 1984a,

1984b). Goldbloom (1982) claimed that insufficient caloric intake is the major etiological factor in NFTT, whereas Holmes (1979) and Skuse (1985) felt that NFTT is a consequence of either psychosocial deprivation or inadequate nutrition. Research by Woolston (1983) revealed three subtypes of NFTT, one in which the child was undernourished and understimulated, one in which the child was undernourished only, and one in which the child refused to consume adequate amounts of food.

According to the DSM-III-R, "in psychosocial dwarfism there rarely is a history of grossly pathogenic care" (p. 93). However, this position does not appear to be supported by the literature. Parental pathology, emotional deprivation, neglect, abuse, disturbed parent–child relationship, and psychosocial stress have been cited by numerous authors as underlying PSD (Bowden & Hopwood, 1982; Ferholt et al., 1985; Green et al., 1984; Kaplan & Sadock, 1985; Money, 1977; Oates, 1984a). According to Oates (1984a), for NFTT and PSD, "family pathology is similar in both conditions" (p. 439). As with NFTT and RAD, PSD children may be inadequately nourished (Oates, 1984a), although PSD may develop in spite of adequate nutrition (Green et al., 1984). For all three diagnostic categories (RAD, NFTT, and PSD), many authors acknowledge the contribution of the child to the attachment process and the caretaker–child relationship, and they recognize that certain child characteristics may negatively affect the relationship.

Mood, Behavioral, and Developmental Correlates

According to the DSM-III-R and Call (1984), apathy is an associated feature of RAD. In addition to apathy, Kaplan and Sadock (1985) noted that infants with RAD may be emotionally disturbed and have developmental delays. Similarly, behavioral and affective disturbances may accompany NFTT (Berkowitz & Senter, 1987), specifically apathy, social withdrawal, and decreased smiling and vocalizations (Goldbloom, 1982). Developmental delays also may be a component of the syndrome of NFTT (Altemeier et al., 1985; Berkowitz & Senter, 1987; Woolston, 1983).

The constellation of symptoms for PSD is more specific and extensive than that described for RAD and NFTT. However, as with RAD and NFTT, apathy (Green et al., 1984; Kaplan & Sadock, 1985) and developmental delay (Bowden & Hopwood, 1982; Green et al., 1984; Kaplan & Sadock, 1985; Money, 1977) are associated with PSD. Children with PSD also evidence bizarre eating behaviors, such as voracious and indiscriminate appetite, pica, hoarding, eating from garbage, drinking from toilet bowls, and in some cases, very selective food preferences

(Bowden & Hopwood, 1982; Green et al., 1984; Kaplan & Sadock, 1985; Money, 1977; Oates, 1984a; Tibbits-Kleber & Howell, 1985; Woolston, 1983). Sleep disturbance is also characteristic of PSD (Bowden & Hopwood, 1982; Gardner, 1972; Green et al., 1984; Guilhaume, Benoit, Gourmelen, & Richardet, 1982; Kaplan & Sadock, 1985; Money, 1977; Tibbits-Kleber & Howell, 1985; Woolston, 1983). A variety of other symptoms may be present in children with PSD including irritability, temper tantrums, encopresis, enuresis, decreased sensitivity to pain, and self-injurious behavior (Bowden & Hopwood, 1982; Green et al., 1984; Money, 1977).

Endocrine Abnormalities

For the majority of children with PSD, growth hormone secretion is suppressed (Bowden & Hopwood, 1982; Gardner, 1972; Green et al., 1984; Guilhaume et al., 1982; Kaplan & Sadock, 1985; Oates, 1984a; Woolston, 1983). According to Gardner (1972) and Guilhaume and associates (1982), this is primarily a consequence of the sleep disturbance that inhibits release of the growth hormone. Most authors consider endrocrine status to be a major symptom differentiating PSD from RAD and NFTT. According to Kaplan and Sadock (1985), endocrine functioning is normal in children diagnosed with RAD. Similarly, Woolston (1983) stated the same is the case for children with NFTT. There is some disagreement on this issue, however, and Tibbits-Kleber and Howell (1985) noted that when RAD children are removed from their emotionally deprived environment, this "results in an increase in growth hormone level" (p. 306).

Age at Onset

According to the majority of authors, age at onset for RAD and NFTT is earlier than that for PSD. However, by no means is there agreement on this issue, and age ranges for onset vary considerably from one source to another. According to the DSM-III-R, the onset for RAD is before age 5, whereas Kaplan and Sadock (1985) specified onset before 8 months. For NFTT, onset is between 0 and 2 years of age (Altemeier et al., 1985; Chatoor, Schaefer, Dickson, & Egan, 1984; Oates, 1984a; Woolston, 1983). In contrast, Woolston (1983) stated that the onset for PSD is between 1.5 and 4.0 years, and Kaplan and Sadock (1985) gave an age range for onset of 2.0 to 3.0 years. A review of publications on PSD by Oates (1984a) revealed that, at the time of the studies, the subjects ranged in age from 2 to 15 years. However, Oates (1984a) noted that "there may be an earlier history of feeding difficulties, irritability and sleep problems during infancy" (p. 442). In contrast to these authors citing a later age of onset for PSD, Bowden and Hopwood (1982) stated that "by history, the onset of symptoms and failure to grow may begin anytime in infancy" (p. 17). Similarly, in a study of four children with PSD (ages 1 to 3 years), the children's short stature had been noted by 6 to 18 months of age (Guilhaume et al., 1982).

Reversal of Symptoms

The three diagnostic categories are linked by the fact that removal from the home to a setting in which care is appropriate results in the reversal of symptoms. This is the case for RAD (DSM-III-R, Tibbits-Kleber & Howell, 1985), NFTT (Gagan et al., 1984; Holmes, 1979), and PSD (Bowden & Hopwood, 1982; Ferholt et al., 1985; Green et al., 1984; Woolston, 1983).

Reconciliation of Diagnostic Categories

According to the literature, RAD is a little recognized and researched diagnostic entity in comparison to NFTT and PSD. A *Medline* search of the literature from 1977 to 1988 disclosed 1 article on RAD, 36 publications on NFTT, and 7 on PSD. No other RAD publications were revealed when the search was extended back 5 additional years. Searching *Psychological Abstracts* yielded one additional article on RAD, bringing the total to two publications that specifically referred to the syndrome as reactive attachment disorder (i.e., Call, 1984; Tibbits-Kleber & Howell, 1985). Furthermore, the instructions regarding subject headings for *Psychological Abstracts* literature searches specify that, for "reactive attachment disorder use failure to thrive" (American Psychological Association, 1988, p. 166).

In the ICD-9-CM, RAD is not mentioned or listed in the index or glossary of mental disorders. In contract, PSD is coded under "dwarfism, not elsewhere classified" (p. 169) and failure to thrive under "lack of expected normal physiological development" (p. 714).

It is evident that the diagnostic labels RAD and NFTT may be applied to the same syndrome. This fact is recognized in the literature. According to Woolston (1983), "the DSM-III . . . calls the syndrome [NFTT] 'Reactive Attachment Disorder of Infancy' " (p. 116). Similarly, the DSM-III-R states that "some severe forms of this disorder [RAD] . . . have been called 'failure to thrive' " (p. 91). Likewise, Call (1984) asserted that the diagnosis of NFTT is subsumed under RAD. According to Tibbits-Kleber and Howell (1985), "RAD . . . represents the nonorganic etiology of the general medical diagnosis of failure-to-thrive" (p. 304). In this respect, NFTT is construed as a medical diagnosis and RAD as a psychiatric diagnosis. However, this does not seem to be a constructive distinction because it causes confusion and inteferes with the integration of knowledge across disciplines.

In the DSM-III-R, Reactive Attachment Disorder of Infancy or Early Childhood is a diagnostic category under the heading Other Disorders of Infancy, Childhood, or Adolescence. Within this diagnosis, if failure to thrive is present, it is coded on Axis III. It is also noted that rumination may be an associated feature of RAD. Psychosocial dwarfism is cited as a disorder that must be ruled out before diagnosing RAD. However, PSD is not listed as a separate diagnostic category in the DSM-III-R.

A comparison of the DSM-III-R categories of RAD and rumination disorder of infancy reveals inconsistencies in the DSM-III-R nosology. According to the literature, rumination in infants is secondary to a disturbance in the caretaker–child relationship. In the case of rumination disorder, rumination is both the symptom and diagnosis, and the impaired relationship is the etiology. Although rumination disorder in infants could thus be construed as a reactive attachment disorder, the DSM-III-R gives it a separate diagnostic category. Similar to the way in which the DSM-III-R classifies rumination, nonorganic failure to thrive could be considered as both the symptom and diagnosis, the etiology of which is the disorder of attachment or, more globally, a disturbance in the caretaker–child relationship. However, the DSM-III-R handles NFTT in a different manner than rumination and does not allot it a separate diagnosis.

It is also evident that more than one type of disorder may result from a disturbance of attachment or an impaired caretaker–child relationship. According to Call (1984), "A review of currently available literature on infant abuse, infantile failure to thrive without organic cause and serious feeding disorders . . . suggests that primary attachment failure of infancy . . . is demonstrable in varying degrees in each of these conditions and should be considered as the primary diagnosis in most such cases" (p. 196). However, RAD is currently an underrecognized and underresearched diagnostic entity, with only two publications on this topic revealed by the computer literature search, and much additional research is needed. At this point in time, it is not known whether RAD can be present without failure to thrive as a component, or vice versa. If the two are inextricably linked, then the different labels refer to one and the same disorder.

The overlap between PSD and NFTT is also recognized in the literature. Cupoli and colleagues (1980) and Oates (1984a) considered PSD to be a subtype of NFTT. A major distinction between PSD and NFTT made by some authors is the later age at onset for PSD. However, this is not definitive and, according to some, PSD can be present and diagnosed in infancy (Bowden & Hopwood, 1982; Guilhaume et al., 1982). Furthermore, the age distinction may be more apparent than real, and PSD may reflect the same underlying disorder as NFTT but at a later age. According to Kaplan and Sadock (1985), many authorities consider PSD to be a continuation of RAD. Several of the PSD behavioral symptoms are not applicable to infancy and cannot be present in infants because of their age-related nature. Therefore, the more extensive behavioral symptomatology of PSD may be a function of age rather than reflecting a disorder that is essentially different from RAD or NFTT.

Clearly, there is a need for diagnostic clarification as well as a comparative integration of research and clinical knowledge on RAD, NFTT, and PSD. It is apparent that these three diagnostic categories represent syndromes that share similar features, etiologies, and treatment strategies. Thus, it may be advisable to consider these syndromes under a single diagnostic heading, subdividing the disorder into separate types if further research warrants such divisions. As currently defined, RAD with failure to thrive, NFTT, and PSD could be incorporated into one diagnostic category under the following conditions:

1. Failure to thrive would be a criterion for diagnosis and defined as weight, height, or both below the third percentile for age.

2. A second criterion for diagnosis would be a disturbance in the caretaker–child relationship, including evidence of pathological care, emotional deprivation, neglect, or a disorder of attachment. In this way, the syndrome would not be limited to the attachment phase. Furthermore, it is not clear from existing research that a disorder of attachment is the primary problem underlying the syndrome or whether its underpinnings relate to broader factors, such as emotional deprivation, pathological care, neglect, or other abnormalities in the caretaker–child relationship. Children who are undernourished only, without evidence of a disordered relationship with the caretaker, would be excluded from this diagnostic category. The criterion would further specify that symptoms improve significantly or are reversible if the child is removed from the environment and adequate care is provided.

3. Age at onset would be broadened to include infancy and childhood, with the upper age limit determined empirically through research studies.

4. A description of mood and behavioral symptoms would take into consideration variations as a function of age. At all age levels, impaired social relatedness, apathy, withdrawal, and possible developmental delay would be evident. In older children, symptoms currently attributa-

ble to PSD may be present, including bizarre eating behavior, sleep disturbance, encopresis, enuresis, irritability, temper tantrums, reduced sensitivity to pain, and self-injurious behavior. Endocrine abnormalities may also be apparent in older children. Further research is needed to determine if this is indeed an age-related phenomenon or whether suppression of growth hormone secretion is also found among younger children, as was demonstrated by Guilhaume and associates (1982) with 1- and 3-year-olds diagnosed with PSD.

If a future revision of the *Diagnostic and Statistical Manual* does not attempt to integrate RAD with failure to thrive, NFTT, and PSD into one diagnostic category, it is advised that the omission of NFTT from the eating disorders category be directly addressed by noting under this section that most cases of NFTT would receive a diagnosis of RAD, as defined in the *Diagnostic and Statistical Manual*. This would serve to reduce continued confusion surrounding the different diagnostic labels used in the literature, promote recognition that these labels may denote the same or similar disorders, and facilitate the integration of research on RAD, NFTT, and PSD across disciplines.

REFERENCES

Albin, J. B. (1977). The treatment of pica (scavenging) behavior in the retarded: A critical analysis and implications for research. *Mental Retardation, 15,* 14–17.

Alford, G. S., Blanchard, E. B., & Buckley, T. M. (1972). Treatment of hysterical vomiting by modification of social contingencies: A case study. *Journal of Behavior Therapy and Experimental Psychiatry, 3,* 209–212.

Altemeier, W. A., III, O'Connor, S. M., Sherrod, K. B., & Vietze, P. M. (1985). Prospective study of antecedents for nonorganic failure to thrive. *Journal of Pediatrics, 106,* 360–365.

American Psychiatric Association. (1987). *Diagnostic and statistical manual of mental disorders* (3rd ed., rev.). Washington, DC: Author.

American Psychological Association. (1988). *Thesaurus of psychological index terms* (5th ed.). Washington, DC: Author.

Arensberg, B. (1956). Loving care does the trick. *American Journal of Nursing, 56,* 622–623.

Ausman, J., Ball, T. S., & Alexander, D. (1974). Behavior therapy of pica with a profoundly retarded adolescent. *Mental Retardation, 12,* 16–18.

Azrin, N. H., & Wesolowski, M. D. (1975). Eliminating habitual vomiting in a retarded adult by positive practice and self-correction. *Journal of Behavior Therapy and Experimental Psychiatry, 6,* 145–148.

Bakwin, H., & Bakwin, R. M. (1972). *Behavior disorders in children* (4th ed.). Philadelphia: Saunders.

Ball, T. S., Hendricksen, H., & Clayton, J. (1974). A special feeding technique for chronic regurgitation. *American Journal of Mental Deficiency, 78,* 486–493.

Barltrop, D. (1966). The prevalence of pica. *American Journal of Diseases of Children, 112,* 116–123.

Barmann, B. C. (1980). Use of contingent vibration in the treatment of self-stimulatory hand-mouthing and ruminative vomiting behavior. *Journal of Behavior Therapy and Experimental Psychiatry, 11,* 307–311.

Barton, L. E., & Barton, C. L. (1985). An effective and benign treatment of rumination. *Journal of the Association for Persons with Severe Handicaps, 10,* 168–171.

Bateson, E. M., & Lebroy, T. (1978). Clay eating by Aboriginals of the Northern Territory. *Medical Journal of Australia, 1* (Suppl. 1), 1–3.

Becker, J. V., Turner, S. M., & Sajwaj, T. E. (1978). Multiple behavioral effects of the use of lemon juice with a ruminating toddler-age child. *Behavior Modification, 2,* 267–278.

Bell, L. S., & Woolston, J. L. (1985). The relationship of weight gain and caloric intake in infants with organic and nonorganic failure to thrive syndrome. *Journal of the American Academy of Child Psychiatry, 24,* 447–452.

Berkowitz, C. D., & Senter, S. A. (1987). Characteristics of mother–infant interactions in nonorganic failure to thrive. *Journal of Family Practice, 25,* 377–381.

Bithoney, W. G. (1986). Elevated lead levels in children with nonorganic failure to thrive. *Pediatrics, 78,* 891–895.

Bithoney, W. G., Snyder, J., Michalek, J., & Newberger, E. H. (1985). Childhood ingestions as symptoms of family distress. *American Journal of Diseases of Children, 139,* 456–459.

Borreson, P. M., & Anderson, J. L. (1982). The elimination of chronic rumination through a combination of procedures. *Mental Retardation, 20,* 34–38.

Bowden, M. L., & Hopwood, N. J. (1982). Psychosocial dwarfism: Identification, intervention and planning. *Social Work in Health Care, 7,* 15–36.

Bright, G. O., & Whaley, D. L. (1968). Suppression of regurgitation and rumination with aversive events. *Michigan Mental Health Research Bulletin, 11,* 17–20.

Bronstein, E. S., & Dollar, J. (1974). Pica in pregnancy. *Journal of the Medical Association of Georgia, 63,* 332–335.

Bruhn, C. M., & Pangborn, R. M. (1971). Reported incidence of pica among migrant families. *Journal of the American Dietetic Association, 58,* 417–420.

Bucher, B., Reykdal, B., & Albin, J. (1976). Brief physical restraint to control pica in retarded children. *Journal of Behavior Therapy and Experimental Psychiatry, 7,* 137–140.

Call, J. D. (1984). Child abuse and neglect in infancy: Sources of hostility within the parent–infant dyad and disorders of attachment in infancy. *Child Abuse and Neglect, 8,* 185–202.

Casey, P. H. (1983). Failure to thrive: A reconceptualization. *Developmental and Behavioral Pediatrics, 4,* 63–66.

Casey, P. H., Bradley, R., & Wortham, B. (1984). Social and nonsocial home environments of infants with nonorganic failure-to-thrive. *Pediatrics, 73,* 348–353.

Cavdar, A. O., Arcasoy, A., Cin, S., Babacan, E., & Gozdasoglu, S. (1983). Geophagia in Turkey: Iron and zinc deficiency, iron and zinc absorption studies and response to treatment with zinc in geophagia cases. In A. S. Prasad, A. O. Cavdar, G. J. Brewer, & P. J. Aggett (Eds.). *Zinc deficiency in human subjects* (pp. 71–97). New York: Alan R. Liss.

Chatoor, I., Dickson, L., & Einhorn, A. (1984). Rumination: Etiology and treatment. *Pediatric Annals, 13,* 924–929.

Chatoor, I., Schaefer, S., Dickson, L., & Egan, J. (1984). Non-organic failure to thrive: A developmental perspective. *Pediatric Annals, 13,* 829–843.

Cohen, D. J., Johnson, W. T., & Caparulo, B. K. (1976). Pica and elevated blood lead level in autistic and atypical children. *American Journal of Diseases of Children, 130,* 47–48.

Conrin, J., Pennypacker, H. S., Johnston, J., & Rast, J. (1982). Differential reinforcement of other behaviors to treat chronic rumination of mental retardates. *Journal of Behavior Therapy and Experimental Psychiatry, 13,* 325–329.

Cooper, M. (1957). *Pica.* Springfield, IL: Charles C. Thomas.

Crump, I. M. (1987). Evaluation of the nutritional status of the handicapped child. In I. M. Crump (Ed.), *Nutrition and feeding of the handicapped child* (pp. 29–39). Boston, MA: College-Hill Press.

Cunningham, C. E., & Linscheid, T. R. (1976). Elimination of chronic infant ruminating by electric shock. *Behavior Therapy, 7,* 231–234.

Cupoli, J. M., Hallock, J. A., & Barness, L. A. (1980). Failure to thrive. *Current Problems in Pediatrics, 10,* 6–42.

Danford, D. E. (1982). Pica and nutrition. *Annual Review of Nutrition, 2,* 303–322.

Danford, D. E. (1983). Pica and zinc. In A. S. Prasad, A. O. Cavdar, G. J. Brewer, & P. J. Aggett (Eds.), *Zinc deficiency in human subjects* (pp. 185–195). New York: Alan R. Liss.

Danford, D. E., & Huber, A. M. (1982). Pica among mentally retarded adults. *American Journal of Mental Deficiency, 87,* 141–146.

Danford, D. E., Smith, J. C., Jr., & Huber, A. M. (1982). Pica and mineral status in the mentally retarded. *American Journal of Clinical Nutrition, 35,* 958–967.

Daniel, W. H. (1982). Management of chronic rumination with a contingent exercise procedure employing topographically dissimilar behavior. *Journal of Behavior Therapy and Experimental Psychiatry, 13,* 149–152.

Davis, P. K., & Cuvo, A. J. (1980). Chronic vomiting and rumination in intellectually normal and retarded individuals: Review and evaluation of behavioral research. *Behavior Research of Severe Devlopmental Disabilities, 1,* 31–59.

Davis, W. B., Wieseler, N. A., & Hanzel, T. E. (1980). Contingent music in management of rumination and out-of-seat behavior in a profoundly mentally retarded institutionalized male. *Mental Retardation, 18,* 43–45.

Demchak, M. A., & Halle, J. W. (1985). Motivational assessment: A potential means of enhancing treatment success of self-injurious individuals. *Education and Training of the Mentally Retarded, 20,* 25–38.

Deveaux, P., Kibel, M. A., Dempster, W. S., Pocock, F., & Formenti, K. (1986). Blood lead levels in preschool children in Cape Town. *South African Medical Journal, 69,* 421–424.

Duker, P. C., & Seys, D. M. (1977). Elimination of vomiting in a retarded female using restitutional overcorrection. *Behavior Therapy, 8,* 255–257.

Eastwell, H. D. (1979). A pica epidemic: A price for sedentarism among Australian ex-hunter-gatherers. *Psychiatry, 42,* 264–273.

Evans, S. L., Reinhart, J. B., & Succop, R. A. (1972). Failure to thrive: A study of 45 children and their families. *Journal of the American Academy of Child Psychiatry, 11,* 440–457.

Favell, J. E., McGimsey, J. F., & Schell, R. M. (1982). Treatment of self-injury by providing alternate sensory activities. *Analysis and Intervention in Developmental Disabilities, 2,* 83–104.

Feldman, M. D. (1986). Pica: Current perspectives. *Psychosomatics, 27,* 519–523.

Ferholt, J., & Provence, S. (1976). Diagnosis and treatment of an infant with psychophysiological vomiting. *Psychoanalytic Study of the Child, 31,* 439–459.

Ferholt, J. B., Rotnem, D. L., Genel, M., Leonard, M., Carey, M., & Hunter, D. E. K. (1985). A psychodynamic study of psychosomatic dwarfism: A syndrome of depression, personality disorder, and impaired growth. *Journal of the American Academy of Child Psychiatry, 24,* 49–57.

Finney, J. W., Russo, D. C., & Cataldo, M. F. (1982). Reduction of pica in young children with lead poisoning. *Journal of Pediatric Psychology, 7,* 197–207.

Fischhoff, J., Whitten, C. F., & Petit, M. G. (1971). A psychiatric study of mothers of infants with growth failure secondary to maternal deprivation. *Journal of Pediatrics, 79,* 209–215.

Flanagan, C. H. (1977). Rumination in infancy—Past and present. *Journal of the American Academy of Child Psychiatry, 16,* 140–149.

Fleisher, D. R. (1979). Infant rumination syndrome: Report of a case and review of the literature. *American Journal of Diseases of Children, 133,* 266–269.

Foxx, R. M., & Martin, E. D. (1975). Treatment of scavenging behavior (coprophagy and pica) by overcorrection. *Behaviour Research and Therapy, 13,* 153–162.

Foxx, R. M., Snyder, M. S., & Schroeder, F. (1979). A food satiation and oral hygiene punishment program to suppress chronic rumination by retarded persons. *Journal of Autism and Developmental Disorders, 9,* 399–412.

Fullerton, D. T. (1963). Infantile rumination: A case report. *Archives of General Psychiatry, 9,* 593–600.

Gagan, R. J., Cupoli, J. M., & Watkins, A. H. (1984). The families of children who fail to thrive: Preliminary investigations of parental deprivation among organic and non-organic cases. *Child Abuse and Neglect, 8,* 93–103.

Galbraith, D. A., Byrick, R. J., & Rutledge, J. T. (1970). An aversive conditioning approach to the inhibition of chronic vomiting. *Canadian Psychiatric Association Journal, 15,* 311–313.

Gallacher, J. E. J., Elwood, P. C., Phillips, K. M., Davies, B. E., & Jones, D. T. (1984). Relation between pica and blood lead in areas of differing lead exposure. *Archives of Disease in Childhood, 59,* 40–44.

Garcia, C., Schulbe, K., Markowitz, R. I., & Young, L. W. (1987). Radiological case of the month: Perforated gastric ulcer in a rock eater. *American Journal of Diseases of Children, 141,* 213–214.

Gardner, L. I. (1972). Deprivation dwarfism. *Scientific American, 227,* 76–82.

Glickman, L. T., Chaudry, I. U., Costantino, J., Clack, F. B., Cypess, R. H., & Winslow, L. (1981). Pica patterns, toxocariasis, and elevated blood lead in children. *American Journal of Tropical Medicine and Hygiene, 30,* 77–80.

Glickman, L. T., Cypess, R. H., Crumrine, P. K., & Gitlin, D. A. (1979). Toxocara infection and epilepsy in children. *Journal of Pediatrics, 94,* 75–78.

Goldbloom, R. B. (1982). Failure to thrive. *Pediatric Clinics of North America, 29,* 151–166.

Gordon, A. H., & Jameson, J. C. (1979). Infant–mother attachment in patients with non-organic failure to thrive syndrome. *Journal of the American Academy of Child Psychiatry, 18,* 251–259.

Green, W. H., Campbell, M., & David, R. (1984). Psychosocial dwarfism: A critical review of the evidence. *Journal of the American Academy of Child Psychiatry, 23,* 39–48.

Griffin, J. B., Jr. (1977). Rumination in a 7-year-old child. *Southern Medical Journal, 70,* 243–245.

Guilhaume, A., Benoit, O., Gourmelen, M., & Richardet, J. M. (1982). Relationship between sleep stage IV deficit and reversible HGH deficiency in psychosocial dwarfism. *Pediatric Research, 16,* 299–303.

Halsted, J. A. (1968). Geophagia in man: Its nature and nutritional effects. *American Journal of Clinical Nutrition, 21,* 1384–1393.

Hawass, N. E. D., Alnozha, M. M., & Kolawole, T. (1987). *Tropical and Geographical Medicine, 39,* 191–195.

Herbst, J., Friedland, G. W., & Zboralske, F. F. (1971). Hiatal hernia and "rumination" in infants and children. *Journal of Pediatrics, 78,* 261–265.

Hogg, J. (1982). Reduction of self-induced vomiting in a multiply handicapped girl by "lemon juice therapy" and concomitant changes in social behaviour. *British Journal of Clinical Psychology, 21,* 227–228.

Hollowell, J. G., & Gardner, L. I. (1965). Rumination and growth failure in male fraternal twin: Association with disturbed family environment. *Pediatrics, 36,* 565–571.

Holmes, G. L. (1979). Evaluation and prognosis in nonorganic failure to thrive. *Southern Medical Journal, 72,* 693–695.

Holvoet, J. F. (1982). The etiology and management of rumination and psychogenic vomiting: A review. In J. H. Hollis & C. E. Meyers (Eds.), *Life threatening behavior: Analysis and intervention* (pp. 29–77). Washington, DC: American Association on Mental Deficiency.

Humphrey, F. J., II, Mayes, S. D., Bixler, E. O., & Good, C. (1989). Variables associated with frequency of rumination in a boy with profound mental retardation. *Journal of Autism and Developmental Disorders, 19,* 435–447.

Iwata, B. A., Dorsey, M. F., Slifer, K. J., Bauman, K. E., & Richman, G. S. (1982). Toward a functional analysis of self-injury. *Analysis and Intervention in Developmental Disabilities, 2,* 3–20.

Jackson, G. M., Johnson, C. R., Ackron, G. S., & Crowley, R. (1975). Food satiation as a procedure to decelerate vomiting. *American Journal of Mental Deficiency, 80,* 223–227.

Kaplan, H. I., & Sadock, B. J. (Eds.) (1985). *Comprehensive textbook of psychiatry* (4th ed.). Baltimore: Williams & Wilkins.

Keith, L., Rosenberg, C., Brown, E., & Webster, A. (1969). Amylophagia during pregnancy: A second look. *Chicago Medical School Quarterly, 28,* 109–114.

Kinnell, H. G. (1985). Pica as a feature of autism. *British Journal of Psychiatry, 147,* 80–82.

Kohlenberg, R. J. (1970). The punishment of persistent vomiting: A case study. *Journal of Applied Behavior Analysis, 3,* 241–245.

Kolandaivelu, G., & Balan, V. (1979). Pica. *Journal of the Indian Medical Association, 73,* 195–196.

Lang, P. J., & Melamed, B. G. (1969). Avoidance conditioning therapy of an infant with chronic ruminative vomiting. *Journal of Abnormal Psychology, 74,* 1–8.

Leibovich, M. A. (1973). Psychogenic vomiting. *Psychotherapy and Psychosomatics, 22,* 263–268.

Libby, D. G., & Phillips, E. (1979). Eliminating rumination behavior in a profoundly retarded adolescent: An exploratory study. *Mental Retardation, 17,* 94–95.

Linscheid, T. R., & Cunningham, C. E. (1977). A controlled demonstration of the effectiveness of electric shock in the elimination of chronic infant rumination. *Journal of Applied Behavior Analysis, 10,* 500.

Lobato, D., Carlson, E. I., & Barrera, R. D. (1986). Modified satiation reducing ruminative vomiting without excessive weight gain. *Applied Research in Mental Retardation, 7,* 337–347.

Lourie, R. S., Layman, E. M., & Millican, F. K. (1963). Why children eat things that are not food. *Children, 10,*143–146.

Luckey, R. E., Watson, C. M., & Musick, J. K. (1968). Aversive conditioning as a means of inhibiting vomiting and rumination. *American Journal of Mental Deficiency, 73,* 139–142.

Madden, N. A., Russo, D. C., & Cataldo, M. F. (1980). Behavioral treatment of pica in children with lead poisoning. *Child Behavior Therapy, 2*, 67–81.

Madison, L. S., & Adubato, S. A. (1984). The elimination of ruminative vomiting in a 15-month-old child with gastroesophageal reflux. *Journal of Pediatric Psychology, 9*, 231–239.

Marholin, D., II, Luiselli, J. K., Robinson, M., & Lott, I. T. (1980). Response-contingent taste-aversion in treating chronic ruminative vomiting of institutionalized profoundly retarded children. *Journal of Mental Deficiency Research, 24*, 47–56.

Matson, J. L., Stephens, R. M., & Smith, C. (1978). Treatment of self-injurious behaviour with overcorrection. *Journal of Mental Deficiency Research, 22*, 175–178.

Mayes, S. D. (1988, June). *Rumination Disorder: Diagnosis, treatment, and associated variables*. Paper presented at the annual meeting of the American Association on Mental Retardation, Washington, DC.

Mayes, S. D. (1989a). [Anxiety-related regurgitation]. Unpublished raw data.

Mayes, S. D. (1989b). [Pica]. Unpublished raw data.

Mayes, S. D., & Humphrey, F. J., II (1989). *Rumination disorder: Treatment*. Manuscript submitted for publication.

Mayes, S. D., Humphrey, F. J., II, Handford, H. A., & Mitchell, J. F. (1988). Rumination disorder: Differential diagnosis. *Journal of the American Academy of Child and Adolescent Psychiatry, 27*, 300–302.

McAlpine, C., & Singh, N. N. (1986). Pica in institutionalized mentally retarded persons. *Journal of Mental Deficiency Research, 30*, 171–178.

McKeegan, G. F., Estill, K., & Campbell, B. (1987). Elimination of rumination by controlled eating and differential reinforcement. *Journal of Behavior Therapy and Experimental Psychiatry, 18*, 143–148.

Menking, M., Wagnitz, J. G., Burton, J. J., Coddington, R. D., & Sotos, J. F. (1969). Rumination—A near fatal psychiatric disease of infancy. *New England Journal of Medicine, 280*, 802–804.

Mestre, J. R., Resnick, R. J., & Berman, W. F. (1983). Behavior modification in the treatment of rumination. *Clinical Pediatrics, 22*, 488–491.

Millican, F. K., Layman, E. M., Lourie, R. S., Takahashi, L. Y., & Dublin, C. C. (1962). The prevalence of ingestion and mouthing of nonedible substances by children. *Clinical Proceedings of Children's Hospital, Washington, D.C., 18*, 207–214.

Minness, P. M. (1980). Treatment of compulsive hand in mouth behaviour in a profoundly retarded child using a sharp pinch as the aversive stimulus. *Australian Journal of Developmental Disabilities, 6*, 5–10.

Mitchell, W. G., Gorrell, R. W., & Greenberg, R. A. (1980). Failure-to-thrive: A study in a primary care setting—Epidemiology and follow-up. *Pediatrics, 65*, 971–977.

Mokhobo, K. P. (1986). Iron deficiency anemia and pica. *South African Medical Journal, 70*, 473–475.

Money, J. (1977). The syndrome of abuse dwarfism (psychosocial dwarfism or reversible hyposomatotropism). *American Journal of Diseases of Children, 131*, 508–513.

Morgan, R. F. (1984). Pica. *Journal of the Royal Society of Medicine, 77*, 1052–1054.

Mulick, J. A., Barbour, R., Schroeder, S. R., & Rojahn, J. (1980). Overcorrection of pica in two profoundly retarded adults: Analysis of setting effects, stimulus, and response generalization. *Applied Research in Mental Retardation, 1*, 241–252.

Mulick, J. A., Schroeder, S. R., & Rojahn, J. (1980). Chronic ruminative vomiting: A comparison of four treatment procedures. *Journal of Autism and Developmental Disorders, 10*, 203–213.

Murray, M. E., Keele, D. K., & McCarver, J. W. (1976). Behavioral treatment of ruminations: A case study. *Clinical Pediatrics, 15*, 591–593, 596.

National Center for Health Statistics. (1978). *International classification of diseases—9th revision—clinical modification* (Vol. 1). Ann Arbor, MI: Commission on Professional and Hospital Activities.

Oates, R. K. (1977). The child who fails to thrive. *Medical Journal of Australia, 1,* 300–302.

Oates, R. K. (1984a). Similarities and differences between nonorganic failure to thrive and deprivation dwarfism. *Child Abuse and Neglect, 8,* 439–445.

Oates, R. K. (1984b). Non-organic failure to thrive. *Australian Paediatric Journal, 20,* 95–100.

O'Neil, P. M., White, J. L., King, C. R., Jr., & Carek, D. J. (1979). Controlling childhood rumination through differential reinforcement of other behavior. *Behavior Modification, 3,* 355–372.

O'Rourke, D. E., Quinn, J. G., Nicholson, J. O., & Gibson, H. H. (1967). Geophagia during pregnancy. *Obstetrics and Gynecology, 29,* 581–584.

Paniagua, F. A., Braverman, C., & Capriotti, R. M. (1986). Use of a treatment package in the management of a profoundly mentally retarded girl's pica and self-stimulation. *American Journal of Mental Deficiency, 90,* 550–557.

Pollitt, E., Eichler, A. W., & Chan, C. (1975). Psychosocial development and behavior of mothers of failure-to-thrive children. *American Journal of Orthopsychiatry, 45,* 525–537.

Posner, L. B., McCottry, C. M., & Posner, A. C. (1957). Pregnancy craving and pica. *Obstetrics and Gynecology, 9,* 270–272.

Pritchard, J. A., MacDonald, P. C., & Gant, N. F. (1985). *Williams obstetrics* (17th ed.). Norwalk, CT: Appleton-Century-Crofts.

Rast, J., Ellinger-Allen, J. A., & Johnston, J. M. (1985). Dietary management of rumination: Four case studies. *American Journal of Clinical Nutrition, 42,* 95–101.

Rast, J., & Johnston, J. M. (1986). Social versus dietary control of ruminating by mentally retarded persons. *American Journal of Mental Deficiency, 90,* 464–467.

Rast, J., Johnston, J. M., Allen, J. E., & Drum, C. (1985). Effects of nutritional and mechanical properties of food on ruminative behavior. *Journal of the Experimental Analysis of Behavior, 44,* 195–206.

Rast, J., Johnston, J. M., & Drum, C. (1984). A parametric analysis of the relationship between food quantity and rumination. *Journal of the Experimental Analysis of Behavior, 41,* 125–134.

Rast, J., Johnston, J. M., Drum, C., & Conrin, J. (1981). The relation of food quantity to rumination behavior. *Journal of Applied Behavior Analysis, 14,* 121–130.

Rast, J., Johnston, J. M., Lubin, D., & Ellinger-Allen, J. (1988). Effects of premeal chewing on ruminative behavior. *American Journal on Mental Retardation, 93,* 67–74.

Richmond, J. B., Eddy, E., & Green, M. (1958). Rumination: A psychosomatic syndrome of infancy. *Pediatrics, 22,* 49–55.

Rojahn, J. (1984). Self-injurious behavior in institutionalized, severely/profoundly retarded adults—Prevalence data and staff agreement. *Journal of Behavioral Assessment, 6,* 13–27.

Rosenn, D. W., Loeb, L. S., & Jura, M. B. (1980). Differentiation of organic from nonorganic failure to thrive syndrome in infancy. *Pediatrics, 66,* 698–704.

Sajwaj, T., Libet, J., & Agras, S. (1974). Lemon-juice therapy: The control of life-threatening rumination in a six-month-old infant. *Journal of Applied Behavior Analysis, 7,* 557–563.

Sauvage, D., Leddet, I., Hameury, L., & Barthelemy, C. (1985). Infantile rumination: Diagnosis and follow-up study of twenty cases. *Journal of the American Academy of Child Psychiatry, 24,* 197–203.

Sayers, G., Lipschitz, D. A., Sayers, M., Seftel, H. C., Bothwell, T. H., & Charlton, R. W. (1974). Relationship between pica and iron nutrition in Johannesburg black adults. *South African Medical Journal, 48,* 1655–1660.

Sayetta, R. B. (1986). Pica: An overview. *American Family Physician, 33,* 181–185.

Severance, H. W., Jr., Holt, T., Patrone, N. A., & Chapman, L. (1988). Profound muscle weakness and hypokalemia due to clay ingestion. *Southern Medical Journal, 81,* 272–274.

Shaheen, E., Alexander, D., Truskowsky, M., & Barbero, G. J. (1968). Failure to thrive—A retrospectrive profile. *Clinical Pediatrics, 7,* 255–260.

Sheagren, T. G., Mangurten, H. H., Brea, F., & Lutostanski, S. (1980). Rumination—A new complication of neonatal intensive care. *Pediatrics, 66,* 551–555.

Sheinbein, M. (1975). Treatment for the hospitalized infantile ruminator: Programmed brief social behavior reinforcers. *Clinical Pediatrics, 14,* 719–721, 724.

Sills, R. H. (1978). Failure to thrive: The role of clinical and laboratory evaluation. *American Journal of Diseases of Children, 132,* 967–969.

Simpson, R. L., & Sasso, G. M. (1978). The modification of rumination in a severely emotionally disturbed child through an overcorrection procedure. *American Association for the Education of the Severely-Profoundly Handicapped Review, 3,* 145–150.

Singer, L. (1987). Long-term hospitalization of nonorganic failure-to-thrive infants: Patient characteristics and hospital course. *Developmental and Behavioral Pediatrics, 8,* 25–31.

Singh, N. N., & Bakker, L. W. (1984). Suppression of pica by overcorrection and physical restraint: A comparative analysis. *Journal of Autism and Developmental Disorders, 14,* 331–341.

Singh, N. N., Manning, P. J., & Angell, M. J. (1982). Effects of an oral hygiene punishment procedure on chronic rumination and collateral behaviors in monozygous twins. *Journal of Applied Behavior Analysis, 15,* 309–314.

Singh, N. N., & Winton, A. S. W. (1984). Effects of a screening procedure on pica and collateral behaviors. *Journal of Behavior Therapy and Experimental Psychiatry, 15,* 59–65.

Singhi, S., & Singhi, P. (1982a). Pica: Not a solitary problem! *Indian Pediatrics, 19,* 615–618.

Singhi, P., & Singhi, S. (1982b). Pica type of "nonfood" articles eaten by Ajmer children and their significance. *Indian Journal of Pediatrics, 49,* 681–684.

Singhi, P., & Singhi, S. (1983). Nutritional status and psycho-social stress in children with pica. *Indian Pediatrics, 20,* 345–349.

Singhi, S., Singhi, P., & Adwani, G. B. (1981). Role of psychosocial stress in the cause of pica. *Clinical Pediatrics, 20,* 783–785.

Skuse, D. H. (1985). Non-organic failure to thrive: A reappraisal. *Archives of Disease in Childhood, 60,* 173–178.

Smith, D. W., & Lyon, R. (1976). Eliminating vomiting behavior in a profoundly retarded resident. *Research and the Retarded, 3,* 24–27.

Spergel, S. M. (1975). Induced vomiting treatment of acute compulsive vomiting. *Journal of Behavior Therapy and Experimental Psychiatry, 6,* 85–86.

Starin, S. P., & Fuqua, R. W. (1987). Rumination and vomiting in the developmentally disabled: A critical review of the behavioral, medical, and psychiatric treatment research. *Research in Developmental Disabilities, 8,* 575–605.

Stein, M. L., Rausen, A. R., & Blau, A. (1959). Psychotherapy of an infant with rumination. *Journal of the American Medical Association, 171,* 2309–2312.

Tibbits-Kleber, A. L., & Howell, R. J. (1985). Reactive attachment disorder of infancy (RAD). *Journal of Clinical Child Psychology, 14,* 304–310.

Tierney, D., & Jackson, H. J. (1984). Psychosocial treatments of rumination disorder: A review of the literature. *Australia and New Zealand Journal of Developmental Disabilities, 10,* 81–112.

Toister, R. P., Condron, C. J., Worley, L., & Arthur, D. (1975). Faradic therapy of chronic vomiting in infancy: A case study. *Journal of Behavior Therapy and Experimental Psychiatry, 6,* 55–59.

Vermeer, D. E., & Frate, D. A. (1979). Geophagia in rural Mississippi: Environmental and cultural contexts and nutritional implications. *American Journal of Clinical Nutrition, 32,* 2129–2135.

Watkins, J. T. (1972). Treatment of chronic vomiting and extreme emaciation by an aversive stimulus: Case study. *Psychological Reports, 31,* 803–805.

White, J. C., Jr., & Taylor, D. J. (1967). Noxious conditioning as a treatment for rumination. *Mental Retardation, 5,* 30–33.

Whitehead, W. E., Drescher, V. M., Morrill-Corbin, E., & Cataldo, M. F. (1985). Rumination syndrome in children treated by increased holding. *Journal of Pediatric Gastroenterology and Nutrition, 4,* 550–556.

Winton, A. S. W., & Singh, N. N. (1983a). Rumination in pediatric populations: A behavioral analysis. *Journal of the American Academy of Child Psychiatry, 22,* 269–275.

Winton, A. S. W., & Singh, N. N. (1983b). Supression of pica using brief-duration physical restraint. *Journal of Mental Deficiency Research, 27,* 93–103.

Woolston, J. L. (1983). Eating disorders in infancy and early childhood. *Journal of the American Academy of Child Psychiatry, 22,* 114–121.

Wortis, H., Rue, R., Heimer, C., Braine, M., Redlo, M., & Freedman, A. M. (1962). Children who eat noxious substances. *Journal of the American Academy of Child Psychiatry, 1,* 536–547.

Wright, D. F., Brown, R. A., & Andrews, M. E. (1978). Remission of chronic ruminative vomiting through a reversal of social contingencies. *Behaviour Research and Therapy, 16,* 134–136.

Wright, M. M., & Menolascino, F. J. (1970). Rumination, mental retardation, and interventive therapeutic nursing. In F. J. Menolascino (Ed.), *Psychiatric approaches to mental retardation* (pp. 205–223). New York: Basic Books.

Wright, L., & Thalassinos, P. A. (1973). Success with electroshock in habitual vomiting: Report of two cases in young children. *Clinical Pediatrics, 12,* 594–597.

CHAPTER 8

Critical Appraisal of the DSM-III-R Diagnostic Criteria for Eating Disorders

David M. Garner
Christine L. Shafer
Lionel W. Rosen
Michigan State University

This chapter reviews the history of classification schemes for anorexia nervosa and bulimia nervosa and then critically evaluates the current diagnostic criteria for both of these disorders with special attention to potential points of controversy. Based on this evaluation, specific recommendations are made for revision to the DSM-III-R (American Psychiatric Association [APA], 1987) diagnostic criteria for the eating disorders. Finally, the range of assessment strategies for measuring eating disorder symptoms, as well as those for determining a diagnosis, are presented.

There are a number of levels at which diagnostic issues are relevant to both the researcher and the clinician. At the most basic level, a clear operational definition leads to a shared observational base that is vital in research, teaching, and clinical practice with eating disorders. Criteria should be neither so restrictive as to exclude cases that may not be prototypical but share essential features nor so broad as to include cases that do not meet a clinically meaningful threshold of severity. At the most sophisticated level, diagnostic schemes reflect the elucidation of etiology that then guides specific interventions. The eating disorder field has not yet achieved this standard; however, recent refinements indicate progress in isolating potential subgroups of eating disorders.

HISTORICAL BACKGROUND

Anorexia Nervosa

Anorexia nervosa has been part of the psychiatric nomenclature for many years but was considered a curious and rare disorder until the relatively recent and dramatic surge in clinical and research reports describing what appears to be a growing problem among young women. Anorexia nervosa has been identified in young children; however, the consensus is that it is very rare in this age group (Jaffe & Singer, 1989). When it is identified in children, the diagnosis is rendered in the same manner as with adults. Although most researchers concur that there has been an actual increased incidence in anorexia nervosa, there are some who favor the view that the base rates have been stable over the last several decades (Lucas, Beard, O'Fallon, & Kurland, 1988). Russell (1985) suggested that the form, expression, or motivational factors underlying anorexia nervosa actually may have evolved over the years so that the modern syndrome may be characteristically different from that which occurred in the past. This view is consistent with that of medical historians who have observed that psychiatric disorders can transform over time (Hare, 1981).

The early description of anorexia nervosa by Morton in 1689, as well as those by Gull and by Lasegue, both in 1873, are remarkably consistent with the current understanding of the disorder as a distinct psychological entity (cf. Beumont, Al-Alami, & Touyz, 1987). Since these initial descriptions, there has been considerable controversy regarding whether anorexia nervosa represents a discrete psychological disorder or simply a manifestation of other illnesses (cf. Garfinkel & Garner, 1982). By misdiagnosing cases of pituitary insufficiency as anorexia nervosa, Simmonds (1914) prompted almost 20 years of diagnostic confusion. The 1940s brought a renewed awareness of anorexia nervosa as a psychological disorder. Nevertheless, there has been continued debate regarding whether anorexia nervosa is a distinct diagnostic entity or simply a manifestation of other psychological disorders. Anorexia nervosa has been considered a variant or subtype of other syndromes such as affective disorder, schizophrenia, obsessional disorder, and "hysteria." These formulations have been understandable, because anorexia nervosa shares symptoms with each of these disorders; however, in recent years there has been a growing recognition of the eating disorders as discrete clinical entities that may be differentiated from other psychological disturbances (Russell, 1978; Szmukler, 1987).

TABLE 8.1
Russell's Criteria for Anorexia Nervosa and Bulimia Nervosa

Criteria for Anorexia Nervosa[a]

1. The patient's behavior leads to a marked loss of body weight.
2. There is an endocrine disorder which manifests itself clinically by cessation of menstruation in females. (In males the equivalent symptom is loss of sexual appetite.)
3. There is a psychopathology characterized by a morbid fear of becoming fat.

Criteria for Bulimia Nervosa[b]

1. The patients suffer from powerful and intractable urges to overeat.
2. They seek to avoid the "fattening" effects of food by inducing vomiting or abusing laxatives or both.
3. They have a morbid fear of becoming fat.

Criteria for Bulimia Nervosa[c]

1. Preoccupations with food, irresistible cravings for food, and repeated episodes of overeating.
2. Devices aimed at countering the "fattening effects" of food.
3. A psychopathology resembling that of classical anorexia nervosa.
4. A previous or cryptic episode of anorexia nervosa.

[a]From "Anorexia Nervosa: Its Identity as an Illness and its Treatment" by G. F. M. Russell, 1970, in J. H. Price (Ed.), *Modern Trends in Psychological Medicine* (Vol. 2, pp. 131–164), London: Butterworths.

[b]From "Bulimia Nervosa: An Ominous Variant of Anorexia Nervosa" by G. F. M. Russell, 1979, *Psychological Medicine, 9*, pp. 429–448.

[c]From "Anorexia Nervosa and Bulimia Nervosa" by G. F. M. Russell, 1983, in G. F. M. Russell & L. Hersov (Eds.), *Handbook of Psychiatry, Vol. 4: The Neuroses and Personality Disorders* (pp. 285–298), Cambridge: Cambridge University Press.

TABLE 8.2a
DSM-III Diagnostic Criteria for Anorexia Nervosa

A. Intense fear of becoming obese, which does not diminish as weight loss progresses.
B. Disturbance in body image, e.g., claiming to "feel fat" even when emaciated.
C. Weight loss of at least 25% of original body weight or, if under 18 years of age, weight loss from original body weight plus projected weight gain from growth charts may be combined to make the 25%.
D. Refusal to maintain body weight over a minimum normal weight for age and height.
E. No known physical illness that would account for the weight loss.

Note. From *Diagnostic and Statistical Manual of Mental Disorders* (3rd ed., p. 69) by American Psychiatric Association, 1980, Washington, DC: Author.

Although there have been differences among the various diagnostic criteria that have emerged over the past 20 years (cf. Garner & Garfinkel, 1988), most have included some variation of the triad of symptoms originally described by Russell (1970) and reproduced in Table 8.1. Other specific criteria for anorexia nervosa have been advanced, including those by Dally (1969), Feighner et al. (1972), Garrow et al. (1975), ICD-10 (1987), Norris (1979), and Rollins and Piazza (1978). The current DSM-III-R criteria for anorexia nervosa (APA, 1987) differ remarkably from those proposed in 1980 (APA, 1980; Table 8.2a). There have been certain points on which the various diagnostic criteria have offered different perspectives, and these are addressed later in the review of the literature related to the DSM-III-R criteria.

Bulimia Nervosa

Over the years, there have been isolated reports of patients who present with uncontrollable bouts of overeating usually followed by behaviors designed to diminish the calorific effects of the binge (Casper, 1983). Typically, this behavior occurred in connection with anorexia nervosa; however, there have been cases reported in connection with obesity (Loro & Orleans, 1981; Stunkard, 1959) and other disorders (cf. Blinder

TABLE 8.2b
DSM-III Diagnostic Criteria for Bulimia

A. Recurrent episodes of binge eating (rapid consumption of a large amount of food in a discrete period of time, usually less than two hours).
B. At least three of the following:
   1. Consumption of high caloric, easily ingested food during a binge.
   2. Inconspicuous eating during a binge.
   3. Termination of such eating episodes by abdominal pain, sleep, social interruption, or self-induced vomiting.
   4. Repeated attempts to lose weight by severely restrictive diets, self-induced vomiting, or use of cathartics or diuretics.
   5. Frequent weight fluctuations greater than 10 pounds due to alternating binges and fasts.
C. Awareness that the eating pattern is abnormal and a fear of not being able to stop eating voluntarily.
D. Depressed mood and self-deprecating thoughts following eating binges.
E. The bulimic episodes are not due to anorexia nervosa or any known physical disorder.

Note. From *Diagnostic and Statistical Manual of Mental Disorders* (3rd ed., rev., pp. 68–69) by American Psychiatric Association, 1987, Washington, DC: Author.

& Cadenhead, 1986). It is only in the last decade that bulimia nervosa has been regarded as a distinct syndrome (Blinder & Cadenhead, 1986; Casper, 1983; Halmi, 1983; Johnson & Connors, 1987), although Beumont (1988) argued recently against acceptance of it as a discrete clinical entity. Epidemiological reports have confirmed that the syndrome of bulimia nervosa is probably more common than anorexia nervosa, and it may be a growing problem among young women. As with anorexia nervosa, bulimia nervosa has been identified in young children; however, most cases lack core diagnostic features and meet the diagnostic criteria for atypical eating disorders (Jaffe & Singer, 1989). Various names for the disorder were proposed in early reports, including *the bulimic syndrome* (Mitchell & Pyle, 1982), *bulimarexia* (Boskind-Lodahl, 1976), the *dietary chaos syndrome* (Palmer, 1979), *the abnormal–normal weight control syndrome* (Crisp, 1980), and *bulimia* (APA, 1980). With the DSM-III-R, however, there appears to be agreement to accept Russell's (1979) original term, *bulimia nervosa,* into the psychiatric nomenclature. As indicated in Table 8.1, Russell's (1979) original diagnostic criteria, as well as the modifications suggested in 1983, are succinct and do capture the essential features.

The original DSM-III criteria (APA, 1980; Table 8.2b) were criticized as being ambiguous, overinclusive, and little more than a description of binge-eating (Fairburn & Garner, 1986; Halmi, 1985), and this has been empirically confirmed (Ben-Tovim, 1988). They failed to differentiate individuals who present simply with the *symptom* of bulimia from those who manifest the full *syndrome,* a criticism that has largely been ameliorated with the introduction of the DSM-III-R criteria (APA, 1987).

Considerable debate has centered on the relationship between bulimia nervosa and depression (Pope & Hudson, 1988; Strober & Katz, 1988; Wilson & Lindholm, 1987). Pope and Hudson (1988) argued that bulimia nervosa is a variant of depression based on evidence that the eating disorder patients exhibit: (a) a high prevalence of depression, (b) a family history of depression, (c) biological markers of depression, and (d) a positive response to antidepressant medications. Detractors from this view argue that "recent attempts to link eating disorders more specifically to affective disorders are premature and have overlooked various noncausal interpretations of their apparent association" (Strober & Katz, 1988, p. 100).

More recent controversy has surrounded the relationship between bulimia nervosa and personality disorders. Some have suggested that personality disorders are overrepresented among bulimia nervosa patients (Johnson, Tobin, & Enright, 1989; Levin & Hyler, 1986; Piran,

Lerner, Garfinkel, Kennedy, & Brouilette, 1988). Others have maintained that the disturbances observed in these patients often reflect secondary elaborations resulting from chaotic eating patterns rather than stable personality attributes (Garner, Olmsted, Davis, et al., 1990; Pope, Frankenburg, Hudson, Jonas, & Yurgelun-Todd, 1987).

In summary, compared to anorexia nervosa, bulimia nervosa has a short history as part of the psychiatric nomenclature. Nevertheless, it has generated active debate regarding the essential requirements for diagnosis, and recent proposals have refined the initial criteria proposed by the DSM-III.

DEFINITIONAL ISSUES: ANOREXIA NERVOSA

The DSM-III-R criteria for anorexia nervosa (APA, 1987) listed in Table 8.3 are presented here in italics; each is followed by a selective review of literature related to its merits. Based on these reviews, recommendations are made for either retaining or changing the existing DSM-III-R criteria. These are summarized in Table 8.3.

A. Refusal to maintain body weight over a minimal normal weight for age and height, e.g., weight loss leading to maintenance of body weight 15% below that expected; or failure to make expected weight gain during a period of growth, leading to body weight 15% below that expected.

Different diagnostic criteria for anorexia nervosa have varied considerably in the amount of weight loss required, if any, and the frame of reference used for measuring weight loss. Dally (1969) specified weight loss of at least 10% of *previous* body weight, whereas Feighner and colleagues (1972) required a 25% loss. Rollins and Piazza (1978) designated 20% weight loss or weight loss to 80% of expectation for age and height. In order to include younger patients who prohibit normal growth by restricting their food intake, the DSM-III and DSM-III-R have stipulated either weight loss or the failure to make *expected* weight. The 1987 ICD-10 (1987) requires a Body Mass Index of 16 or less. Some criteria require weight loss without stipulating any quantitative value (Fairburn & Garner, 1986; Russell, 1970), whereas Norris (1979) did not include weight loss for a diagnosis of anorexia nervosa.

The DSM-III-R Criterion A represents a departure from the earlier DSM-III criteria, which specified a *weight loss* of 25% of original body weight. The revision has a number of advantages. First, the weight loss of 25% is rather extreme and would preclude a positive diagnosis of clear cases that are rather early in their course. Furthermore, in the

TABLE 8.3
DSM-III-R Criteria for Anorexia Nervosa and Recommended Revisions

DSM-III-R Diagnostic Criteria for Anorexia Nervosa[a]

A. Refusal to maintain body weight over a minimal weight for age and height, e.g., weight loss leading to maintenance of body weight 15% below that expected; or failure to make expected weight gain during a period of growth, leading to body weight 15% below that expected.
B. Intense fear of gaining weight or becoming fat, even though underweight.
C. Disturbance in the way in which one's body weight, size, or shape is experienced, e.g., the person claims to "feel fat" even when emaciated, believes that one area of the body is "too fat" even when obviously underweight.
D. In females, absence of at least three consecutive menstrual cycles when otherwise expected to occur (primary or secondary amenorrhea). (A woman is considered to have amenorrhea if her periods occur only following hormone, e.g., estrogen administration.)

Recommended Diagnostic Criteria for Anorexia Nervosa

A. Refusal to maintain body weight over a minimal normal weight for age and height, e.g., weight loss leading to maintenance of body weight 15% below that expected; or failure to make expected weight gain during a period of growth, leading to body weight 15% below that expected.
B. Disturbance in the way in which one's body weight, size, or shape is experienced. This may take the form of extreme concerns about body weight or shape or distorted beliefs or perceptions related to weight, shape, or size (e.g., intense fear of gaining weight or becoming fat, even though underweight; the person claims to "feel fat" even when emaciated or believes that one area of the body is "too fat" even when obviously underweight; weight or body shape are used as the sole or predominant criterion for self-evaluation).
C. Behavior designed to control body weight. The person regularly engages in either self-induced vomiting, use of laxatives or diuretics, strict dieting or fasting, or vigorous exercise in order to lose weight or prevent weight gain.

Bulimic Subtype: When the individual experiences recurrent episodes of binge eating (binge eating is defined by the consumption of an amount of food that the individual considers excessive and is accompanied by feelings of loss of control) *and* when this is followed by self-induced vomiting or laxative abuse at least once a month for the past three months, then a diagnosis of anorexia nervosa, bulimia subtype is given.

Restrictor Subtype: Anorexia nervosa patients who fail to meet the bulimic subtype diagnosis are given a diagnosis of restrictor subtype.

[a]DSM-III-R diagnostic criteria for Anorexia Nervosa from *Diagnostic and Statistical Manual of Mental Disorders* (3rd ed., rev., pp. 68–69) by the American Psychiatric Association, 1987, Washington, DC: Author.

earlier standard there were two separate criteria related to weight that have been modified and consolidated in the DSM-III-R. Finally, the DSM-III-R weight criterion reflects sensitivity to the clinical observation that younger patients may not lose body weight but may simply interrupt gaining at the expected rate during a period of growth.

There is a major problem with this criterion as it stands, because it may be overly lenient in that "expected weights" are typically derived from population mean weights with considerable variation around this index of central tendency. It is not known what proportion of young individuals lose and then maintain a body weight that is more than 15% below the statistical average through normal dieting. On the other hand, there is no consensus regarding whether body weight should fall below a certain point or how much weight should be lost before there are serious medical consequences or secondary symptoms related to starvation (Pirke & Ploog, 1987). Thus, the specificity of the DSM-III-R weight criterion adds an apparent precision but actually includes so many individuals who fall within the normal distribution of body weights in the population that it is of limited value. It may be argued that Russell's (1970) simple requirement of the patient's behavior leading to "marked weight loss" is just as informative, because it is unlikely that patients presenting for a diagnosis of anorexia nervosa would meet all other criteria but be excluded by Criterion A as it is currently worded. Nevertheless, in our view, the more liberal nature of Criterion A does not present serious problems, and there are not adequate data on which to make recommendations for change (Table 8.3).

B. Intense fear of gaining weight or becoming fat, even though underweight.

This criterion is similar to that proposed by Russell (1970) requiring that "there is a psychopathology characterized by a morbid fear of becoming fat" (Table 8.1). Perhaps the most conspicuous problem with Criterion B is that it overlaps considerably with Criterion C. It is our view that these two criteria should be combined in the interests of simplicity and in the absence of convincing data justifying their distinction. With this recommendation in mind, the conceptual and empirical merits of both criteria are discussed in the following section.

C. Disturbance in the way in which one's body weight, size, or shape is experienced, e.g., the person claims to "feel fat" even when emaciated, believes that one area of the body is "too fat" even when obviously underweight.

It is evident from clinical descriptions representing very different orientations (e.g., Bruch, 1982; Crisp, 1980; Goodsitt, 1985; Russell, 1970) that concerns about body weight, size, and shape are central to anorexia nervosa and, as is argued later, to bulimia nervosa. Their importance is amplified by the fact that they are not integral to, or even associated with, most psychiatric syndromes and, in this sense, have been described as "distinct or core psychopathology" for the eating disorders (Fairburn, 1987; Fairburn & Garner, 1986; Russell, 1979). Although virtually all of the recent sets of diagnostic criteria refer to these characteristic extreme concerns about weight, there are striking differences in the descriptions used to define this area of psychopathology (Fairburn & Garner, 1988). Nevertheless, the clinical significance of these attitudes and fears has been confirmed by research findings demonstrating that anorexia nervosa patients report extreme concerns about weight and shape on relevant scales of various standardized self-report measures (Garner & Garfinkel, 1979; Garner & Olmsted, 1984; Slade, 1973) and structured interviews (Cooper & Fairburn, 1987; Palmer, Christie, Cordle, Davies, & Kenrick, 1987).

The *experience* of size, weight, or shape may include aberrations in perceptions, attitudes, or feelings. It could be argued that Criterion B refers to the more emotional aspects of disturbed bodily awareness, in contrast to more attitudinal or perceptual aspects connoted in Criterion C. There has been research indicating that subjects may respond differently when asked to respond to the way that they feel versus the way that they think about their body (Thompson, Dolce, Spana, & Register, 1987); however, it remains uncertain whether this is a semantic or a fundamental distinction.

One of the most noteworthy and perhaps controversial aspects of the DSM-III-R criteria for anorexia nervosa is that they do not include the term *body image disturbance,* as did the 1980 version of the DSM-III (Table 8.2b). This may be due to studies that have operationally defined the body image construct in terms of size overestimation and found that there are some anorexic patients who do not overestimate their own size and that overestimation is not unique to those with the disorder (Hsu, 1982). It has been argued that it may be premature to dismiss size estimation as an operational measure of body image, because it may have different meaning and prognostic significance for eating disorder patients and controls (cf. Garner, Garfinkel, & Bonatto, 1987). Current operational measures of body image, when taken alone, appear to have little diagnostic value.

Criteria B and C avoid the ambiguity associated with the term *body image* and appear to favor the affective and attitudinal dimensions of body dissatisfaction, which have also been described as representing forms of body image disturbance (Garner & Garfinkel, 1981). Although it has been argued largely on a priori grounds, several authors have emphasized the central role of body dissatisfaction in the development and maintenance of anorexia nervosa (Bruch, 1962, 1973; Casper, 1982;

Garner & Bemis, 1982; Slade, 1982). Despite its theoretical appeal, there has been surprisingly little systematic research on the role of body dissatisfaction in anorexia nervosa. Several standardized measures have been introduced for assessing this construct in eating disorders (Cooper, Taylor, Cooper, & Fairburn, 1987; Garner, Olmsted, & Polivy, 1983; Slade & Dewey, 1986); however, the specificity argument applies to this construct as well as size estimation, because body dissatisfaction is very common in those without formal eating disorders (Garner, Olmsted, Polivy, & Garfinkel, 1984; Huon, Brown, & Morris, 1988; Lindholm & Wilson, 1988). Lindholm and Wilson (1988) reported that eating disorder subjects were different from nondieters, but they were similar to dieters on both self-estimation and body dissatisfaction tasks. Huon et al. (1988) found that "dieting when already thin" and "intense fear of gaining 2 to 3 pounds" were viewed as neither uncommon nor abnormal in a survey of adult men and women. Thus, these and associated concerns about weight and shape may be relatively common among members of the general public, and research is needed to determine qualitative or quantitative features specific to eating disorders. Perhaps the way that these concerns have been stated underemphasizes their extreme nature among those with clinical eating disorders. On clinical grounds, it has been suggested that it is the anorexia nervosa patient's use of weight or shape as the sole or the predominant criterion for judging self-worth is distinctive (Garner & Bemis, 1982). This connection between shape and self-evaluation is specifically rated on Cooper and Fairburn's (1987) structured clinical interview (the Eating Disorder Examination), and there is empirical support for clinical differences between eating disorder patients and dieters on this interview measure (Wilson & Smith, 1989). Even if the form that attitudes, feelings, or perceptions about weight or shape take may not be specific to eating disorders, it may be that their *intensity, as well as the specific behaviors that some may resort to in order to achieve their ends of weight loss*, distinguishes those with clinical eating disorders from the more benign intense dieter. In this regard, individual diagnostic criteria may not be necessarily weakened because they include those without the disorder (i.e., false positives), inasmuch as it may be assumed that other criteria will be exclusionary. It is disturbance in the way that the body is experienced *within the context of a weight below a healthy threshold* that is required for a diagnosis of anorexia nervosa. Either criterion alone is insufficient for a diagnosis.

In summary, in spite of the evidence that extreme concerns about weight and shape are common in nonclinical samples, the prevailing view still holds that disturbances in body experience are central if not pathognomonic for anorexia nervosa. They have diagnostic value because they exclude others who have achieved a low weight for reasons other than self-imposed starvation. It is our view that criteria B and C should be combined because of their conceptual overlap and because we are not aware of data that justify considering them separately (revised Criterion B, Table 8.3). Because of the similarity in the body shape and weight concerns for both anorexia nervosa and bulimia nervosa, the wording of the revised Criterion B in Table 8.3 has been modified to make it parallel to the relevant criterion for bulimia nervosa (as is presented later). Further discussion regarding the specificity and importance of this area of psychopathology is presented later in relation to Criterion E for bulimia nervosa.

D. In females, absence of at least three consecutive menstrual cycles when otherwise expected to occur (primary or secondary amenorrhea). (A woman is considered to have amenorrhea if her periods occur only following hormone, e.g., estrogen, administration.)

This requirement is a departure from the DSM-III criteria for anorexia nervosa, and it represents a return to earlier diagnostic schemes originally advocated by Dally (1969) and Russell (1970). It is based on the observation of amenorrhea as a common symptom and the findings in some studies that disturbances in hypothalamic-pituitary-gonadal axis depend only in part on weight or nutritional status. Russell (1977) summarized three possible causes of the hypothalamic dysfunction as follows: (a) weight loss "damages" the hypothalamus; (b) the mental disturbance, or those events which are considered of psychogenic importance ("psychic stress"), interfere with hypothalamic function; and (c) the endocrine manifestations and the psychopathological features are relatively independent expressions of a primary hypothalamic deficit of unknown etiology.

On the one hand, Criterion D does not really pose practical limitations, because few cases of anorexia nervosa present without primary or secondary amenorrhea. On the other hand, in the absence of evidence to suggest that this criterion demarcates a group with a distinctive natural history or response to treatment, no convincing case has been made for its retention (Fairburn & Garner, 1988). It is our recommendation that the requirement of amenorrhea be eliminated from the diagnostic criteria for anorexia nervosa (Table 8.3).

Other Issues in the Diagnosis of Anorexia Nervosa

There are several issues that should be addressed in considering possible revisions of the diagnostic criteria for anorexia nervosa. These include the relevance of specific behaviors designed to control weight as well as the merits of designating subtypes based on age, restricting or binging symptoms, and psychological features.

Specific Behaviors Designed to Produce Weight Loss. It is well recognized from most clinical descriptions of anorexia nervosa that the weight loss observed is a consequence of certain idiosyncratic behaviors, such as food avoidance, severe dieting, self-induced vomiting, abuse of purgatives, and excessive exercise. These behaviors are not required in most sets of diagnostic criteria and are not specified for the DSM-III-R. The requirement of "an intense fear of gaining weight or becoming fat" (Criterion B) separates anorexia nervosa from other physical, psychiatric, or social reasons for weight loss; however, it could be argued that the requirement of specific behaviors designed to produce weight loss would be desirable. First, in the absence of accepted criteria for measuring or quantifying the "intense fear of gaining weight or becoming fat," behavioral criteria allow clear differentiation of anorexia nervosa from other emotional disorders that may present with weight loss, such as depression and schizophrenia (Garfinkel, Garner, Kaplan, Rodin, & Kennedy, 1983). Furthermore, as is presented later, this approach would make the diagnostic criteria for anorexia nervosa more parallel to those for bulimia nervosa in which weight controlling behaviors are required. As illustrated in Table 8.3, our recommended revised Criterion C requires weight controlling behavior for a diagnosis of anorexia nervosa to be made.

Subtypes Based on Age. The most recent diagnostic criteria do not stipulate age requirements for anorexia nervosa; however, Dally (1969) specified age of onset between 11 and 35 years, and Feighner et al. (1972) required onset prior to 25. Norris (1979) was even more restrictive, with an age of onset between 13 and 15 years. Cases of adult onset are common, and there have been reports of clear cases in the elderly (Hsu & Zimmer, 1988; Kellett, Trimble, & Thorley, 1976; Launer, 1978). In the absence of evidence that the pathogenesis of pediatric cases is different from those who have adult onset, it may be premature to introduce specific age restrictions. Nevertheless, there is evidence that the response to treatment is different for pediatric and adult patient groups. A review of outcome studies in which the patient samples are predominately young indicates that recovery can be expected for between 75% and 85% of cases, with very few deaths. In older patient samples, most studies report recovery in only 35% to 50% of the cases (Garfinkel & Garner, 1932). It is not known whether these differential outcome rates reflect inherent distinctions in the age groups or simply that the older sample consists of the residual of young, recalcitrant patients.

There is also evidence that the treatment of choice may be different for adult and adolescent patients. It has been the clinical impression of some that family therapy is most beneficial in younger patients and individual therapy is preferred for older patients (Minuchin, Rosman, & Baker, 1978; Strober & Yager, 1985). In a controlled comparison of family and individual therapy for anorexia nervosa, Russell, Szmukler, Dare, and Eisler (1987) provided empirical support for this opinion. Although there may be some merit in considering distinguishing patients who are 14 years of age or younger from their older counterparts on the basis of response to treatment and provisional treatment of choice, we believe that this radical departure from the DSM-III-R criteria should await further research to determine if age distinguishes meaningful subgroups of anorexia nervosa patients.

Subtypes Based on Restricting/Binging Symptoms. A relatively convincing case can be made for distinguishing between anorexia nervosa patients who lose weight by rigidly restricting their food intake (restricting subtype) from those whose stringent attempts to limit intake are interrupted by episodes of binge eating (bulimic subtype). A number of studies have indicated that anorexia nervosa patients with the complication of bulimia tend to present at a heavier weight with more frequent premorbid and family obesity than restrictor patients (Garfinkel, Moldofsky, & Garner, 1980; Garner, Garfinkel, & O'Shaughnessy, 1985a; Strober, 1981). Bulimic anorexics also present with a consistently longer duration of illness than restrictors (Andersen, 1985; Garfinkel et al., 1980; Garner et al., 1985; Holmgren et al., 1983; Vandereycken & Pierloot, 1983). Of even greater significance, the bulimic anorexia nervosa patients report greater impulsivity, social/sexual activity, family dysfunction, depression, and generally more conspicuous emotional disturbance (Casper, Eckert, Halmi, Goldberg, & Davis, 1980; Garfinkel et al., 1980; Garner et al., 1985; Laessle, Wittchen, Fichter, & Pirke, 1989; Mickalide & Andersen, 1985; Strauss & Ryan, 1988; Strober, 1981; Strober, Salkin, Burroughs, & Morrell, 1982; Vandereycken & Pierloot, 1983). Whether the reported symptoms represent a fundamental disturbance or simply discomfort associated with bulimic behaviors is not known. Eckert, Halmi, Marchi, and Cohen (1987) indicated that many of the reported differences in overall psychopathology between restricting and bulimic groups disappear with hospital treatment.

The original recommendation for distinguishing between subtypes of anorexia nervosa patients based on very similar elements was proposed by Beumont, George, and Smart (1976), who advocated dividing anorexic patients into "dieters" and "vomiters" based on differences between the two groups on many of the dimensions previously indicated. Because approximately 20% of restricting patients also report vomiting (Garfinkel et al., 1980; Garner et al., 1985), it is evident that the dieting and vomiting subgroups proposed by Beumont and associates (1976) overlap with, but are not identical to, the binging and restricting subtypes. Unfortunately, the respective merit of these two systems has not received adequate attention in empirical studies. In later discussion related to bulimia nervosa, a case is made for placing greater diagnostic emphasis on purging rather than binging, and these same arguments could be applied to anorexia nervosa.

An option that is consistent with the evidence presented for distinguishing between bulimic and restricting subtypes is the proposal by Fairburn and Garner (1986), which specifies that the diagnosis of anorexia nervosa and bulimia nervosa should be based on the presence or absence of certain core features (see Table 8.4). According to this scheme, the diagnosis of bulimia nervosa should be made *irrespective of weight*, with the diagnosis of anorexia nervosa reserved for the restricting patients described earlier. In other words, the diagnosis of bulimia nervosa takes priority over, or trumps, that of anorexia nervosa. It is argued that this solution is preferable to the diagnostic distinction based solely on weight, because studies that have compared bulimic patients with different weights and weight histories have failed to find meaningful differences, whereas all of these bulimic groups tend to differ from the restricting anorexia nervosa patients (Andersen, 1985; Garner et al., 1985; Garner, Olmsted, & Garfinkel, 1985b; Laessle et al., 1989). Moreover, similar treatment strategies are recommended for interrupting the binging and associated pathogenic weight control behaviors, regardless of the patient's weight.

Although data from most studies support dividing patients into *restrictor* and *bulimic* subtypes, this nominal distinction may be a problematic oversimplification for several reasons. First, although studies

TABLE 8.4
Relationship Between the Principal Clinical Features of Anorexia Nervosa and Bulimia Nervosa

	Anorexia Nervosa	*Bulimia Nervosa*
Characteristic extreme concerns about shape and weight	+[a]	+
Behavior designed to control body weight	+	+
Episodes of bulimia	−[b]	+
Low weight according to population norms	+	+ or −

Note. From "The Diagnosis of Bulimia Nervosa" by C. G. Fairburn & D. M. Garner, 1986, *International Journal of Eating Disorders, 5*, 403–419.
[a] + present
[b] − *absent*

have indicated between-group differences on some variables, there is extraordinary variability *within* each of these subgroups on a wide range of demographic, clinical, and psychological dimensions (Garner et al., 1985). These two groups of patients tend to be more alike than different, and it is advisable to resist the inclination to draw specific psychological or dynamic inferences from the simple observation of binging or restricting behaviors. By far the most parsimonious interpretation of binging purports that it is a biologically mediated "normal" response to the caloric deprivation and is experienced by eating disorder patients as well as other who engage in less extreme dietary restraint (Garner, Rockert, Olmsted, Johnson, & Coscina, 1985; Polivy & Herman, 1985). Moreover, the same patients have been observed to move between these two subtypes at different points in time (Russell, 1979; Vandereycken & Pierloot, 1983).

In summary, there is merit in distinguishing between restricting and binging anorexia nervosa patients, and there are two reasonable options for doing so. The first is the more controversial alternative but one that is most consistent with existing data. It involves applying the term *bulimia nervosa* to all patients who binge, regardless of weight, and reserving the term *anorexia nervosa* for emaciated patients who do not experience episodes of binge eating (Fairburn & Garner, 1986; Garner & Fairburn, 1988). It could be argued that this approach does not emphasize sufficiently the importance of the complications associated with a low body weight; however, there may be theoretical and proctical advantages in thinking about both bulimia nervosa as well as anorexia nervosa as being associated with possible aberrations in body weight regulation (Garner & Fairburn, 1988; Russell, 1979).

Despite these arguments, we favor the second alternative, which involves preserving this distinction within the anorexia nervosa population as presently defined by the DSM-III-R by specifying restricting and bulimic subtypes for the disorder, because it requires the least change to the existing criteria. Thus, the criteria for anorexia nervosa should be changed in a manner that is similar to the recommendations of Halmi (1985) to stipulate bulimic and restrictor subtypes for a diagnosis of anorexia nervosa (see Table 8.3). It is specified that episodes of binge eating involve the consumption of an amount of food that the individual considers excessive *and* that is followed by self-induced vomiting or laxative abuse (this is consistent with the criteria for bulimia nervosa and is discussed fully later in this chapter). A minimum criterion for frequency has been recommended requiring binging and purging at least once a month for the past 3 months. This is an arbitrary frequency criterion and one that is quite "liberal" in the sense that it favors placing patients in the bulimic anorexic subgroup even though they binge at a frequency well below that required for a diagnosis of bulimia nervosa. This frequency criterion has a very different purpose from that used in diagnosing bulimia nervosa, where it is designed to exclude subclinical cases. In anorexia nervosa, it is aimed at ensuring that the restricting subgroup is relatively homogeneous so that it cannot be said to be characterized by the symptoms of binging and purging except as incidental behaviors.

Psychological Topologies. The DSM-III-R addresses the issue of primary diagnostic entities and personality with the multiaxial model, and this system seems to be as suitable for eating disorders as for others. Nevertheless, it is noteworthy that several prominent theorists have proposed subtypes of anorexia nervosa based on personality features (Dally, 1969; Janet, 1919). Perhaps the most elegant subtyping of anorexia nervosa would involve empirically derived or validated psychological profiles that would have significance in terms of the etiology, course, or treatment of the disorder. Strober (1983) was able to differentiate three subtypes of anorexia nervosa patients using the MMPI and cluster analysis methods. The Eating Disorder Inventory (EDI) was introduced with the specific aim of identifying subgroups of patients based on psychological features rather than simple behavioral symptoms (Garner et al., 1983; Garner & Olmsted, 1984). The EDI-2 adds three new subscales (Asceticism, Impulse Regulation, and Interpersonal Sensitivity) to the original instrument, and all of the subscales may be used to identify subgroups of patients on the basis on prominant psychological features (Garner, 1991). Despite the admirable goal of identifying psychological topologies of eating disorder patients, and some empirical support for the idea, there are not yet compelling data to support changes in existing criteria based on personality organization.

DEFINITIONAL ISSUES: BULIMIA NERVOSA

The original DSM-III (see Table 8.2b) criteria were published at a time when researchers and clinicians were just beginning to recognize that a significant number of patients without anorexia nervosa were presenting with a disorder involving recurrent episodes of binge eating. Perhaps because so little was known about the disorder at the time, the original diagnostic criteria proved inadequate (Halmi, 1985). The revised criteria of the DSM-III-R (APA, 1987) represented a major advancement over the original DSM-III; however, many key terms remain vague or undefined. The following sections review the scientific and theoretical issues pertaining to each of the revised criteria; the reader is encouraged to consult Pope, Hudson, Spitzer, and Williams (1988) for a detailed account of the rationale for the development of the revisions to the DSM-III.

A. Recurrent episodes of binge eating (rapid consumption of a large amount of food in a discrete period of time).

Although binge eating is the key symptom identifying bulimia nervosa, agreement has not been achieved regarding the definition, measurement, or relative significance of this behavior in the disorder. Criterion A identifies binge eating but leaves all key terms undefined. Although it is probably not the most controversial aspect of the current criterion, it is not clear why "rapid" consumption is required, and it is also not obvious what constitutes a rapid pace. The original DSM-III criteria suggested a time frame of "usually less than two hours," but this was dropped because the committee was not convinced that there should be any specific time limit to a binge (Pope et al., 1988). Certainly, it would be inconsistent with clinical wisdom to exclude a patient who meets all other elements of the criteria for bulimia nervosa but consumes large amounts of food at a more moderate pace, punctuated by episodes of vomiting.

The current specification of "discrete" episodes presents similar practical difficulties. For patients who binge and vomit more or less without interruption for prolonged periods, it is often virtually impossible for either the patient or the trained interviewer to determine when one "episode" stops and another begins. During these chaotic periods, the entire experience may be clouded by intense affect and mental stupor. We recommend deleting the words "rapid" and "discrete" from the diagnostic criteria for bulimia nervosa (Table 8.5). Although it could be argued that the existing criteria should be modified only if there is compelling empirical support for doing so, we believe that the initial inclusion of these terms lacked empirical justification and that they have continued to be a source of unnecessary confusion.

One of the most troublesome aspects of this criterion relates to the term *large* in specifying the amount of food required to define a binge. Delimiting a binge by amount eaten is complicated by potential estimation error and by the fact that the same food may have different connotations for different individuals or for the same individual over time. Nevertheless, several authors have attempted to provide objective standards by defining a binge as the consumption of more than 1,200 calories (Katzman & Wolchik, 1984) or 1,000 calories (Fairburn, 1987). This must be reconciled with the fact that it is not uncommon for a patient to view consuming even a small amount of food as a binge. Rosen, Leitenberg, Fisher, and Khazam (1986) reported that almost half of the episodes labeled as binges involved less than 1,000 calories and that there was no relationship between the amount of food eaten and the rating of

TABLE 8.5
DSM-III-R Diagnostic Criteria for Bulimia Nervosa and Recommended Revisions

DSM-III-R Diagnostic Criteria For Bulimia Nervosa[a]

A. Recurrent episodes of binge eating (rapid consumption of a large amount of food in a discrete period of time).
B. A feeling of lack of control over eating during the eating binges.
C. The person regularly engages in either self-induced vomiting, use of laxatives or diuretics, strict dieting or fasting, or vigorous exercise in order to prevent weight gain.
D. A minimum average of two binge eating episodes per week for at least three months.
E. Persistent overconcern with body weight and shape.

Recommended Revisions in the Criteria for Bulimia Nervosa

A. Recurrent episodes of binge eating (binge eating is defined by the consumption of an amount of food that the individual considers excessive and is accompanied by feelings of lack of control).
B. Behavior designed to control body weight. The individual engages in a minimum average of two purging episodes (i.e., self-induced vomiting or laxative abuse) per week for at least three months.
C. Disturbance in the way in which one's body weight, size, or shape is experienced. This may take the form of extreme concerns about body weight or shape or distorted beliefs or perceptions related to weight, shape, or size (e.g., intense fear of gaining weight or becoming fat, even though normal weight; intense fear of "being fat" even when normal weight, or the intense fear that one area of the body is "too fat" even if it is of normal size; weight or body shape are used as the sole or predominant criterion for self-evaluation).

[a]DSM-III-R diagnostic criteria for Bulimia Nervosa from *Diagnostic and Statistical Manual of Mental Disorders* (3rd ed., rev., pp. 65–69) by the American Psychiatric Association, 1987, Washington, DC: Author.

anxiety. Davis, Freeman, and Garner (1988) reported that the mean caloric intake of a binge was just over 1,300 calories, but there was substantial within-subjects variability, with average minimum and maximum caloric values of 669 and 2,327, respectively. Using the 7-day self-monitoring records of 32 bulimia nervosa patients, Rossiter and Agras (1990) found that the average binge amounted to about 1,200 calories and that 28% of the binge episodes consisted of fewer than 500 calories. Clearly, it is incongruous to define a binge as "large" if it constitutes fewer calories than are contained in a modest meal consisting of a hamburger and milk shake. In the absence of clear data indicating that there are fundamental differences in the nature of binges based on their size, we believe that the distinction between large and small binge episodes should be dropped from the diagnostic criteria for bulimia nervosa.

The basic questions remain as to who should define what constitutes a binge, the patient or the observer, and should this definition be quantitative or qualitative? Fairburn (1987) maintained that the binge should be defined in quantitative terms and that the interviewer should make this determination according to specific guidelines. Even with the added precision, the interviewer still has to base the judgment on "what might be the usual amount eaten under such circumstances" (Fairburn, 1987, p. 4). This normative approach has value but may not take into account the ordinary variation in eating experienced by many individuals (Lacey, Chadbund, Crisp, & Whitehead, 1978). Moreover, is the attempt at quantification of a binge really getting at the most important aspect of the behavior? It could be argued that the patient interpreting the consumption of an objectively *small* amounts of food as a binge might reflect even *greater* psychopathology (Criterion D) than if this label were reserved for larger amounts. The requirement of *objective binges* has posed a major diagnostic dilemma regarding the classification for patients who engage in self-induced vomiting or abuse laxatives after eating *small* amounts of food. These individuals often experience their behavior as a binge in that they feel that the amount of calories consumed is excessive and that their eating is out of control. Even if some of their eating episodes qualify as an objective binge and they are vomiting many times daily, they may fail to meet the frequency criterion of an average of two binge episodes a week (see Criterion D). These patients are currently relegated to the diagnosis of an *atypical eating disorder*, yet they closely resemble those who meet the current criteria related to binge eating.

Regardless of the amount of food used to define a bulimic episode, there are two features that almost invariably characterize the behavior. The individual regards the amount of food as excessive, and it is associated with a subjective sense of loss of control (as now covered in Criterion B of the DSM-III-R). Thus, it is our view that it is the quality of a binge rather than the quantity that makes the behavior distinctive. In the presence of rather convincing data indicating that a significant proportion of "binges" reported by bulimia nervosa patients involve small amounts of food, and in the absence of a compelling rationale for distinguishing between these experiences and those involving the consumption of over 1,000 calories, we recommend that the term *large* be dropped from Criterion A for bulimia nervosa (Table 8.5).

Vomiting and Laxative Abuse as Target Symptoms

Even with these modifications, there are both practical and theoretical reasons for targeting vomiting and laxative abuse, rather than binging, as key symptoms in the diagnosis of bulimia nervosa. First, on an entirely practical level, some of the problems attributed earlier to defining binge episodes do not apply to vomiting and laxative abuse, because they tend to be a more discrete events with distinct terminations. This has apparently prompted some investigators to stipulate vomiting, rather than binging, as the dependent variable of choice in treatment studies (cf. Garner, 1987; Garner, Fairburn, & Davis, 1987).

Secondly, on clinical grounds, it could be argued that the vomiting and laxative abuse, as well as other drastic weight-losing behaviors, are more closely tied to the psychopathology of the disorder than is binge eating. A number of investigators have emphasized that the reliance on self-induced vomiting perpetuates the disorder by keeping weight at a reduced level and by diminishing anxiety associated with consuming foods perceived as fattening (Garner et al., 1985; Rosen & Leitenberg, 1982; Rosen, Leitenberg, Gross, & Willmuth, 1985; Russell, 1979). This view was clearly summarized by Rosen and Leitenberg (1982) as follows:

> Binge eating and self-induced vomiting in bulimia nervosa seem to be linked in a vicious circle by anxiety. Vomiting is an escape response that is reinforced by the subsequent reduction in anxiety about weight . . . Binge eating usually only occurs in anticipation of vomiting, and binge eating becomes more severe as vomiting increases in frequency. In other words, binge eating in bulimia nervosa is more a consequence of vomiting than vomiting is a consequence of binge eating. (pp. 196–197)

In our view, the dominant role given to vomiting in this model is accurate, but we believe that it is incomplete without recognizing that bouts of overeating, increased hunger, and food preoccupations are biologically mediated by weight loss and dieting to maintain a suboptimal weight (Garner et al., 1985; Polivy & Herman, 1985; Russell, 1979; Wardle, 1980).

If drastic weight-control behaviors directly stem from the core psychopathology of bulimia nervosa, and the urge to engage in binge eating (which patients resist with varying degrees of success) may be explained as a *by-product* of chronic dieting, then it could be predicted that patients who gain temporary control over their binge eating but fail to curb their vomiting would be no better off over time than those who are binging *and* vomiting. This assumption is supported by follow-up data for 47 bulimia nervosa patients who participated in a comparative psychotherapy outcome study conducted at the University of Toronto (Garner, 1989). At the end of the treatment and at follow-up 1 year later, the frequencies of binging and vomiting were assessed by structured interview. Following 4 months of treatment, 9 patients had brought their binging under control but had failed to control their vomiting, 27 patients were binging and vomiting, 11 patients were abstinent from both of these symptoms, and no patients were binging without vomiting. As indicated in Table 8.6, all patients were assigned a good, moderate, or poor outcome status at follow-up based on binging and vomiting frequency. Those requiring further treatment during the follow-up period were assigned a poor outcome irrespective of symptom frequency. Although the sample size is small, it is evident that vomiting alone at the end of treatment confers just as poor a prognosis as binging *and* vomiting. These results conform to our clinical impressions with this subgroup of highly treatment-resistant patients who adopt what may be considered to be a "restricting anorexic stance" in that they suppress binging temporarily but continue to diet, vomit, and engage in other extreme weight-controlling behaviors. If dieting, vomiting, and other weight-controlling behaviors are truly tied to the core disturbance in bulimia nervosa, then the entire cluster of behavioral and attitudinal symptoms must be addressed for treatment to be successful.

Furthermore, there is convincing evidence that demarcating bulimia nervosa in terms of purging rather than binging defines a more homogenous subgroup of individuals who have a more severe form of the disorder. Willmuth, Leitenberg, Rosen, and Cado (1988) compared 20 purging and 20 nonpurging bulimics on a range of behavioral and psychological measures and found that the purging bulimics consumed less during a test meal, indicated greater anxiety while eating, and displayed greater disturbance on standardized body image and eating attitudes measures than the nonpurging bulimics. Although the non-

TABLE 8.6
What Happens to Patients Who Vomit But Do not Binge at the End of Treatment

Outcome at One year (Number of Episodes of Binging or Vomiting)	*Vomiting but not Binging (%) (N=9)*	*Binging and Vomiting (%) (N=27)*	*Not Binging or Vomiting (%) (N=11)*
Good (< 2)	1 (11%)	5 (19%)	8 (73%)
Moderate (2–7)	2 (22%)	5 (19%)	1 (9%)
Poor (> 7 or treatment required during follow-up)	6 (67%)	17 (63%)	2 (18%)

Note. Data from the Toronto comparative psychotherapy study, in *A Comparison Between Cognitive-behavioral and Psychodynamic Psychotherapy for Bulimia Nervosa* by D. M. Garner, June 1989, Oxford, England: World Congress of Cognitive Therapy. Six-month follow-up data were used for two patients on whom 1-year follow-up data were not available.

purging bulimics scored higher than normal on many of these measures, they were never significantly more maladjusted than the purging bulimics on any of the measures. Similar findings were reported by Prather and Williamson (1988), who compared 16 purging and 16 nonpurging bulimics on eating disorder symptom scales, the MMPI, the SCL-90R, and the Beck Depression Inventory (BDI). The purging bulimics had as high or higher mean scores on all measures of psychopathology, and the group differences were significant on the Eating Attitudes Test (EAT) and two MMPI scales.

Some researchers have examined both binging and vomiting as predictors of outcome, and the findings are less clear. A number of reports have failed to find a relationship between pretreatment levels of binging or vomiting and response to treatment (Abraham, Mira, & Llewellyn-Jones, 1983; Fairburn, Kirk, O'Connor, & Cooper, 1986; Hsu & Holder, 1986; Mitchell, Davis, Goff, & Pyle, 1986; Ordman & Kirschenbaum, 1985; Wooley & Kearney-Cook, 1986); however, two recent studies found binge frequency related to outcome (Garner et al. 1990; Mitchell, Fletcher, et al., 1989). Mitchell and associates (1989) followed 91 patients 2 to 5 years after treatment and reported that those in the worst outcome group had significantly higher levels of pretreatment binging and vomiting than those with the best outcome. The association between these symptoms was stronger for vomiting than binging: 57% of those in the treatment failure group were binge eating more than once a day at baseline compared to 26% in the best outcome group; 70% of those in the treatment failure group were vomiting several times a day compared to 32% of the best outcome group. Garner and colleagues (1990) found that bulimia nervosa patients with a poor outcome at the end of a 4-month treatment trial had an average pretreatment binge frequency that was almost twice as high as those with a poor outcome (M = 34.4, SD = 29.8 versus M = 16.3, SD = 14.6). Vomiting was not significantly related to outcome at the end of treatment, but a more recent analysis has indicated that it is a more potent predictor of outcome at 1 year than binging frequency (Garner, 1989). Thus, recent studies that have examined the symptoms of binging and vomiting, largely in patients who engage in both, indicate that these symptoms are related to outcome for the disorder. In the two studies that directly compared purging and nonpurging bulimic patients, the data were clear in indicating that the purging defined a more disturbed subgroup of patients. It can be concluded that defining the disorder of bulimia nervosa in terms of vomiting rather than binging would appear to enhance the homogeneity of the clinical entity.

Finally, the serious physical health consequences and metabolic abnormalities reported in bulimia nervosa are more directly related to the various pathogenic weight control methods than to binge eating

(Mitchell, Pomeroy, & Huber, 1988). In assessing the severity of the disorder, it would seem that vomiting would be a more meaningful index because of its relationship to these health risks. In questioning the validity of bulimia nervosa as a diagnostic entity, Beumont (1988) emphasized the need for the diagnostic formulation to highlight these potentially dangerous compensatory behaviors.

A final caveat is in order before concluding that purging behaviors uniformly define the clinical syndrome of bulimia nervosa. Olmsted and Garner (1986) found that most women selected from a nonclinical sample who report that they currently engaged in self-induced vomiting for weight control only superficially resembled bulimia nervosa patients. However, most of the women in subgroups that did not resemble clinical bulimia nervosa patients were vomiting relatively infrequently.

In summary, DSM-III-R Criterion A defines bulimia nervosa in terms of recurrent episodes of binge eating; however, there are serious concerns regarding the definition, measurement, and relative significance of this behavior. We have offered a rather protracted discussion of this criterion because of our view that there is merit in considering purging in addition to, (and perhaps in preference to) binging in defining the diagnostic entity under consideration. We fully recognize the theoretical problem that this solution poses; namely, how can a patient be assigned a diagnosis of bulimia nervosa in the possible absence of the symptom of bulimia? It would seem to contradict the pre-eminence of the behavior around which the disorder bulimia nervosa has come to be recognized! Although it does not completely address this theoretical dilemma, we recommend that Criterion A be modified to require *recurrent episodes of binging* and to define binge eating episodes subjectively as indicated previously (i.e., "the amount of food that the individual considers excessive" in which there is a feeling of lack of control over eating; see Table 8.5). In addition, and as is described later, we recommend that purging on average of twice a week for 3 months be required to fulfill the diagnosis of bulimia nervosa. Patients who do not engage in purging or who fail to meet this frequency criteria are to be given the diagnosis of *atypical eating disorder, bulimic type*. As indicated earlier, although the term *bulimia nervosa* and the historical parameters for definition have highlighted binge eating, it is of interest that one of the original reports identifying subtypes of anorexia nervosa did so on the basis of purging rather than binging (Beaumont et al., 1976).

B. A feeling of lack of control over eating during the eating binges.

This is similar to Criterion C of the original DSM-III and, as indicated earlier, most patients report this experience. However, there are some patients who describe all other features of bulimia nervosa but specifically state that they do not feel a lack of control over the behavior and, in fact, report that it is quite calculated. It is not immediately obvious that these individuals differ remarkably from those who report the feeling of lack of control. Sometimes the "planned" nature of eating binges is a function of chronicity in that these patients admit that they once felt a lack of control over their behavior, but now it is predictable and even pleasurable on occasion (Fairburn, 1987).

Fairburn (1987) suggested that if the lack of control is denied, the interviewer should determine if the subject believes that he or she could have prevented or interrupted the binge once eating had begun and, if this would have been difficult or impossible, then the criterion for lack of control is met. This is a useful guideline, but it alludes to the significance of "voluntary control" that was part of the original DSM-III criteria and was dropped because it was ambiguous (Pope et al., 1988).

Loss of control during binge eating is not required according to Russell's (1979, 1983) criteria for bulimia nervosa. It is not known whether those who present with this complaint have a different course to their disorder than those who do not. Johnson and Love (1985) reported that feeling out of control when binge eating was the best predictor of life impairment in a self-selected mail survey of individuals reporting concerns about bulimia. This is an interesting finding that needs to be replicated with a clinical sample and with measures of life impairment that are not exclusively attitudinal.

Intuitively, it would seem that patients who feel that their behavior is "under control" and ego-syntonic might be less likely to seek treatment and, consequently, be more resistent to intervention. In the subgroup of patients that we have seen who fit this description, it is our impression that they overlap in most regards with the more typical patient who freely reports a loss of control during binge eating. Nevertheless, loss of control denotes the subjective distress of the patient and, in the absence of compelling data indicating that there are large numbers of patients who would be disqualified by this criterion, it is our recommendation that it be incorporated in Criterion A, as indicated earlier and in Table 8.5.

C. The person regularly engages in either self-induced vomiting, use of laxatives or diuretics, strict dieting or fasting, or vigorous exercise in order to prevent weight gain.

This criterion represented a substantial improvement over the DSM-III that did not make these behaviors mandatory for diagnosis. Considerable attention was devoted earlier to the importance of certain of these behaviors in bulimia nervosa; therefore, the discussion here is limited. It is our view that these behaviors are paramount for a diagnosis of bulimia nervosa because they usually indicate the intensity of concern about body shape and weight (Criterion E), and they have serious medical consequences. Fairburn (1987) maintained that these behaviors should be regarded as interchangeable in determining whether or not these behaviors occur regularly. This is a reasonable solution for ascertaining presence of the cluster of symptoms, but it raises the question of their relative importance in the diagnosis of bulimia nervosa.

These behaviors may not be equivalent in the degree to which they are viewed as uncommon or abnormal in society. One study has indicated that self-induced vomiting and purgative abuse are regarded as both uncommon and abnormal among most members of the general public in contrast to strict dieting, fasting, and vigorous exercise in order to prevent weight gain, which are not seen as uncommon or particularly abnormal (Huon et al., 1988). As indicated earlier, they also may have different medical consequences, with serious risks being associated with self-induced vomiting and laxative or diuretic abuse (Mitchell & Boutacoff, 1986; Mitchell et al., 1988). Although we have seen patients presenting with strict dieting or vigorous exercise as the exclusive weight-control method and warranting immediate clinical consideration because of the intensity of their distress, it is our general impression that their disorder is less severe. According to the changes that we are recommending to the diagnostic criteria for bulimia nervosa, individuals who engage in weight-losing behaviors in the absence of vomiting or laxative abuse should receive a diagnosis of atypical eating disorder, bulimic type. Although Criterion C was useful within the context of the DSM-III-R, it is no longer required in its present form, because it has been subsumed under the next criterion to form a severity index for purging behavior required for a positive diagnosis.

D. A minimum average of two binge eating episodes per week for at least 3 months.

This criterion was aimed at addressing a major deficiency of the DSM-III that failed to set a threshold for severity for the diagnosis of bulimia nervosa. The original criteria could have been met by individuals who might engage in occasional eating binges but who would clearly not qualify as having a clinically significant syndrome as specified in the introduction to the DSM-III (APA, 1980, p. 6). In describing the rationale of the DSM-III-R Committee in selecting this particular threshold, Pope and colleagues (1988) admitted that different degrees of severity were preferred and that the minimum average frequency and the duration were arbitrary.

The advantage of the criterion requiring an *average* number of episodes per week takes into account the fluctuating nature of the disorder. An obvious disadvantage is that an individual reporting a regular pattern of binge eating of two times a week over a 3-month period would meet the same threshold for chronicity as someone who had just under 5 episodes a day for a week. Fairburn (1987) provided guidelines for greater uniformity by requiring no more than 2 weeks of abstinence unless environmental factors have prevented binge episodes.

The arguments presented earlier in support for purging defining a more homogeneous and more severe form of the disorder, along with the data from studies that have compared purging and nonpuring bulimics (Prather & Williamson, 1988; Willmuth et al., 1988), form the basis for our recommendation that purging, rather than binging, should be used in determining the threshold of severity for bulimia nervosa. Accordingly, we recommend that Criterion D be modified to require that the individual engage in a minimum average of two purging episodes (i.e., self-induced vomiting or use of laxatives) per week for at least 3 months.

E. Persistent overconcern with body weight and shape.

After considerable debate among the DSM-III-R Committee members, this criterion was included primarily because it made the DSM-III-R criteria more compatible with those used most often in Europe (Pope et al., 1988). Some Committee members voiced the primary objection that the criterion was redundant because it would be unlikely for an individual to exhibit behaviors designed to prevent weight gain without displaying an overconcern with body weight and shape. It was acknowledged that these attitudes are characteristic of those with eating disorders, and further research is needed to determine their possible role in the development and maintenance of bulimia nervosa. A detailed presentation of the rationale for considering this criterion as fundamental for the diagnosis of bulimia nervosa is not presented here, because it has been the subject of several recent reviews (Fairburn & Garner, 1986, 1988; Garner & Fairburn, 1988). The salient points are quite straightforward. First, persistent overconcerns with weight and shape are prominent clinical features of bulimia nervosa. In addition, these attitudes are significant because they are a common feature of both anorexia nervosa and bulimia nervosa. Existing diagnostic criteria for anorexia nervosa stipulate that some variant of persistent overconcern for weight and shape is required, and, thus, incorporating these overconcerns in the criteria for bulimia nervosa maintains an important parallel between these two disorders. Furthermore, as indicated earlier, the behaviors designed to control eating and weight are a logical consequence of these attitudes. Finally, it has been suggested that modification of these concerns is important for lasting recovery. Although treatments that do not focus on changing these attitudes have produced positive outcomes (Fairburn et al., 1986), this does not diminish the diagnostic significance of overconcern with body weight and shape, because these attitudes are prominent when patients are symptomatic and disappear upon recovery.

Perhaps the most pointed argument against making persistent overconcern with body weight and shape an essential criterion relates to findings from a study mentioned earlier by Huon and colleagues (1988), which indicates that intense fear of gaining 2 to 3 pounds, being upset about having even a small amount of fat on one's body, feeling fat even when one is objectively not fat, being preoccupied with one's weight, having a strong desire for a flat stomach, being dissatisfied with one's body, weighing oneself daily, wanting to be extremely thin, and other attitudes were judged as neither uncommon nor abnormal by many men and women surveyed. This observation prompted Beumont (1988) to question the proposal by Russell (1983) and others that the bulimic patient's concern about weight and shape is the psychopathology underlying the disorder in the same way that organic pathology underlies a physical disease.

It is clear that the forms of the concerns about weight and shape are common among many women in society, and careful research must be done to determine if there are particular attitudes that are specific to individuals who clearly meet the diagnoses for eating disorders. Nevertheless, clinical experience suggests that there are at least some features that separate the normal dieter from the bulimic patient who has pursued drastic dieting for many months and who uses self-induced vomiting and laxatives in the desperate attempt to prevent weight gain. We believe that further delineation of the specific nature of these concerns is useful. As indicated in Table 8.5, they may be manifest by an intense fear of gaining weight or becoming fat, even though normal weight; an intense fear of being "too fat" when at a normal weight; or using weight or body shape as the sole or predominant criterion for self-evaluation. Even if research were to fail to show reliable differences between normal dieters and those with a clinical eating disorder *in the form of their concerns about weight and shape, it may be that important differences lie in their intensity and the lengths that the individual will go to alleviate them*. Similarly, most would not question the intense ambition for greater financial prosperity except when the intensity of this desire or its behavioral expression grossly interferes with personal health, social adjustment, and psychological functioning. Nevertheless, the concerns of Beumont (1988) and Huon et al.

(1988) should not be dismissed lightly, because there is real danger in failing to appreciate fully the social context within which the eating disorders are understood. Even though the DSM-III-R Criterion E for bulimia nervosa may not be specific to the disorder, it does exclude individuals who may engage in binge eating and self-induced vomiting but who do not appear overly concerned with weight and shape (Olmsted & Garner, 1986). Thus, the most compelling argument for retaining Criterion E may not be that these attitudes are specific to eating disorders but that there are some individuals who could meet the other criteria and not have bulimia nervosa (Garfinkel et al., 1983). Following the sometimes sharp criticisms of certain DSM-III-R diagnostic criteria, it is important to remain aware of the fact that it is not the intention for any of the criteria to stand on their own for the purpose of making a diagnosis. They must be evaluated as a set where each component has incremental value. The wording of the recommended Criterion D has been modified to make it consistent with the related criterion for anorexia nervosa (Table 8.3).

Other Issues in the Diagnosis of Bulimia Nervosa

As discussed earlier, rather than subdivide anorexia nervosa into binging and restricting subtypes, we recommend that the diagnosis of bulimia nervosa be given regardless of body weight. This change should be indicated in a description of the essential features for both disorders. Two issues that have not been covered within the context of the DSM-III-R criteria warrant brief discussion. These are the relevance of the history of anorexia nervosa to diagnosis and the possible addition of a diagnostic category of compulsive overeating.

History of Anorexia Nervosa. Russell (1983, 1988) has contended that a history of frank or "cryptic" anorexia nervosa is an essential feature for bulimia nervosa because it identifies a clinically homogeneous subgroup of patients who presumably have a more severe form of the disorder. The term *cryptic* has been operationally defined as a weight loss of 3 to 5 kg and three missed menstrual periods (Russell, 1988). Again, Beumont (1988) questioned the specificity of these "cryptic" episodes of anorexia nervosa by suggesting that loss of this amount of weight is a common experience for women in our society.

Until recently, there has been little data to support the potential value of differentiating subgroups of bulimia nervosa patients on the basis of their history of anorexia nervosa, because most studies have indicated that there are few clinical or psychometric differences between patients with and without such a history (Garner et al., 1985; Mickalide & Andersen, 1985). Outcome studies that have examined this variable have generally failed to link it to prognosis, although there are several recent reports indicating that patients with a poor outcome have significantly lower past weights than those with a favorable outcome (Wilson, Rossiter, Kleifield, & Lindholm, 1986). The preliminary results from the Toronto comparative psychotherapy study described earlier indicate that, regardless of which treatment was received, patients who had a probable history of anorexia nervosa had a significantly poorer outcome than those who had never attained a low weight (Garner, 1989).

Although it may be that the members of the subgroup who have had a history of anorexia nervosa or greater weight loss may be more resistent to treatment, this marker may be a rather indirect or crude index of severity. To exclude someone who is exhibiting protracted and severe symptoms from a diagnosis of bulimia nervosa because of their weight history does not seem warranted at this time. Nevertheless, results from several studies provide convincing evidence that should compel researchers to determine carefully if patients have had a probable history of anorexia nervosa, and comparative studies should stratify groups on this variable.

Compulsive Overeating. The term *compulsive overeating* is widely used by the Overeaters Anonymous (OA) program, which was founded in 1960 and has become popular in certain settings to describe binge eating in the absence of self-induced vomiting or purgative abuse. Several studies have indicated that this pattern of binge eating is common among obese individuals (Gormally, Black, Daston, & Rardin, 1982; Loro & Orleans, 1981; Marcus, Wing, & Lamparski, 1985; Telch, Agras, & Rossiter, 1988). Because of the popularity of the term and the apparent pervasiveness of the problem that it identifies, it is appropriate to question whether "compulsive overeating" should be formally adopted as part of the eating disorder nomenclature. In our view, this would be a mistake, because attributing bouts of overeating to a compulsion provides it with surplus meaning that is misleading and unjustified. According to the DSM-III-R, obsessive compulsive disorder (300.30) is specifically precluded if the content of the obsession relates to food in the presence of an eating disorder. Typically, the individual experiencing bouts of binge eating only superficially resembles someone with an obsessive compulsive disorder. In this connection, "the preoccupations with food, cravings, voracious appetite, or the 'drive' to eat in the absence of the subjective experience of hunger may be much more readily understood as a consequence of dieting and/or maintenance of a suboptimal weight than resulting from . . . compulsive overeating" (Garner, 1985, p. 714).

In addition, the term *compulsive overeating* makes it difficult to separate the label from the OA model of treatment. Although OA self-help groups are undoubtedly helpful to some individuals (Malenbaum, Herzog, Eisenthal, & Wyshak, 1988), their formulation of the problem of binge eating and their abstinence model of treatment have been the subject of rather vigorous criticism (Bemis, 1985; Garner, 1985). To suggest, as some of the influential OA writings do, that bulimic individuals are "sick people" who suffer from a "progressive illness which cannot be cured but . . . can be arrested" (Overeaters Anonamous, 1979, p. 2) is a disheartening message that is inconsistent with the emergent data on treatment effectiveness (Fairburn et al., 1986). Thus, it is our view that individuals who report binge eating in the absence of purgation or who fail to meet the severity threshold for bulimia nervosa should be given the diagnosis of *atypical eating disorder* or *atypical eating disorder, bulimic type.*

SUMMARY

The recommended diagnostic criteria for both anorexia nervosa and bulimia nervosa have been presented in Tables 8.3 and 8.5. They are based on reviews of the literature and theoretical arguments. Some of the recommended changes are relatively minor. One aim has been to increase the correspondence between the respective criteria for both eating disorders. Another goal has been to eliminate terms that appear to needlessly exclude patients from a positive diagnosis (e.g., patients excluded from a diagnosis of bulimia nervosa because binge episodes do not involve the *rapid* consumption of *large amounts* of food). Although it may be argued that these criteria should be dropped *only* if there are convincing data to justify their elimination, we believe that their initial inclusion was unwarranted and not empirically based. Moreover, bulimia nervosa is a relatively "new" diagnostic entity, and the criteria were originally put into place in the absence of a strong empirical base. Thus, we believe that there should be less resistance to changing diagnostic features that are inconsistent with the current understanding of the disorder than there might be for disorders that have been part of the diagnostic nomenclature for many years.

Several more radical changes also have been recommended. First, patients who experience episodes of binging and vomiting at a low weight would previously have been diagnosed as anorexia nervosa, but according to the recommended revisions would receive a diagnosis of anorexia nervosa, bulimic subtype. Furthermore, for anorexia nervosa, the requirement of amenorrhea has been dropped. Finally, in the diagnosis of bulimia nervosa, purging is given a more prominent role in defining the disorder and in determining the necessary threshold for severity.

DIAGNOSTIC AND ASSESSMENT PROCEDURES

A comprehensive review of diagnostic and assessment procedures is not the intention of this section, because recent reviews of these topics are available (Fairburn, 1987; Garner & Davis, 1986; Garner & Rosen, in press; Halmi, 1985; Johnson & Connors, 1987; Swift, 1985; Williamson, Goreczny, & Duchmann, 1987; Wilson, 1987). Several approaches to gathering this information have been designed for eating disorders, including the semistructured interview, interviewer ratings, standardized self-report measures, nonstandardized symptom checklists, self-monitoring, and standardized test meals. Table 8.7 provides a selective

TABLE 8.7
Assessment Methods for Eating Disorders

Semistructured Interviews
Eating Disorder Examination (EDE; Cooper & Fairburn, 1987)
Clinical Eating Disorder Rating Instrument (CEDRI; Palmer, Christie, Cordle, Davies, & Kendrick, 1987)
Interviewer Ratings
Anorectic Attitudes Questionnaire (Goldberg et al., 1980)
Anorexic Behavior Scale (Slade, 1973)
Standardized Self-Report Measures Derived from Clinical Samples
Bulimia Test (BULIT; Smith & Thelen, 1984)
Eating Attitudes Test (Garner, Olmsted, Bohr, & Garfinkel, 1982)
Eating Disorder Inventory (EDI; Garner, 1991)
Screening Instrument for Identifying Individuals at Risk of Developing Anorexia Nervosa or Bulimia Nervosa (SCANS; Slade & Dewey, 1986)
Non-Standardized Symptom Checklists
Bulimia Interview Form (Walsh & Gladis, 1985)
Eating Disorders Questionnaire (Mitchell et al., 1985)
Diagnostic Survey for Eating Disorders (Johnson, 1985)
Self-Monitoring
Mitchell, Pyle, & Eckert (1981)
Fairburn (1985)
Wilson (1987)
Standardized Test Meals
Rosen, Leitenberg, Gross, & Willmuth (1985)
Ordman & Kirschenbaum (1985)

summary of these methods as well as a key reference that provides further descriptive material.

For the purpose of diagnosis and referral, several areas should be covered in a clinical interview, and these include: (a) assessment of the symptom picture, including weight, weight history, eating patterns, weight-losing methods, and attitudes toward weight and shape; (b) determination of the present as well as premorbid psychological, social, and family functioning; (c) careful evaluation of the physical complications; and (d) assessment of the motivation for change. Information relevant to a positive diagnosis may be derived from an unstructured interview; however, Fairburn (1987) added strength and precision to this process by suggesting specific guidelines and probes for each of the DSM-III-R criteria for bulimia nervosa. Cooper and Fairburn (1987) also developed a structured interview for the assessment of specific symptoms of anorexia nervosa and bulimia nervosa.

Psychometric assessment of eating disorders may be divided into two broad areas. The first is measurement of attitudes or behaviors that are characteristic of eating disorders. As indicated in Table 8.7, there have been a number of measures developed in recent years, and only those that have been validated on clinical cases of eating disorder patients have been listed. The second area for assessment relates to associated psychological or personality features that may indicate overall functioning or may elucidate certain themes relevant to treatment. The range of options should include measures of mood, psychological distress, self-esteem, personality, and social functioning. Because starvation, severe dieting, and the chaotic eating patterns exhibited by most patients with eating disorders may influence test scores in these areas, the interpretation must be cautious (Garner et al., 1990).

There is a growing debate regarding the respective value of self-report and interview methods in the assessment of eating disorders (Cooper, Cooper, & Fairburn, 1985; Wilson & Smith, 1989). This debate has centered around certain criticisms of self-report measures that may reflect, in part, a failure to appreciate the very different aims of self-report and interview assessment procedures. For example, Wilson and Smith (1989) found that the semistructured interview, the Eating Disorder Examination (EDE), was superior to the self-report measure, the Eating Disorder Inventory (EDI), in differentiating bulimia nervosa patients from restrained eaters. They concluded that the EDE should be considered in outcome studies "as a superior measure of the core pathology of bulimia nervosa than standardized [self-report] questionnaires" (p. 173). This conclusion implies that these measurement strategies should be competitive rather than complimentary. It also disregards the fact that self-reports have corresponded closely with other measures of clinical improvement in a rather large number of outcome studies (cf. Garner et al., 1987). Clearly, the semistructured interview is the gold standard for diagnosing an eating disorder and evaluating the salient components of the core psychopathology as it is currently understood. It has the advantages of a more fine-grained appraisal of specific psychopathology, the opportunity for probing, and clarification of the meaning behind certain responses. On the negative side, however, it can take 60 to 90 minutes, and it requires a trained interviewer to administer, which makes it unsuitable for many situations. Repeated administration during the course of treatment may be impractical with a semistructured interview, and the repeated interpersonal interactions may increase the risk of experimenter and respondent expectancy bias. Self-report instruments have the advantages of economy, standard administration, minimal interpersonal contact, potential for mass administration, actuarial scoring, and brief administration time. They may be useful in predicting meaningful group differences in certain populations.

Some of the criticisms of self-report measures stem from their inappropriate use as diagnostic instruments in certain populations. The first author of this chapter reports that prospective users of the EAT or EDI frequently ask some variation of the following question: What is the cut-off score for diagnosing eating disorders in a nonclinical sample? Just as it would be inappropriate to diagnose major affective disorder with the Beck Depression Inventory or schizophrenia using the MMPI, it is improper to diagnose eating disorders solely with self-report measures and, in particular, those measures that assess attitudes or traits rather than the specific features stipulated by the DSM-III-R diagnostic criteria. Despite the fact that self-report measures are not appropriate for diagnosing cases in nonclinical populations, it is of interest that high scores on certain simple instruments like the EAT are able to distinguish the vast majority of women who do not meet diagnostic criteria for an eating disorder from a smaller subgroup (about 10% of the total in nonclinical samples) who either have an eating disorder (true positives) or who may be classified as "normal dieters" (false positives) (Mann et al., 1983; Williams, Hand, & Tarnopolsky, 1982). This point has been highlighted with the use of the EAT as a screening instrument for identifying eating disorders in different populations (Szmuckler, 1985; Williams et al., 1982).

In the absence of an incredibly precise measure, the best estimate of the true incidence of the disorder would be to predict that it does not exist; this would lead to an error rate equal to the incidence of the disorder. However, there may be circumstances where it is desirable to identify suspected cases who then may be interviewed to determine if they meet diagnostic standards (Garner, Garfinkel, Rockert, & Olmsted, 1987; Mann et al., 1983; Szmuckler, Eisler, Gillies, & Hayward, 1985). Moreover, multivariate procedures may yield screening procedures that dramatically improve the accuracy of discrimination of eating disorder in nonclinical populations. Williams, Schaefer, Shisslak, Gronwaldt, and Comerci (1986) used a linear discriminant analysis to derive a set of items from the EAT and the EDI that accurately classified 86% of normals, dieters, and suspected bulimics identified by interview. Thus, it is inappropriate to use self-report measures to arrive at a clinical diagnosis; however, they may constitute an effective and economical initial step in a two-stage screening process in which individuals with elevated scores participate in an interview designed to arrive at a clinical diagnosis. Inferences regarding validity should be cautious, because the efficiency of the EAT in detecting possible "cases" varies with different populations (Szmukler, 1985). It is evident from other studies that concerns about weight are common among young women and that the majority of these weight-preoccupied individuals only superficially resemble those with eating disorders (Garner et al., 1984; Lindholm & Wilson, 1988). However, self-report measures, when properly used, can be a valuable source for hypothesis testing in populations that may not be accessible by interview. For example, Rippon, Nash, Myburgh, and Noakes (1988) reported that the EAT was superior to physical activity and body mass in predicting menstrual dysfunction in models, ballet dancers, and runners.

In summary, it is our view that the most appropriate measurement strategy for eating disorders is to employ convergent methods to assess the features that have been described as characteristic of anorexia nervosa and bulimia nervosa as well as those to assess the broad range of associated features related to mood, psychological state, and personality. In most cases, with knowledge of the DSM-III-R criteria, diagnosis of both anorexia nervosa and bulimia nervosa is relatively straightforward from an interview. Self-report measures are useful for tracking symptoms over time, as initial screening tools in some populations, as outcome measures, and as anchors for comparing different samples.

SUMMARY AND FUTURE DIRECTIONS

This chapter has reviewed the history of the classification systems for eating disorders and has provided a critical appraisal of the current DSM-III-R diagnostic criteria. Specific recommendations have been made for revisions to both sets of criteria. One goal has been to make both diagnostic schemes parallel to one another, because the bulk of evidence indicates tremendous overlap between syndromes. Empirical and theoretical support has been provided for several rather controversial recommendations for change to the current criteria for both disorders. For example, it was proposed that the requirement that binge episodes be "large" and that they occur over a "discrete" period of time be dropped from diagnostic criteria for bulimia nervosa. It was also suggested that vomiting and laxative abuse, rather than binging, be considered the target symptoms for bulimia nervosa. Further research will determine the relative merit of these and other recommendations.

There will, undoubtedly, be further refinements to the diagnostic criteria in the future. Several issues will probably be important in this regard. First, there will always be a push toward developing diagnostic criteria that provide meaningful differentiation of subgroups based on response to treatment. At this time, little is known regarding the predictors of outcome for bulimia nervosa, and even less is apparent for anorexia nervosa. If subgroups can be reliably discriminated from one another on the basis of outcome, this will have a major impact on future diagnostic formulations. Similarly, if subgroups can be differentiated on the basis of etiological pathways, this will set the stage for modifications to existing diagnostic schemes. A second direction for future research relates to comorbidity and its effect on shaping the manifestation of the eating disorder. The current multiaxial nature of the DSM-III-R diagnostic system may accommodate the issue of comorbidity in a satisfactory manner, but there is the possibility that there are meaningful differences in groups with certain combinations of symptoms, and this may impact the entire diagnostic picture for eating disorders. Moreover, there has been the suggestion that the presentation of eating disorders has changed considerably over time. It must be remembered that diagnostic entities are not static phenomenon but are moving targets. Future diagnosis formulations for anorexia nervosa and bulimia nervosa must take this fact into consideration. The result will be adaptations to the new or altered forms of expression for eating disorders in the future.

The fundamental relationship between diagnosis, etiology, and treatment assures that advancements made in each of these areas lead to corresponding refinements in the others. The development of more precise and more useful diagnostic criteria for the eating disorders promises to be a fruitful area for future research and theoretical discussion.

REFERENCES

Abraham, S. F., Mira, M., & Llewellyn-Jones, D. (1983). Bulimia: A study of outcome. *International Journal of Eating Disorders, 2,* 175–180.

American Psychiatric Association. (1980). *Diagnostic and statistical manual of mental disorders* (3rd ed.). Washington, DC: Author.

American Psychiatric Association. (1987). *Diagnostic and statistical manual of mental disorders* (3rd ed., rev.). Washington, DC: Author.

Andersen, A. E. (1985). *Practical comprehensive treatment of anorexia nervosa and bulimia*. Baltimore, MD: Johns Hopkins Press.

Bemis, K. M. (1985). "Abstinence" and "nonabstinence" models for the treatment of bulimia. *International Journal of Eating Disorders, 4,* 389–406.

Ben-Tovim, D. I. (1988). DSM-III, draft DSM-III-R, and the diagnosis and prevalence of bulimia in Australia. *American Journal of Psychiatry, 145,* 1000–1002.

Beumont, P. J. V. (1988). Bulimia: It is an illness entity? *International Journal of Eating Disorders, 7,* 167–176.

Beumont, P. J. V., Al-Alami, M. S., & Touyz, S. W. (1987). The evolution of the concept of anorexia nervosa. In P. V. Beumont, G. D. Burrows, & R. C. Casper (Eds.), *Handbook of eating disorders, part 1: anorexia and bulimia nervosa* (pp. 105–116). New York: Elsiver.

Beumont, P. J. V., George, G. G., & Smart, D. E. (1976). "Dieters" and "vomiters and purgers" in anorexia nervosa. *Psychological Medicine, 6,* 617–622.

Blinder, B. J., & Cadenhead, K. (1986). Bulimia: A historical overview. In S. C. Feinstein, A. H. Esman, J. G. Looney, A. Z. Schwartzberg, A. D. Sorosky, & M. Sugar (Eds.), *Adolescent psychiatry: Developmental and clinical studies* (pp. 231–240). Chicago: The University of Chicago Press.

Boskind-Lodahl, M. (1976). Cinderella's stepsisters: A feminist perspective on anorexia nervosa and bulimia. *Signs: Journal of Women in Culture and Society, 2,* 342–356.

Bruch, H. (1962). Perceptual and conceptual disturbances in anorexia nervosa. *Psychosomatic Medicine, 24,* 187–194.

Bruch, H. (1973). *Eating disorders: Obesity, anorexia nervosa and the person within.* New York: Basic Books.

Bruch, H. (1982). Anorexia nervosa: Therapy and theory. *American Journal of Psychiatry, 139,* 1531–1538.

Casper, R. C. (1982). Treatment principles in anorexia nervosa. *Adolescent Psychiatry, 10,* 86–100.

Casper, R. C. (1983). On the emergence of bulimia nervosa as a syndrome: A historical view. *International Journal of Eating Disorders, 2,* 3–16.

Casper, R. C., Eckert, E. D., Halmi, K. A., Goldberg, S. C., & Davis, J. M. (1980). Bulimia. Its incidence and clinical importance in patients with anorexia nervosa. *Archives of General Psychiatry, 37,* 1030–1034.

Cooper, Z., Cooper, P. J., & Fairburn, C. G. (1985). The specificity of the Eating Disorder Inventory. *British Journal of Clinical Psychology, 24,* 129–130.

Cooper, Z., & Fairburn, C. G. (1987). The Eating Disorder Examination: A semi-structured interview for the assessment of the specific psychopathology of eating disorders. *International Journal of Eating Disorders, 6,* 1–8.

Cooper, P. J., Taylor, M. J., Cooper, Z., & Fairburn, C. G. (1987). The development of validation of the Body Shape Questionnaire. *International Journal of Eating Disorders, 6,* 485–494.

Crisp, A. H. (1980). *Anorexia nervosa*. New York: Grune & Stratton.

Dally, P. J. (1969). *Anorexia nervosa*. New York: Grune & Stratton.

Davis, R., Freeman, R. J., & Garner, D. M. (1988). A naturalistic investigation of eating behavior in bulimia nervosa. *Journal of Consulting and Clinical Psychology, 56,* 273–279.

Eckert, E. D., Halmi, K. A., Marchi, P., & Cohen, J. (1987). Comparison of bulimic and non-bulimic anorexia nervosa patients during treatment. *Psychological Medicine, 17,* 891–898.

Fairburn, C. G. (1985). Cognitive-behavioral treatment for bulimia. In D. M. Garner & P. E. Garfinkel (Eds.), *Handbook of psychotherapy for anorexia nervosa and bulimia* (pp. 160–192). New York: Guilford Press.

Fairburn, C. G. (1987). The definition of bulimia nervosa: Guidelines for clinicians and research workers. *Annals of Behavioral Medicine, 9*, 3–7.

Fairburn, C. G., & Garner, D. M. (1986). The diagnosis of bulimia nervosa. *International Journal of Eating Disorders, 5*, 403–419.

Fairburn, C. G., & Garner, D. M. (1988). Diagnostic criteria for anorexia nervosa and bulimia nervosa: The importance of attitudes to shape and weight. In D. M. Garner & P. E. Garfinkel (Eds.), *Diagnostic issues in anorexia nervosa and bulimia nervosa* (pp. 36–55). Monograph Series. New York: Brunner/Mazel.

Fairburn, C. G., Kirk, J., O'Connor, M., & Cooper, P. J. (1986). A comparison of two psychological treatments for bulimia nervosa. *Behaviour Research and Therapy, 24*, 629–643.

Feighner, J. P., Robins, E., Guze, S. B., Woodruff, R. A., Jr., Winokur, G., & Munoz, R. (1972). Diagnostic criteria for use in psychiatric research. *Archives of General Psychiatry, 26*, 57–63.

Garfinkel, P. E., & Garner, D. M. (1982). *Anorexia nervosa: A multidimensional perspective*. New York: Brunner/Mazel.

Garfinkel, P. E., Garner, D. M., Kaplan, A. S., Rodin, G., & Kennedy, S. (1983). Differential diagnosis of emotional disorders that cause weight loss. *Canadian Medical Association Journal, 129*, 939–945.

Garfinkel, P. E., Moldofsky, H., & Garner, D. M. (1980). The heterogeneity of anorexia nervosa. *Archives of General Psychiatry, 37*, 1036–1040.

Garner, D. M. (1985). Iatrogenesis in anorexia nervosa and bulimia nervosa. *International Journal of Eating Disorders, 4*, 701–726.

Garner, D. M. (1987). Psychotherapy outcome research with bulimia nervosa. *Psychotherapy and Psychosomatics, 48*, 129–140.

Garner, D. M. (1989, June). *A comparison between cognitive-behavioral and psychodynamic psychotherapy for bulimia nervosa*. World Congress of Cognitive Therapy, Oxford, England.

Garner, D. M. (1991). *Eating Disorder Inventory-2: Professional Manual*. Odessa, Florida: Psychological Assessment Resources.

Garner, D. M., & Bemis, K. M. (1982). A cognitive-behavioral approach to anorexia nervosa. *Cognitive Therapy and Research, 6*, 123–150.

Garner, D. M., & Davis, R. (1986). The clinical assessment of anorexia nervosa and bulimia nervosa. In P. A. Keller & L. Ritt (Eds.), *Innovations in clinical practice: A source book* (pp. 5–28). Sarasota, FL: Professional Resource Exchange.

Garner, D. M., & Fairburn, C. G. (1988). Relationship between anorexia nervosa and bulimia nervosa: Diagnostic implications. In D. M. Garner & P. E. Garfinkel (Eds.), *Diagnostic issues in anorexia nervosa and bulimia nervosa* (pp. 56–79). New York: Brunner/Mazel.

Garner, D. M., Fairburn, C. G., & Davis, R. (1987). Cognitive-behavioral treatment of bulimia nervosa: A critical appraisal. *Behavior Modification, 11*, 398–431.

Garner, D. M., & Garfinkel, P. E. (1979). The Eating Attitudes Test: An index of the symptoms of anorexia nervosa. *Psychological Medicine, 9*, 273–279.

Garner, D. M., & Garfinkel, P. E. (1981). Body image in anorexia nervosa: Measurement, theory and clinical implications. *International Journal of Psychiatry in Medicine, 11*, 263–284.

Garner, D. M., & Garfinkel, P. E. (1988). *Diagnostic issues in anorexia nervosa and bulimia nervosa*. New York: Brunner/Mazel.

Garner, D. M., Garfinkel, P. E., & Bonato, D. (1987). Body image measurement in eating disorders. In G. A. Fava & T. N. Wise (Eds.), *Advances in psychosomatic medicine* (pp. 119–133). Basel: Karger.

Garner, D. M., Garfinkel, P. E., & O'Shaughnessy, M. (1985). The validity of the distinction between bulimia with and without anorexia nervosa. *American Journal of Psychiatry, 142*, 581–587.

Garner, D. M., Garfinkel, P. E., Rockert, W., & Olmsted, M. P. (1987). A prospective study of eating disturbances in the ballet. *Psychotherapy and Psychosomatics, 48*, 170–175.

Garner, D. M., & Olmsted, M. P. (1984). *The eating disorder inventory manual*. Odessa, FL: Psychological Assessment Resources.

Garner, D. M., Olmsted, M. P., Bohr, Y., & Garfinkel, P. E. (1982). The Eating Attitudes Test: Psychometric features and clinical correlates. *Psychological Medicine, 12*, 871–878.

Garner, D. M., Olmsted, M. P., Davis, R., Rockert, W., Goldbloom, D., & Eagle, M. (1990). The association between bulimic symptoms and reported psychopathology. *International Journal of Eating Disorders, 9*, 1–15.

Garner, D. M., Olmsted, M. P., & Garfinkel, P. E. (1985). Similarities among bulimic groups selected by different weights and weight histories. *Journal of Psychiatric Research, 19*, 129–134.

Garner, D. M., Olmsted, M. P., & Polivy, J. (1983). The Eating Disorder Inventory: A measure of cognitive-behavioral dimensions of anorexia nervosa and bulimia. In P. L. Darby, P. E. Garfinkel, D. M. Garner, & D. V. Coscina (Eds.), *Anorexia Nervosa: Recent developments in research* (pp. 173–184). New York: Alan R. Liss.

Garner, D. M., Olmsted, M. P., Polivy, J., & Garfinkel, P. E. (1984). Comparison between weight-preoccupied women and anorexia nervosa. *Psychosomatic Medicine, 46*, 255–266.

Garner, D. M., Rockert, W., Olmsted, M. P., Johnson, C. L., & Coscina, D. V. (1985). Psychoeducational principles in the treatment of bulimia and anorexia nervosa. In D. M. Garner, & P. E. Garfinkel (Eds.), *Handbook of psychotherapy for anorexia nervosa and bulimia* (pp. 513–572). New York: Guilford Press.

Garner, D. M., & Rosen, L. W. (in press). Anorexia nervosa and bulimia nervosa. In A. S. Bellack, M. Hersen, & A. E. Kazdin (Eds.), *International handbook of behavior modification and therapy*. New York: Plenum Publishing.

Garrow, J. S., Crisp, A. H., Jordon, H. A., Meyer, J. E., Russell, G. F. M., Silverstone, T., Stunkard, A. J., & Van Itallie, T. B. (1975). Pathology of eating, group report. In T. Silverstone (Ed.), *Dahlem konferenzen, Life sciences research report 2*. Berlin.

Goldberg, S. C., Halmi, K. A., Eckert, E. D., Casper, R. C., Davis, J. M., & Roper, M. (1980). Attitudinal dimensions in anorexia nervosa. *Journal of Psychiatry Research, 15*, 239–251.

Goodsitt, A. (1985). Self psychology and the treatment of anorexia nervosa. In D. M. Garner, & P. E. Garfinkel (Eds.), *Handbook of psychotherapy for anorexia nervosa and bulimia* (pp. 55–84). New York: Guilford Press.

Gormally, J., Black, S., Daston, S., & Rardin, D. (1982). The assessment of binge eating severity among obese persons. *Addictive Behavior, 7*, 47–55.

Halmi, K. A. (1983). The state of research in anorexia nervosa and bulimia. *Psychiatric Developments, 3*, 247–262.

Halmi, K. A. (1985). Classification of the eating disorders. *Journal of Psychiatric Research, 19*, 113–119.

Hare, E. (1981). The two manias: A study of the evolution of the modern concept of mania. *British Journal of Psychiatry, 138*, 88–89.

Holmgren, S., Humble, K., Norring, C., Roos, B. E., Rosmark, B., & Sohlberg, S. (1983). The anorectic bulimic conflict: An alternative diagnostic approach to

anorexia nervosa and bulimia. *International Journal of Eating Disorders, 2,* 3–14.
Hsu, L. K. G. (1982). Is there a disturbance in body image in Anorexia nervosa? *International Journal of Eating Disorders, 2,* 11–20.
Hsu, L. K. G., & Holder, D. (1986). Bulimia nervosa: Treatment and short-term outcome. *Psychological Medicine, 16,* 65–70.
Hsu, L. K. G., & Zimmer, B. (1988). Eating disorders in old age. *International Journal of Eating Disorders, 7,* 133–138.
Huon, G. F., Brown, L., & Morris, S. (1988). Lay beliefs about disordered eating. *International Journal of Eating Disorders, 7,* 239–252.
I.C.D.-10 (1986). *Draft of Chapter V: Mental, behavioural and developmental disorders. Clinical descriptions and diagnostic guidelines.* World Health Organization, Division of Mental Health, Geneva, 1987.
Jaffe, A. C., & Singer, L. T. (1989). Atypical eating disorders in young children. *International Journal of Eating Disorders, 8,* 575–582.
Janet, P. (1919). *Les obsessions et la psychasthenie.* Paris: Felix Alcan.
Johnson, C. (1985). Initial consultation for patients with bulimia and anorexia nervosa. In D. M. Garner & P. E. Garfinkel (Eds.), *Handbook of psychotherapy for anorexia nervosa and bulimia* (pp. 19–51). New York: Guilford Press.
Johnson, C., & Connors, M. E. (1987). Treatment of bulimia: A review. In P. J. V. Beaumont, G. D. Burrows, & R. C. Casper (Eds.), *Handbook of eating disorders Part 1: Anorexia and bulimia nervosa* (pp. 299–317). New York: Elsevier.
Johnson, C. L., & Love, S. Q. (1985). Bulimia: Multivariate predictors of life impairment. *Journal of Psychiatric Research, 19,* 343–347.
Johnson, C. L., Tobin, D., & Enright, A. (1989). Prevalence and clinical characteristics of borderline patients in an eating disorder population. *Journal of Clinical Psychiatry, 50,* 9–15.
Katzman, M. A., & Wolchik, S. A. (1984). Bulimia and binge eating in college women: A comparison of personality and behavioral characteristics. *Journal of Consulting and Clinical Psychology, 52,* 423–438.
Kellett, J., Trimble, M., & Thorley, A. (1976). Anorexia nervosa after the menopause. *British Journal of Psychiatry, 128,* 555–558.
Lacey, J. H., Chadbund, C., Crisp, A. H., & Whitehead, J. (1978). Dietary patterns in normal schoolgirls. *British Journal of Human Nutrition, 32,* 419.
Laessle, R. G., Wittchen, H. U., Fichter, M. M., & Pirke, K. M. (1989). The significance of subgroups of bulimia and anorexia nervosa: Lifetime frequency of psychiatric disorders. *International Journal of Eating Disorders, 8,* 569–574.
Launer, M. A. (1978). Anorexia nervosa in late life. *British Journal of Medical Psychology, 51,* 375–377.
Levin, A. P., & Hyler, S. E. (1986). DSM-III personality diagnosis in bulimia. *Comprehensive Psychiatry, 27,* 47–53.
Lindholm, L., & Wilson, G. T. (1988). Body image assessment in patients with bulimia nervosa and normal controls. *International Journal of Eating Disorders, 7,* 527–539.
Loro, A. D., & Orleans, C. S. (1981). Binge eating in obesity: Preliminary findings and guidelines for behavioral analysis and treatment. *Addictive Behaviors, 6,* 155–166.
Lucas, A. R., Beard, C. M., O'Fallon, W. M., & Kurland, L. T. (1988). Anorexia nervosa in Rochester, Minnesota: A 45-year study. *Mayo Clinic Proceedings, 63,* 433–442.
Malenbaum, R., Herzog, D., Eisenthal, S., & Wyshak, G. (1988). Overeaters Anonymous: Impact on bulimia. *International Journal of Eating Disorders, 7,* 139–143.
Mann, A. H., Wakeling, A., Wood, K., Monck, E., Dobbs, R., & Szmukler, G. (1983). Screening for abnormal eating attitudes and psychiatric morbidity in an unselected population of 15-year-old schoolgirls. *Psychological Medicine, 13,* 573–580.

Marcus, M. D., Wing, R. R., & Lamparski, D. M. (1985). Binge eating and dietary restraint in obese patients. *Addictive Behavior, 10,* 163–168.

Mickalide, A. D., & Anderson, A. E. (1985). Subgroups of anorexia nervosa and bulimia: Validity and utility. *Journal of Psychiatric Research, 19*(2/3), 121–128.

Minuchin, S., Rosman, B. L., & Baker, L. (1978). *Psychosomatic families: anorexia nervosa in context.* Cambridge, MA: Harvard University Press.

Mitchell, J. E., & Boutacoff, M. A. (1986). Laxative abuse complicating bulimia: Medical and treatment implications. *International Journal of Eating Disorders, 5,* 325–334.

Mitchell, J. E., Davis, L., Goff, G., & Pyle, R. (1986). A follow-up study of patients with bulimia. *International Journal of Eating Disorders, 5,* 441–450.

Mitchell, J. E., Fletcher, L., Pyle, R., Eckert, E., Hatsukami, D., & Pomeroy, C. (1989). The impact of treatment on meal patterns in patients with bulimia nervosa. *International Journal of Eating Disorders, 8,* 167–172.

Mitchell, J. E., Hatsukami, D., Goff, G., Pyle, R. L., Eckert, E. D., & Davis, L. E. (1985). Intensive outpatient group treatment for bulimia. In D. M. Garner & P. E. Garfinkel (Eds.), *Handbook of psychotherapy for anorexia nervosa and bulimia* (pp. 240–256). New York: Guilford Press.

Mitchell, J. E., Pomeroy, C., & Huber, M. (1988). A clinician's guide to the eating disorders medicine cabinet. *International Journal of Eating Disorders, 7,* 211–233.

Mitchell, J. E., & Pyle, R. L. (1982). The bulimic syndrome in normal weight individuals: A review. *International Journal of Eating Disorders,* 61–73.

Mitchell, J. E., Pyle, R. L., & Eckert, E. D. (1981). Frequency and duration of binge-eating episodes in patients with bulimia. *American Journal of Psychiatry, 138,* 835–836.

Mitchell, J. E., Pyle, R. L., Hatsukami, D., Goff, G., Glotter, D., & Harper, J. (1989). A 2–5 year follow-up study of patients treated for bulimia. *International Journal of Eating Disorders, 8,* 157–165.

Norris, D. (1979). Clinical diagnostic criteria for primary anorexia nervosa. *AUX* (South African medical journal), *56,* 987–992.

Olmsted, M. P., & Garner, D. M. (1986). Application of the Eating Disorder Inventory to a sample of Black, White, and mixed race schoolgirls in Zimbabwe. *International Journal of Eating Disorders, 5,* 161–168.

Ordman, A. M., & Kirschenbaum, D. S. (1985). Cognitive-behavioral therapy for bulimia: An initial outcome study. *Journal of Consulting and Clinical Psychology, 53,* 305–313.

Overeaters Anonymous. (1979). (Pamphlet) Torrance, CA: Author.

Palmer, R. L. (1979). The dietary chaos syndrome: A useful new term? *British Journal of Medical Psychology, 52,* 187–190.

Palmer, R., Christie, M., Cordle, C., Davies, D., & Kenrick, J. (1987). The Clinical Eating Disorder Rating Instrument (CEDRI): A preliminary description. *International Journal of Eating Disorders, 6,* 9–16.

Piran, N., Lerner, P., Garfinkel, P. E., Kennedy, S. H., & Brouilette, C. (1988). Personality disorders in anorexia patients. *International Journal of Eating Disorders, 5,* 589–599.

Pirke, K. M., & Ploog, D. (1987). Biology of human starvation. In P. J. V. Beumont, G. D. Burrows, & R. C. Casper (Eds.), *Handbook of eating disorders part 1: Anorexia and bulimia nervosa* (pp. 79–102). New York: Elsevier.

Polivy, J., & Herman, C. P. (1985). Dieting and bingeing: A causal analysis. *American Psychologist, 40,* 193–201.

Pope, H. G., Frankenburg, F. R., Hudson, J. I., Jonas, J. M., & Yurgelun-Todd, D. (1987). Is bulimia associated with borderline personality disorder? A controlled study. *Journal of Clinical Psychiatry, 48,* 181–184.

Pope, H. G., & Hudson, J. I. (1988). Is bulimia nervosa a heterogeneous disorder? Lessons from the history of medicine. *International Journal of Eating Disorders, 7,* 155–166.

Pope, H. G., Hudson, J. I., Spitzer, R. L., & Williams, J. B. (1988). Revisions in the DSM-III Criteria for bulimia nervosa. In D. M. Garner & P. E. Garfinkel (Eds.), *Diagnostic issues in anorexia nervosa and bulimia nervosa* (pp. 26–35). New York: Brunner/Mazel.

Prather, R. C., & Williamson, D. A. (1988). Psychopathology associated with Bulimia, binge eating, and obesity. *International Journal of Eating Disorders, 7*, 177–184.

Rippon, C., Nash, J., Myburgh, K. H., & Noakes, T. (1988). Abnormal Eating Attitude Test scores predict menstrual dysfunction in lean females. *International Journal of Eating Disorders, 7*, 617–624.

Rollins, N., & Piazza, E. (1978). Diagnosis of anorexia nervosa. A critical reappraisal. *Journal of Child Psychology and Psychiatry and Allied Disciplines, 17*, 126–137.

Rosen, J. C., & Leitenberg, H. (1982). Bulimia nervosa: Treatment with exposure and response prevention. *Behavior Therapy, 13*, 117–124.

Rosen, J. C., & Leitenberg, H. (1985). Exposure plus response prevention treatment of bulimia. In D. M. Garner & P. E. Garfinkel (Eds.), *Handbook of psychotherapy for anorexia nervosa and bulimia* (pp. 193–209). New York: Guilford Press.

Rosen, J. C., Leitenberg, H., Fisher, C., & Khazam, C. (1986). Binge-eating episodes in bulimia nervosa: The amount and type of food consumed. *International Journal of Eating Disorders, 5*, 255–267.

Rosen, J. C., Leitenberg, H., Gross, J., & Willmuth, M. (1985). Standardized test meals in the assessment of bulimia nervosa. *Advances in Behavior Research and Therapy, 7*, 181–197.

Rossiter, E. M., & Agras, W. S. (1990). An empirical test of the DSM-III-R definition of binge. *International Journal of Eating Disorders, 9*, 513–518.

Russell, G. F. M. (1970). Anorexia nervosa: Its identity as an illness and its treatment. In J. H. Price (Ed.), *Modern trends in psychological medicine* (Vol. 2, pp. 131–164). London: Butterworths.

Russell, G. F. M. (1977). Editorial: The present status of anorexia nervosa. *Psychological Medicine, 7*, 363–367.

Russell, G. F. M. (1978). Letter to the editor. Differential diagnosis of anorexia nervosa. *Journal of the Royal Society of Medicine, 71*, 71–72.

Russell, G. F. M. (1979). Bulimia nervosa: An ominous variant of anorexia nervosa. *Psychological Medicine, 9*, 429–448.

Russell, G. F. M. (1983). Anorexia nervosa and bulimia nervosa. In G. F. M. Russell & L. Hersov (Eds.), *Handbook of psychiatry, Vol. 4: The neuroses and personality disorders* (pp. 285–298). Cambridge: Cambridge University Press.

Russell, G. F. M. (1985). The changing nature of anorexia nervosa: An introduction to the conference. *Journal of Psychiatric Research, 19*, 101–109.

Russell, G. F. M. (1988). The diagnostic formulation in bulimia nervosa. In D. M. Garner & P. E. Garfinkel (Eds.), *Diagnostic issues in anorexia nervosa and bulimia nervosa* (pp. 3–25). Monograph Series. New York: Brunner/Mazel.

Russell, G. F. M., Szmukler, G. I., Dare, C., & Eisler, I. (1987). An evaluation of family therapy in anorexia nervosa and bulimia nervosa. *Archives of General Psychiatry, 44*, 1047–1056.

Simmonds, M. (1914). Ueber embolische prozesse in des hypophysis. *Archives of Pathology and Anatomy, 21*, 226–239.

Slade, P. D. (1973). A short anorexic behavior scale. *British Journal of Psychiatry, 122*, 83–85.

Slade, P. D. (1982). Towards a functional analysis of anorexia nervosa and bulimia. *British Journal of Clinical Psychology, 21*, 167–179.

Slade, P. D., & Dewey, M. E. (1986). Development and preliminary validation of SCANS: A screening instrument for identifying individuals at risk of developing anorexia and bulimia nervosa. *International Journal of Eating Disorders, 5*, 517–536.

Smith, M. C., & Thelen, M. H. (1984). Development and validation of a test for Bulimia. *Journal of Consulting and Clinical Psychology, 52*, 863–872.

Strauss, J., & Ryan, R. M. (1988). Cognitive dysfunction in eating disorders. *International Journal of Eating Disorders, 7*, 19–27.

Strober, M. (1981). A comparative analysis of personality organization in juvenile anorexia nervosa. *Journal of Youth and Adolescence, 10*, 285–295.

Strober, M. (1983). An empirically derived typology of anorexia nervosa. In P. Darby, P. Garfinkel, D. Garner, & D. Coscina (Eds.), *Anorexia nervosa: recent developments in research* (pp. 185–198). New York: Alan R. Liss.

Strober, M., & Katz, J. (1988). Depression in the eating disorders: A review and analysis of descriptive, family, and biological findings. In D. M. Garner & P. E. Garfinkel (Eds.), *Diagnostic issues in anorexia nervosa and bulimia nervosa* (pp. 88–111). New York: Brunner/Mazel.

Strober, M., Salkin, B., Burroughs, J., & Morrell, W. (1982). Validity of the bulimia-restrictor distinction in anorexia nervosa: Parental personality characteristics and family psychiatric morbidity. *The Journal of Nervous and Mental Disease, 170*, 345–351.

Strober, M., & Yager, J. (1985). A developmental perspective on the treatment of anorexia nervosa in adolescents. In D. M. Garner & P. E. Garfinkel (Eds.), *Handbook of psychotherapy for anorexia nervosa and bulimia* (pp., 363–390). New York: Guilford Press.

Stunkard, A. J. (1959). Eating patterns and obesity. *Psychiatric Quarterly, 33*, 284–295.

Swift, W. J. (1985). Assessment of the bulimic patient. *American Journal of Orthopsychiatry, 55*, 384–396.

Szmukler, G. I. (1985). The epidemiology of anorexia nervosa and bulimia. *Journal of Psychiatric Research, 19*(2/3), 143–153.

Szmukler, G. (1987). Some comments on the link between anorexia nervosa and affective disorder. *International Journal of Eating Disorders, 6*, 181–189.

Szmukler, G. I., Eisler, I., Gillies, C., & Hayward, M. E. (1985). The implications of anorexia nervosa in a ballet school. *Journal of Psychiatric Research, 19*, 177–181.

Telch, C. F., Agras, W. S., & Rossiter, E. M. (1988). Binge eating increases with increasing adiposity. *International Journal of Eating Disorders, 7*, 115–119.

Thompson, J. K., Dolce, J. J., Spana, R. E., & Register, A. (1987). Emotionally versus intellectually based estimates of body size. *International Journal of Eating Disorders, 6*, 507–513.

Vandereycken, W., & Pierloot, R. (1983). The significance of subclassification in anorexia nervosa: A comparative study of clinical features in 141 patients. *Psychological Medicine, 13*, 543–549.

Walsh, B. T., & Gladis, M. (1985). Bulimia Interview Form. *Psychopharmacology Bulletin, 21*(3), 1017–1023.

Wardle, J. (1980). Dietary restraint and binge eating. *Behavioral Analysis and Modification, 4*, 201–209.

Williams, P., Hand, D., & Tarnopolsky, A. (1982). The problem of screening for uncommon disorders—a comment on the Eating Attitudes Test. *Psychological Medicine, 12*, 431–434.

Williams, R. L., Schaefer, C. A., Shisslak, C. M., Gronwaldt, V. H., & Comerci, G. D. (1986). Eating attitudes and behaviors in adolescent women: Discrimination of normals, dieters, and suspected bulimics using the Eating Attitudes Test and Eating Disorder Inventory. *International Journal of Eating Disorders, 5*, 879–894.

Williamson, D. A., Goreczny, M. A., & Duchmann, E. G. (1987). Behavioral and psychophysiological assessment of bulimia. *Annals of Behavioral Medicine, 9*, 8–11.

Willmuth, M. E., Leitenberg, H., Rosen, J. C., & Cado, S. (1988). A comparison of purging and nonpurging normal weight bulimics. *International Journal of Eating Disorders, 7*, 825–835.

Wilson, G. T. (1987). Assessing treatment outcome in bulimia nervosa: A methodological note. *International Journal of Eating Disorders, 6,* 339–348.

Wilson, G. T., & Lindholm, L. (1987). Bulimia nervosa and depression. *International Journal of Eating Disorders, 6,* 725–732.

Wilson, G. T., Rossiter, E., Kleifield, E. I., & Lindholm, L. (1986). Cognitive-behavioral treatment of bulimia nervosa: A controlled evaluation. *Behavior Research and Therapy, 24,* 277–288.

Wilson, G. T., & Smith, D. (1989). Assessment of bulimia nervosa: An evaluation of the eating disorders examination. *International Journal of Eating Disorders, 8,* 173–179.

Wooley, S. C., & Kearney-Cooke, A. (1986). Intensive treatment of bulimia and body image disturbance. In K. D. Brownell & J. P. Foreyt (Eds.), *Handbook of eating disorders* (pp. 476–502). New York: Basic Books.

CHAPTER 9

Gender Identity Disorder

Kenneth J. Zucker
Clarke Institute of Psychiatry

The first edition of the *Diagnostic and Statistical Manual* (DSM; American Psychiatric Association, 1952) contained only two diagnoses specifically for children—adjustment reaction and schizophrenic reaction, childhood type. The second edition (American Psychiatric Association, 1968) contained nine diagnoses for children. Neither of these editions included a disorder pertaining to childhood gender identity problems. This situation changed in the third edition (American Psychiatric Association, 1980), which introduced the diagnosis gender identity disorder of childhood (GIDC); it may, however, have been given a kind of outlaw status by making it the only disorder for children not located in the section of DSM-III entitled Disorders Usually First Evident in Infancy, Childhood, or Adolescence. Perhaps because of this separation, a number of recent texts devoted exclusively to child psychiatric diagnoses (Frame & Matson, 1987; Ollendick & Hersen, 1983) have omitted the GIDC from discussion. The revised third edition of the DSM (DSM-III-R; American Psychiatric Association, 1987) placed the GIDC in the same section as other child psychiatric disorders, so perhaps its previous neglect will become nothing more than a dim memory. The present chapter provides the reader with a critical overview regarding the common terminology used in the study of psychosexual development and its disorders, the reliability and validity of various approaches to diagnostic classification, available assessment procedures, and directions for future clinical research in the areas of assessment and diagnosis.

HISTORICAL BACKGROUND

Descriptive Terminology

Current thinking about psychosexual development suggests the use of, at minimum, a tripartite conceptual scheme whose components are *gender identity, gender role,* and *sexual orientation* (Green, 1974; Money, 1973; Stoller, 1968a). *Gender identity* can be defined as children's recognition or awareness that they are a member of one sex and not the other. At a more affective level, there is a valuing of this knowledge, such that children express pride or "positive prejudice" about their gender (Etaugh, Levine, & Mennella, 1984). *Gender role* can be defined as those behaviors, attitudes, and personality traits that a society, in a given culture and historical period, designates as masculine or feminine. Assessment techniques typically evaluate the extent to which a child prefers to engage in, or to adopt, masculine or feminine gender roles. *Sexual orientation* can be defined as a person's preferred mode of erotic fantasy and behavior. The most salient dimensions of sexual orientation seem to be the sex and age of one's partner, though reliance on fetishistic stimuli and paraphilic fantasy for sexual arousal also needs to be considered.

Children who meet the DSM-III-R diagnostic criteria for GIDC manifest deviations with regard to the first two components of psychosexual development. These children either perceive themselves as of the opposite sex or express a dislike about their status as a boy or as a girl and desire to change sex. Second, in a variety of behavioral domains these children show gender role preferences that are typical of the opposite sex.

The idea that children can show a marked anomaly in their gender identity development has been a controversial one. The reasons for this are, no doubt, multiple and diverse. Historically, the idea that gender identity represents a unique aspect of the self is relatively recent, at least in scientific circles. Freud (1925), for example, claimed that prior to the "oedipal" phase (i.e., about ages 4–5), boys and girls were essentially similar in their psychological makeup and made little differentiation among the components of psychosexual development as they are now understood.

In the 1950s, Money's (1952, 1985; Money, Hampson, & Hampson, 1955) seminal work with physically hermaphroditic children demonstrated the importance of conceptualizing gender identity as a distinct psychological variable. A hermaphroditic child born with genital anomalies illuminates the salience of gender as a biosocial category—should the "sex of assignment" be announced as male or female? Despite the anomalous sexual biology of hermaphroditic children, Money, Hampson, and Hampson (1957) concluded that these children could, in fact, develop an unconflicted gender identity if they were assigned to one gender or the other early in life and then reared in an "unambiguous" manner. Later, Stoller (1964) pointed out that continual uncertainty about a child's gender status often led to the development of a "hermaphroditic identity." Other studies, including moving personal accounts (Barbin, 1980), illustrated the damage that resulted from trying to change a hermaphrodite's gender status on the basis of arbitrary biological criteria.

The ubiquity of gender as a dimension of social behavior and social life has received increasing recognition (Cucchiari, 1981; Maccoby, 1988). Infants as young as 5 months have been shown to use gender-linked cues as discriminative stimuli (Dirks & Gibson, 1977; Fagan & Singer, 1979), though it is unlikely that they are consciously aware of this.

Between the second and third year of life, children develop the capacity for a more conscious type of gender discrimination that seems to serve an organizing function for the expression of at least some sex-typed behaviors. Fagot, Leinbach, and Hagan (1986), for example, tested toddlers between the ages of 21 and 40 months on a gender-labeling task in which they were required to discriminate between pictures of boys and girls. Over a 4-week period, these toddlers were then observed in a naturalistic play setting in which the occurrence of a number of sex-typed behaviors was assessed. Fagot and colleagues (1986) found that the toddlers (mean age = 30 mos) who "passed" the gender-labeling task spent more time playing with same-sex peers than the toddlers (mean age = 26 mos) who "failed" the task; the girls who passed the task were also less aggressive than the girls who failed it, even after controlling for age. These findings point to the important role of cognition as an organizing variable in the display of sex-dimorphic behaviors.

While the psychology of hermaphroditism was being explored and the concept of gender identity articulated, the adult syndrome of transsexualism began to attract notice. A major scientific watershed was the publication of the Christine Jorgensen case by the Danish endocrinologist Hamburger (1953; Hamburger, Sturup, & Dahl-Iverson, 1953). Other personal and scientific reports along the same lines appeared at about the same time (e.g., Benjamin, 1954; Cauldwell, 1949; Cowell, 1954), but the Jorgensen case helped crystallize the notion that the discontent with their gender identity experienced by some adults might impel them to seek radical physical transformations. The relevance of this adult syndrome for the study of children was disclosed by life history interviews, from which it appeared that the patient's gender dysphoria, or discontent, originated in childhood. Many transsexual adults recalled an extensive childhood history of behaving like, and wishing to be of, the opposite sex. Such recollections served as one rationale for the idea that children "at risk" for transsexualism could be identified and studied *in statu nascendi* (Green, 1968; Stoller, 1968b).

At present, gender identity has been fairly well accepted as an important psychological construct, though its scope and functional properties are still being debated (Bem, 1981; Deaux & Major, 1987; Freimuth & Hornstein, 1982; Spence, 1984, 1985; Unger, 1979). The notion that children can have a gender identity disorder, however, remains somewhat controversial. For example, it is not uncommon for professionals to interpret a child's wish to be of the opposite sex and preference for cross-gender role behaviors as only a phase (Stoller, 1967). Although normative data suggest that extensive cross-gender behavior is uncommon at all ages (Zucker, 1985), the significance of the behaviors is minimized and interpreted as something that all children go through. At a more theoretical level, there is debate as to whether, for example, a boy who engages in extensive feminine behaviors should be considered deviant in a pathological sense, as opposed to a mere statistical one, given efforts in some quarters to expand the boundaries of acceptable gender role behaviors for boys and girls.

Clinical Features

Accounts of children whose behavior patterns corresponded to the DSM-III-R diagnosis of GIDC were provided in three early clinical papers (Bender & Paster, 1941; Friend, Schiddle, Klein, & Dunaeff, 1954; MacDonald, 1938), but the authors of these papers lacked the descriptive terminology that has proved so useful in organizing the clinical picture. More systematic accounts of such children appeared in reports published during the 1960s (Bakwin, 1960; Green & Money, 1960; Stoller, 1968b; Zuger, 1966). A number of behavioral characteristics cut across these reports. Among boys, these included verbal statements that he was or would like to be a girl, cross-dressing in girls' or women's clothing, a preference for culturally stereotypical feminine toys and activities, emulation of females in fantasy play, admiration of females, a preference for girls as playmates, display of feminine or effeminate motor movements, a high-pitched effeminate voice, expression of dislike of his sexual anatomy (e.g., hiding his penis in order to simulate the female genital configuration, sitting to urinate), and an aversion to rough-and-tumble play and group sports. Much less was written about girls during the 1960s, but subsequent reports (Bradley, 1980; Green, 1974; Meyer & Dupkin, 1985; Rekers & Mead, 1979, 1980; Zucker, 1989) have revealed a similar, albeit inverted, clinical picture: verbal statements that she was or would like to be a boy, a preference for masculine clothing co-occurring with an aversion to culturally stereotypical girls' clothing (e.g., dresses), a preference for culturally stereotypical masculine toys and activities, emulation of males in fantasy play, admiration of males, a preference for boys as playmates, display of exaggerated masculine motoric movements, attempts to speak in a "deep" or gruff voice, expression of dislike of her sexual anatomy (e.g., wanting to have a penis, standing to urinate), and an intense interest in rough-and-tumble play and group sports with boys.

There was no formal diagnosis of such behavior, so individual authors invented their own terms to characterize it. Some of these terms were closely tied to certain theoretical preconceptions, others less so. The terms included *atypical gender development* (Rekers, 1977a), *atypical gender identity* (Green, 1973), *childhood transsexualism* (Stoller, 1968b), *cross-gender behavior* (Green, 1979), *cross-gender identification* (Green, 1968), *deviant gender role behavior* (Bakwin, 1968), *effeminacy* (Green & Money, 1961), *effeminate behavior* (Zuger, 1966), *feminine behavior* (Green, 1975), *feminoid*[ism] (Rekers & Yates, 1976), *gender aberrations* (Stoller, 1978), *gender deviance* (Bates, Bentler, & Thompson, 1973), *gender disturbance* (Rekers, Bentler, Rosen, & Lovaas, 1977), *gender-dysphoric* (Rosen, Rekers, & Brigham, 1982), *gender identity confusion* (Schultz, 1979), *gender identity disorder* (Green, 1971), *gender incongruity syndrome* (Higham, 1976), *gender-problem* (Skilbeck, Bates, & Bentler, 1975), *gender role abnormalities* (Bates, Skilbeck, Smith, & Bentler, 1974), *incongruous gender role* (Green & Money, 1960), *pre-transsexual* (Rekers & Varni, 1977), *sexual identity conflict* (Green, 1974), *sexual identity disorder* (Rekers & Milner, 1978), and *transvestism* (Bakwin, 1960). DSM-III used Green's (1971) term, *gender identity disorder,* to represent the basic phenomenology that had been described prior to 1980.

Previous Classification Approaches

Prior to DSM-III, a few attempts were made to include gender identity problems in behavioral classification systems, which varied greatly in the extent to which they relied on theory. Empirically derived classification systems, such as those based on factor analysis, occasionally identified behavioral traits suggestive of gender identity problems. Dreger's Children's Behavior Classification Project contained a factor variously termed *homoerotic affectation versus hysteric apprehensiveness* (Dreger, 1970), *identity problem* (Baker & Dreger, 1973), and *gender confusion* (Dreger, 1981). Behaving like the opposite sex (e.g., cross-dressing) and acting in an effeminate manner seemed to be the items most relevant.

Perhaps the most well known classification system of this kind is the

Child Behavior Checklist (CBCL; Achenbach, 1978). This parent-report inventory of child behavior problems contains 118 items, each of which is rated on a 0–2 point scale for frequency of occurrence. The CBCL has been factor-analyzed by sex for three age groupings (4–5, 6–11, 12–16) (Achenbach & Edelbrock, 1981, 1983). "Behaves like opposite sex" and "wishes to be of opposite sex" are the items most relevant for identifying potential gender identity problems.

For both boys and girls in the 4–5 age group, a factor labeled Sex Problems emerged; that factor contained the two CBCL items most closely related to possible gender identity problems. "Behaves like opposite sex" also loaded on the Obese subscale for girls. None of the other four sex-by-age groupings contained a similar factor, though "behaves like opposite sex" loaded on the Schizoid subscale in the 12–16 age group for boys and on the Cruel subscale in the 6–11 age group for girls.

Both Achenbach (1980) and Dreger (1981) suggested that their gender-related factors corresponded to the DSM-III diagnosis of GIDC. In our own research experience, we have found that the majority of the parents of gender-referred children rate the two CBCL items as either a 1 or a 2. In contrast, these items have rarely been endorsed among our control groups. Therefore, it could be argued that the items show adequate sensitivity and specificity (Vecchio, 1966). Whether variations in parental ratings on these items show any within-group sensitivity remains to be demonstrated. This might be particularly important in unselected populations where the risk of a false positive diagnosis could occur only if the CBCL items are used as screens (Pleak, Meyer-Bahlburg, O'Brien, Bowen, & Morganstein, 1989).

Classification systems like the CBCL are relatively atheoretical, though the empirical returns that such systems generate have been used to develop theory and new hypotheses (Achenbach, 1985, 1988). In contrast, Stoller (1968b) proposed a more theoretically based classification system that relied not only on phenomenology but also on putative dynamic and etiological variables. He attempted to differentiate boys whom he viewed as "transsexual" (or pretranssexual) from other boys (and men) engaging in feminine behaviors (Stoller, 1968b). At some times, Stoller seemed to have taken the position that transsexual boys differed qualitatively from other feminine boys, both in their behavior and in the etiological factors that led to their disorder. At other times, Stoller (1985) took a more spectrum or quantitatively oriented point of view: "The simplest form of the hypothesis: in boys . . . the more mother and the less father, the more femininity" (p. 25).

In an early paper based on a sample of three boys, Stoller (1968b) argued that the symptom most unique to the transsexual boy was the "fixed belief that [he] is a member of the opposite sex and will grow up and develop the anatomical characteristics of the opposite sex" (p. 92). In addition, he noted that "these boys do not only wish at times that they were girls . . . [but also] maintain . . . they are . . . females" (p. 97). In the absence of these behaviors, Stoller would not make the diagnosis of male childhood transsexualism.

In a critique, Zucker (1982) suggested that there were at least two main problems with Stoller's diagnostic criteria. First, Stoller was inconsistent with regard to the defining feature of boyhood transsexualism in that he did not always distinguish between *wishing* and *believing*. For example, Stoller (1968b) wrote that "this condition is called childhood transsexualism because its most obvious manifestation is the boy's *feeling* he is a girl" (p. 196, emphasis added). Given the difference between believing and feeling that one is of the opposite sex, it cannot be certain that the key diagnostic criterion is, in fact, the child's "fixed belief that [he] is a member of the opposite sex" (cf. Stoller & Newman, 1971). In addition, Stoller's three subjects were all quite young at assessment. It is therefore conceivable that the putative misclassification of gender was heavily influenced by developmental factors.

Zucker, Bradley, and Kuksis (1988) studied patterns of gender constancy development in a sample of 70 gender-referred children. On Slaby and Frey's (1975) gender constancy interview, for example, it was found that only 3 out of 70 gender-referred children incorrectly labeled themselves as of the opposite sex, a percentage that did not differ from that of control subjects. Even among the youngest children (ages 3–4 years) with extreme cross-gender identification, misclassification of gender was more the exception than the rule. At more advanced levels of gender constancy development, however, there was some evidence that the gender-referred children performed more poorly than the controls. Thus, there appears to be some evidence that "cognitive gender confusion" is part of the clinical picture, but not the overwhelmingly decisive part of it as reported by Stoller.

It should also be noted that Stoller has never made clear the means by which his data were collected (e.g., whether the data came from the mother, the child, therapy sessions, etc.) and has never published comprehensive transcripts of child interviews.

Despite these difficulties, the extent of cross-gender-identification could still be utilized as a frame of reference in trying to decide whether a particular case might correspond to the extremes observed by Stoller. There is a problem in this connection, however, because Stoller (1975) reported having evaluated a boy who was "as feminine as any seen," yet was not, in his view, a transsexual. His basis for this claim was etiological; that is, he felt that the variables associated with his other cases were not present in their full form and that consideration of etiological factors was therefore necessary to confirm the diagnosis of male childhood transsexualism. This scheme conflates descriptive and putative etiological variables in making a diagnostic decision.

Despite the problems with Stoller's proposed classification, one can glean from it the high probability that there is some type of spectrum with regard to verbal gender-dysphoric statements. At one extreme of this continuum might be children who insist that they are of the opposite sex. At less extreme points along the continuum might be children who vacillate in their capacity to identify themselves correctly as boys or girls, children who know they are of one sex but wish to be of the other sex, and children who are ambivalent and do not know what their sex should be. Obviously, in order to determine the extent to which the child's behavior is influenced by cognitive immaturity, such a spectrum approach would have to take into account developmental norms for the ability to self-label.

Another classification scheme has been offered by Rekers, Rosen, and their colleagues (Bentler, Rekers, & Rosen, 1979; Rosen, Rekers, & Friar, 1977). Rosen and associates (1977) stated that two distinct syndromes—*cross-gender identification* and *gender behavior disturbance*—were detectable among boys referred for potential gender identity problems. They based the differential diagnosis on three characteristics: (a) only boys in the first group have a "preference for a feminine identity," as inferred, for example, from verbal statements about wanting to be a girl; (b) these boys also engage in more extreme and persistent cross-dressing; and (c) these boys are more likely to have an extremely close and dependent relationship with their mothers. Rosen and colleagues did not feel that other characteristics, such as cross-gender toy play and cross-gender peer preferences, differentiated the two diagnostic types.

Conceptually, this scheme was based on the idea that one's gender identity (sense of maleness or femaleness) need not be correlated with one's preference for same-sex or cross-sex behavior (Rosen et al., 1977). Clinically, the scheme provided a diagnostic category for youngsters who engage in extensive cross-gender behavior but do not verbalize the wish to be of the opposite sex.

To test for the distinctiveness of the two syndromes, Bentler and colleagues (1979) utilized some extremely complex data sources to make severity ratings on two 5-point scales—one for "sex-role identity disturbance" and the other for "sex-role behavior disturbance"—in a sample of gender-referred children. The correlation between the two ratings was .71; thus, Bentler and colleagues (1979) concluded that the two syndromes "were not entirely synonymous" and there was "a basis of differentiation of these concepts in individual cases" (p. 277).

Unfortunately, Rosen and associates (1977) and Bentler and colleagues (1979) provided rather cryptic accounts of their procedures, including the decision rules they utilized to make their ratings; in addition, they gave no evidence for interrater reliability. More important, however, their studies lacked empirical evidence for the existence of two syndromes. Rosen and associates (1977) and Bentler and colleagues (1979) did not show that the traits they claimed were of relevance for differential diagnosis "hung together," as might have been demonstrated through factor analysis, nor did they show this on a case-by-case basis. They also failed to provide other validity tests, such as differential response to treatment or differences in natural history.

Rosen and colleagues (1977) seemed to be struggling with the conceptual question of how to think about a youngster who engages in extensive cross-gender behavior but does not voice the desire to change sex. They also seemed to be striving for some type of system that could deal with general variation in severity, much as this issue has been struggled with in other areas of child psychopathology, such as depression and hyperactivity. In this respect, their proposed system has heuristic value (Coates & Zucker, 1988; Zucker, 1982, 1985).

DEFINITIONAL ISSUES

This section considers the adequacy of the DSM-III-R diagnostic criteria for the GIDC, which are presented in Table 9.1. For both sexes, two criteria (Points A and B) are required for the diagnosis. Point A seems to index children's sense of discomfort with their assigned sex and their desire to change sex. Descriptively, this point appears to be most directly tied to the concept of gender identity. Point B-1 seems to emphasize children's preference for cross-gender roles and activities and, at the same time, the children's aversion to roles and clothing more typically associated with their own sex. These characteristics seem to be most directly related to the concept of gender role. Point B-2 emphasizes the children's dislike of and aversion to their sexual anatomy. It would appear that the framers of DSM-III-R believed that such behavior was more relevant for gender role than for gender identity, though the empirical justification for this is scant.

A few issues with respect to the Point A criterion deserve comment. For both sexes, the child must show a "persistent and intense distress" about being a boy or a girl. This phrase did not appear in the DSM-III criteria for either sex. Unfortunately, DSM-III-R does not specify how one assesses such distress or in what ways the distress might be distinct

TABLE 9.1
DSM-III-R Diagnostic Criteria for Gender Identity Disorder of Childhood

For females:

A. Persistent and intense distress about being a girl, and a stated desire to be a boy (not merely a desire for any perceived cultural advantages from being a boy), or insistence that she is a boy.
B. Either (1) or (2);
    (1) persistent marked aversion to normative feminine clothing and insistence on wearing stereotypical masculine clothing, e.g., boys' underwear and other accessories
    (2) persistent repudiation of female anatomic structures, as evidenced by at least one of the following:
        (a) an assertion that she has, or will grow, a penis
        (b) rejection of urinating in a sitting position
        (c) assertion that she does not want to grow breasts or menstruate
C. The girl has not yet reached puberty.

For males:

A. Persistent and intense distress about being a boy and an intense desire to be a girl or, more rarely, insistence that he is a girl.
B. Either (1) or (2):
    (1) preoccupation with female stereotypical activities, as shown by a preference for either cross-dressing or simulating female attire, or by an intense desire to participate in the games and pastimes of girls and rejection of male stereotypical toys, games, and activities
    (2) persistent repudiation of male anatomic structures, as indicated by at least one of the following repeated assertions:
        (a) that he will grow up to become a woman (not merely in role)
        (b) that his penis or testes are disgusting or will disappear
        (c) that it would be better not to have a penis or testes
C. The boy has not yet reached puberty

Note. From *Diagnostic and Statistical Manual of Mental Disorders* (3rd ed., rev., pp. 73–74) by American Psychiatric Association, 1987, Washington, DC: Author. Reprinted by permission.

from other operationalized components in the criteria. The phraseology that follows this portion of the Point A criterion then shows a subtle difference between the sexes. For girls, there must be a "*stated* desire to be a boy" (emphasis added), whereas for boys, there must be an "*intense* desire to be a girl" (p. 73, emphasis added). For girls, then, the desire must be expressed verbally, but this is not explicitly required for boys. In addition, the phraseology for girls does not address the issue of intensity or some other variable pertaining to chronicity. Why these two distinctions appeared in DSM-III-R is not clear, because the phraseology for the two sexes was identical in DSM-III: "strongly and persistently *stated* desire to be a boy [girl]" (emphasis added). For boys, the issue of how one infers such desire independent of other aspects of the criteria (e.g., the "preoccupation with female stereotypical activities" in Point B-1) is paramount if specific reliance is not placed on verbal statements.

Furthermore, for girls a cross-sex wish cannot be "merely a desire for any perceived cultural advantages from being a boy." This exclusion rule presents a couple of difficulties. First, it makes an etiological or motivational assumption about a girl's verbal desire to be a boy—for example, that one type of desire is based on a perception of cultural bias, whereas at least one other unspecified type is not. Although this distinction might have relevance for such parameters as natural history and response to treatment, it is unclear why it should be used diagnostically. Second, there is no similar exclusion rule for boys. This is puzzling because, in principle, a boy may wish to be a girl because of a similar perception of cultural bias. The "manifest" reasons that clinic-referred boys give for wishing to be girls include: girls get to wear dresses, wear lipstick, are not yelled at as much, do not play rough, and so on (Coates, 1985; Green, 1974). If such rationales are construed in cultural terms, the potential for bias should apply equally to both sexes.

It should also be noted that the Point A criterion requires a clinical judgment in determining what qualifies as "persistent and intense distress" or an "intense desire" to be of the opposite sex. What criteria should clinicians utilize in deciding whether the desire to change sex is persistent and intense? To some extent, the answer to this question hinges on what is known about the prevalence and intensity of cross-sex wishes in the general population. Achenbach and Edelbrock's (1981, 1983) CBCL study, among others, provided some information with regard to the prevalence of wishing to be of the opposite sex in referred and nonreferred samples. The percentage of nonreferred boys and girls, ages 4–13, grouped at 2-year intervals, rated positive ("sometimes" or "often") on the item "wishes to be of opposite sex" never exceeded 5% (median = 2.1%). The median percentage was higher among referred children (median = 5.4%; range = 1.1–15.5%), with referred boys ages 4–5 showing an outlier percentage of 15.5. In both groups, the percentages were higher for girls than for boys and, at least for boys, negatively related to age (cf. Pleak et al., 1989). Generally, the CBCL data suggest that the desire to change sex is fairly uncommon, particularly among boys. Nevertheless, one probably has to be cautious, as Meyer-Bahlburg (1985) pointed out, in demarcating the "zone of transition between clinically significant cross-gender behavior and mere statistical deviations from the gender norm" (p. 682).

The Point B-1 criterion included some of the cross-gender behaviors commonly observed in cross-gender-identified boys, such as cross-dressing and cross-gender toy play. In addition, this criterion included an aversion to culturally typical masculine activities. Thus, there is a cross-gender preference, and not an equal attraction for both masculine and feminine activities, which would be somewhat more difficult to interpret. For example, some theorists might conceptualize such a pattern as "androgynous," whereas others might interpret it as a reflection of gender role confusion or ambivalence. Interestingly, the examples provided did not include a preference for female roles in fantasy play or a preference for female playmates, which are also extremely common traits among cross-gender-identified boys (Green, 1976).

DSM-III did not include a similar criterion for girls; that is, it made no reference to the gender-disturbed girl's intense preoccupation with cross-dressing and involvement in masculine stereotypical activities. In DSM-III-R, however, a new criterion was included (i.e., B-1) that emphasized the gender-disturbed girl's aversion to normative feminine clothing and involvement in cross-dressing. The inclusion of this criterion was based, in part, on clinical observation that an aversion to normative feminine clothing may distinguish gender-disturbed girls from girls who engage in masculine behavior but are not necessarily gender dysphoric (Zucker, 1982).

The Point B-2 criterion for boys captured the concept of "anatomic dysphoria," that is, the dislike of one's sexual anatomy. The behavioral manifestations remained unchanged from those given in DSM-III. The wording of the criteria for girls, however, has changed substantially from that of DSM-III. The DSM-III criteria required either "delusional" (e.g., that "she has . . . a penis") or "immature" thinking but did not include feelings of dislike toward one's sexual anatomy (Zucker, 1982). This has changed in DSM-III-R, whose criteria for girls are more similar to the criteria for boys.

SELECTIVE REVIEW OF THE LITERATURE

Reliability and Validity of Diagnosis

Although a number of authors use DSM-III criteria in describing their samples (Coates & Person, 1985; Davenport, 1986; Green, 1987; Kosky, 1987), only one study has actually attempted to determine whether the criteria can be reliably diagnosed. Zucker, Finegan, Doering, and Bradley (1984) had two raters read the chart histories of 36 consecutive referrals (31 boys, 5 girls) to a child clinic that specialized in gender identity problems. Part of each history focused on seven aspects of the child's gender identity development: cross-gender identity statements, toy preferences, peer preferences, sex-typed mannerisms, cross-dressing, involvement in rough-and-tumble play, and anatomic dysphoria.

One rater was familiar with the details of the case, whereas the other rater knew nothing about the case except what was available from the history. The history data were used to decide whether the child met the DSM-III criteria for GIDC. Only Point A was evaluated because of our disagreement with the Point B criteria for girls (as noted earlier). According to the first rater, 16 of the boys met both Points A and B of the DSM-III criteria, and all 5 girls met Point A. For Point A, the second rater agreed with the first rater in 34 of the 36 cases (19 present, 15 absent); for Point B, the second rater agreed with the first rater in 28 of the 31 cases (16 present, 12 absent). The kappa values for these two ratings were .89 and .80, respectively (both *ps* $< .001$).

These data suggest that achieving good reliability in diagnosis is not particularly difficult, though a few caveats should be mentioned. First, our concerns about the accuracy of the Point B criteria for girls in DSM-III led us to ignore it on the ground that it would lead to a false negative diagnosis. (Incidentally, all five girls would meet the revised Point B criteria in DSM-III-R.) Moreover, our study was conducted by individuals "interested" in this particular disorder, and thus more complete information may have been documented in the histories than might have ordinarily been available. This raises the question of what information is actually used in making a diagnostic decision, a point not addressed in the Zucker and associates (1984) study. It would be interesting to know what threshold of information a clinician requires before making such a decision. For example, suppose an analogue case history of a boy included information regarding cross-dressing, cross-sex toy play, and affiliation with female peers (behaviors relevant for the Point B-1 criteria) but contained no specific information with regard to Point A. Would a clinician recognize that the available information was insufficient to make a diagnostic decision? Similarly, suppose a history indicated the presence of some cross-gender behavior but not enough to fulfill the DSM-III criteria. Would a clinician overdiagnose simply because of the presence of some cross-gender behavior in the history?

In the Zucker and associates (1984) study, the validity of the DSM-III criteria was assessed by comparing the two diagnostic groups on a number of demographic variables and sex-typed behaviors. It should be noted that, by and large, the children who did not meet the complete DSM-III criteria showed at least some characteristics of cross-gender-identification and were not necessarily inappropriate referrals. In fact, some of the non-DSM-III cases had met the complete criteria at an earlier age but not at the time of the assessment.

Table 9.2 (Cohort 1) shows the demographic data for the DSM-III and non-DSM-III subgroups. It can be seen that the DSM-III subjects were significantly younger than their non-DSM-III counterparts but did not differ with regard to sex, full-scale IQ, and parents' social class and

TABLE 9.2
Demographic Characteristics as a Function of Diagnostic Status for Gender Identity Disorder of Childhood

		Diagnostic Status by Cohort											
		Cohort 1			*Cohort 2*			*Cohort 3*			*Combined*		
Variables		*DSM-III* (N=21)		*Non-DSM-III* (N=15)	*DSM-III* (N=18)		*Non-DSM-III* (N=18)	*DSM-III* (N=15)		*Non-DSM-III* (N=21)	*DSM-III* (N=54)		*Non-DSM-III* (N=54)
Sex of child													
Male	N	16		15	15		16	14		20	45		51
Female	N	5		0	3		2	1		1	9		3
	p		ns			ns			ns			ns	
Age (in years)	M	6.6		9.7	6.6		8.9	6.2		8.6	6.4		9.0
	SD	2.2		2.8	2.4		2.5	2.0		2.9	2.1		2.7
	p		.000			.006			.008			.000	
Full-scale IQ	M	104.6		104.0	111.8		109.9	109.1		101.2	108.3		104.9
	SD	20.8		11.6	17.3		13.1	13.6		23.0	17.8		17.4
	p		ns			ns			ns			ns	
Social class	M	39.8		32.1	44.7		38.8	47.6		36.7	43.6		36.1
	SD	13.8		17.5	16.9		14.1	18.1		15.8	16.2		15.7
	p		ns			ns			.065			.016	
Family status													
Both parents	N	17		10	13		8	13		12	39		30
Mother only/ reconstituted	N	4		5	5		10	2		9	15		24
	p		ns			ns			ns			ns	

marital status. Among the boys, the DSM-III subjects were more likely to be singletons and less likely to have a sister. Moreover, the sisters of the DSM-III boys were significantly younger than the sisters of the non-DSM-III boys. The two subgroups did not differ with regard to the percentage who had brothers or with regard to the age of their brothers (Zucker et al., 1984).

Table 9.2 shows the same demographic data for Cohorts 2 and 3, each consisting of 36 consecutive referrals to our gender identity clinic. In both cohorts, the DSM-III subjects were, again, significantly younger, but there were no differences with regard to sex, IQ, and social class and marital status of the parents, apart from a marginal effect for social class in Cohort 3. The sibling effect observed in Cohort 1 was not found for the second and third cohorts. When collapsed across the three cohorts, both age and social class were significantly different (Table 9.2).

These data show quite clearly that younger children are more likely than older children to meet the complete DSM-III criteria for GIDC. In the total sample, children with higher social class backgrounds were more likely to meet the complete criteria. Correlational analyses indicated that the variables of age, IQ, and social class and marital status of the parents were all significantly correlated with one another (absolute rs ranged from .29 to .55). To test which variables contributed to the correct classification of the subjects in the two diagnostic groups, a discriminant function analysis was performed. Age and IQ contributed to the discriminant function, with age showing the greatest power. In the DSM-III group 81.5% were correctly classified, and in the non-DSM-III group 66.7% were correctly classified.

In the Zucker and colleagues (1984) study, the two diagnostic subgroups also were compared on 10 measures of sex-typed behavior (e.g., play behavior in the clinic setting, parent-report on standardized questionnaires). The DSM-III subgroup showed more cross-gender behavior or less same-sex behavior than the non-DSM-III subgroup on all 10 measures; on 6 of these measures, the difference was statistically significant. Covarying age did not substantially alter the pattern. Thus, there seemed to be at least some genuine behavioral differences between the two diagnostic subgroups in the degree of same-sex or cross-sex-typed behavior, even with age controlled. Whether this diagnostic distinction is related to other differences (e.g., etiology, long-term follow-up) remains to be seen.

Influence of Informant

In our research, we have relied primarily on parents to act as *informants* during the clinical interview in making a diagnostic decision. We have not formally relied on what the children had to say. The degree of informant concordance in reporting psychiatric symptomatology in children has become a topic of increasing interest over the past few years (Edelbrock & Costello, 1988; Gutterman, O'Brien, & Young, 1987). There is some evidence that better concordance (e.g., between mother and child) is found for symptoms that are concrete, observable, and unambiguous (e.g., Herjanic & Reich, 1982). For example, the Diagnostic Interview for Children and Adolescents contains two items related to gender identity: cross-dressing and wishing to be of the opposite sex. Herjanic and Reich (1982) reported a kappa of .33 for cross-dressing but a kappa of only .10 for wishing to change sex. The low kappa values for both items can be partially explained by their relatively low frequency of occurrence, but the difference between the two values seems consistent with Herjanic and Reich's general finding regarding the influence of certain characteristics of their items, such as relative observability.

In our experience with a gender-referred population, we have encountered a few cases in which parents claimed never to have heard their child verbalize a desire to change sex, though significant others (teachers, siblings) and the child clearly indicated such a desire. In these cases, making the diagnosis of GIDC would be informant-dependent. We are currently employing a structured gender dysphoria interview with the child that will enable us to evaluate parent–child discrepancies more formally. Preliminary results suggest that children diagnosed as GIDC based on parent interview data are more likely to report the desire to be of the opposite sex or to show gender identity confusion on the structured interview than are children who do not meet the full criteria for GIDC. Thus, at least within an extreme population, the degree of parent–child concordance seems promising. Nevertheless, the identification of instances of discrepancies will probably prove useful for case formulation and management strategies.

Assessment Techniques

Over the years, a number of assessment tools have been developed for use with cross-gender-identified children. These assessment tools have included structured parent interviews regarding specific sex-typed behaviors (Green, 1987; Roberts, Green, Williams, & Goodman, 1987), parent-report on questionnaires dealing with sex-typed play and behavior (Bates & Bentler, 1973; Bates et al., 1973; Green, 1976, 1987; Zucker, Bradley, Doering, & Lozinski, 1985), measurement of overt (Green, Fuller, Rutley, & Hendler, 1972b; Rekers & Yates, 1976; Zucker et al., 1982) and covert (Green & Fuller, 1973; Zucker, Doering, Bradley, Alon, &

Lozinski, 1984) sex-typed play in standardized situations, observation of sex-typed motoric behavior (Bates, Bentler, & Thompson, 1979; Green, Neuberg, & Finch, 1983), assessment of gender constancy development (Zucker et al., 1988), and sex-typed indices on the Draw-a-Person (Green, Fuller, & Rutley, 1972a; Skilbeck et al., 1975; Zucker, Finegan, Doering, & Bradley, 1983) and Rorschach (Lozinski, 1988; Tuber & Coates, 1985) tests. These techniques are presented in Table 9.3.

Generally, the studies cited have shown significant differences between the index group of gender-referred children and controls, the latter of which have included siblings, children with psychiatric problems, and normal children. Based on parent interview data, for example, Green (1987) found that a discriminant function analysis required 6 of 16 sex-typed behaviors to classify correctly all boys as members of either the feminine group or the male control group. Green also utilized a variety of psychological tests in his research, and these tests also discriminated the probands from controls; however, he has not yet provided information with regard to the power of the tests in group classification.

In our research, psychological testing using some of the assessment strategies already noted has proved useful in distinguishing gender-referred children from controls, though the discriminating power of individual tests is clearly not perfect. For example, consider the Draw-a-Person (DAP) test, a relatively simple and probably crude marker of gender identification. On this test, children are asked to draw a person and then to identify its sex. Normative research has long shown that a large proportion of both boys and girls draw a person of their own sex first in response to this request (Brown, 1979; Heinrich & Triebe, 1972; Jolles, 1952; Tolor & Tolor, 1974). In contrast, three studies with gender-problem children have shown that these subjects are more likely than control subjects to draw an opposite-sex person first (Green et al., 1972a; Skilbeck et al., 1975; Zucker et al., 1983). The percentage of gender-problem and control subjects in each of the three studies who drew an opposite-sex person first was 57% versus 24%, 32% versus 6%, and 61% versus 20%, respectively.

Although significant in each case, the false negative rate was considerably higher than the false positive rate. The high rate of false negatives may be interpreted in several ways. First, given the nominal nature of the measure, the probability of an "incorrect" response is 50% by chance alone. It is also likely that gender-referred children vary in the degree to which they are cross-gender-identified, and this may contribute to more variance on psychological testing. In the Zucker and associates (1984) study, 76% of the gender-referred children who met the complete DSM-III criteria for GIDC drew an opposite-sex person

TABLE 9.3
Description of Assessment Measures

Reference	*Measure*	*Content*	*Original/Additional References*
Green (1976, 1987)	Parent-report	Gender identity, gender role behaviors	Roberts et al. (1987)
Green et al. (1982)	Parent-report	Gender identity, gender role behaviors	
Bates & Bentler (1973)	Parent-report	Sex-typed games and activities	Doering (1981); Klein & Bates (1980); Meyer-Bahlburg, Feldman & Ehrhardt (1985); Pleak et al. (1989); Zucker et al. (1985)
Bates et al. (1973)	Parent-report	Gender role behaviors	Bates et al. (1979); Meyer-Bahlburg et al. (1985); Pleak et al. (1989); modified version reported by Zucker, Bradley, Corter, Doering, & Finegan (1980)
Green et al. (1972b)	Free play	Masculine and feminine sex-typed play	
Rekers & Yates (1976)	Free play	Masculine and feminine sex-typed play	Zucker et al. (1982, 1985)
Green & Fuller (1973)	Fantasy play	Masculine and feminine fantasy play (stories)	
Zucker et al. (1984)	Fantasy play	Masculine and feminine fantasy play and content analysis of stories	Cramer & Hogan (1975); Erikson (1951)
Green et al. (1972a)	Draw-a-Person	Sex of first figure drawn; heights of same-sex and opposite sex persons; content analysis	Skilbeck et al. (1975); Zucker et al. (1983)
Zucker et al. (1988)	Gender constancy	"Stages" of gender constancy development	Slaby & Frey (1975)
Lozinski (1988)	Rorschach	Sex-typed responses; gender confusion	Tuber & Coates (1985)

Note. These assessment measures are the most readily accessible for clinical assessment. All have shown at least some discriminant validity, that is, they have distinguished gender-referred children from normal, sibling, and/or psychiatric controls. Some of the measures are appropriate for both boys and girls, whereas others (e.g., Bates et al., 1973) have been validated only for boys.

first, in contrast to only 40% of the gender-referred children who did not meet the complete criteria; thus, the false negative rate seems to have been reduced among the more extreme group of gender-referred children. Moreover, the nominal nature of the DAP precludes any type of quantitative trait assessment (Serbin, 1980). Although this holds true for the particular response under consideration, other potential indices of sex-typing on the DAP are amenable to more refined analyses. Zucker and associates (1983), for example, found that gender-referred children drew taller opposite-sex persons than same-sex persons, whereas controls tended to draw taller same-sex persons than opposite-sex persons. Skilbeck and colleagues (1975) found that gender-problem boys provided more details in their drawings of females than in their drawings of males, which is a common observation noted in therapy with these boys (Coates, 1985).

Despite the discriminant validity of the DAP, the rate of false negatives in particular should warn against using the test in isolation. This appears to hold true for other behavioral tests as well (Rekers & Yates, 1976; Zucker et al., 1982). In our unit, we are currently attempting to determine what combination of psychological tests and parent-report questionnaires contributes most to the correct classification of gender-problem children as judged by discriminant function analysis.

Most of the aforementioned measures have been applied almost exclusively to gender-referred boys. This is due primarily to the rather large male-to-female sex ratio in clinic referrals, reported in three different settings to be 6:1, 17:1, and 30:1, respectively (Coates & Zucker, 1988); thus, the putative discriminant validity of the DSM-III criteria has been verified primarily for males.

Green, Williams, and their colleagues (Green, Williams, & Goodman, 1982; Green, Williams, & Harper, 1980: Williams, Goodman, & Green, 1985; Williams, Green, & Goodman, 1979), however, generated a sample of 50 masculine-behaving girls ("tomboys") by means of newspaper advertisement. This method of recruitment differed from that used in Green's earlier study of feminine boys, in which the boys were referred primarily through professional channels (Green, 1970). In terms of their gender-role preferences, these girls appeared to show behavioral patterns similar to those observed in girls referred for clinical assessment (e.g., Green, 1974; Meyer & Dupkin, 1985; Rekers & Mead, 1980, Zucker, 1989), and they were significantly more masculine than female controls.

There are, however, a few issues that require clarification. It is not clear, for example, whether a majority of the girls studied by Green would meet the DSM-III-R criteria for GIDC. Although Williams and colleagues (1979) reported that 81% of the girls in their study either "frequently" or "once in a while" expressed the wish to be a boy, Green

(1980) stated elsewhere that these girls were "generally *content being female*" (p. 262, emphasis in original). Green and his colleagues reported that the majority of their female subjects preferred "casual" or "functional" clothing as opposed to conventionally "feminine" clothing, though it was not clear whether these girls had an aversion to the latter, which is now a symptom in DSM-III-R and is invariably observed among clinic-referred females (Zucker, 1989). In addition, Green and his colleagues did not provide information on anatomic dysphoria, which is another symptom in the DSM-III-R and another behavioral marker potentially important for differential diagnosis. In summary, then, it is probable that girls seen clinically show patterns of cross-gender-identification similar to those found for boys. Green's study with non-clinic-referred girls showed extensive cross-gender role preferences, though such girls, as a whole, may have been at a less extreme point along the spectrum of cross-gender-identification.

A final issue that needs to be discussed with regard to assessment is the mediating role of age. Clinical observation has suggested that cross-gender behavior shows a reduction with age (Green, 1975; Zuger, 1978), and, indeed, there is some empirical evidence of such a reduction (Bates et al., 1974; Zucker et al., 1984). The interpretive issue revolves around the explanation of the reduction. Does the reduction reflect a bona fide shift in the child's cross-gender-identification? Does it mean that the children's cross-gender behavior is going "underground" as they become more aware of negative social responses by significant others? Is the problem a measurement issue in that the techniques used to assess gender identity and gender role in older children are either inappropriate or too transparent to elicit valid responses?

It may well be that to some extent all of these explanations are correct. In our research, for example, we have found that some measures are strongly affected by age (e.g., overt sex-typed play in a structured clinic setting), whereas others are much less affected (e.g., sex-typed fantasy play and other projective measures). This suggests that some measures of gender-role preference are probably more valid than others for use with older children. Given these findings, it should be somewhat easier to work around the problem of faking. Many clinicians have noted that older children are less likely than younger children to acknowledge the desire to be of the opposite sex (cf. Zucker et al., 1984), even though they continue to manifest other signs of cross-gender-identification. This has been the case even for some children who had previously expressed cross-sex wishes.

Clinically, the issue is whether, given the absence of cross-sex wishes, such children can be considered to still have a gender identity disorder. For girls, the absence of a "stated desire" to be a boy precludes this diagnosis. The peculiar change in the criteria for boys (an "intense desire," not a stated desire, to be a girl) could probably be inferred from the child's fantasy and behavior, but this would seem redundant with the criteria for Point B (see Table 9.1). In any case, if the clinician keeps in mind that what is probably being dealt with is a spectrum of cross-gender-identification, the residual diagnosis, Gender Identity Disorder Not Otherwise Specified, can be used for children who fall short of meeting the complete criteria for GIDC.

As noted by Rutter (1978), demonstration of differences between groups with regard to presenting characteristics is only a first step in validating a psychiatric syndrome. There is, however, other evidence that GIDC is a discrete syndrome. Perhaps the most compelling evidence so far has been the strong concordance of the GIDC with subsequent sexual orientation, with the majority of GIDC boys developing a bisexual or homosexual orientation (Green, 1987; Money & Russo, 1979; Zuger, 1984). Some evidence also links the GIDC with subsequent gender dysphoria or transsexualism, particularly when there is little change in the condition by late childhood (Bradley & Zucker, 1984; Davenport, 1986; Green, 1987; Zucker & Bradley, 1989).

Green (1987) and his colleagues (Roberts et al., 1987) also provided some evidence that the degree of femininity within their group of feminine boys bore some relation to external variables. Based on parent-report data at the time of initial assessment, Green (1987) derived a statistical composite of the extent of femininity. As measured by Kinsey ratings for fantasy and behavior (see Green, 1987), the extent of femininity at assessment was not related to subsequent sexual orientation; however, the continuation of certain cross-gender behaviors through late childhood was associated with subsequent homosexuality. Green (1987) and Roberts and associates (1987) also reported that the degree of femininity within the feminine boy group was moderately correlated with a few variables of potential etiological relevance, such as the mother's degree of initial approval of the cross-gender behavior.

Proposed Changes in DSM-III-R Criteria

Table 9.4 provides a summary of proposed changes to the DSM-III-R criteria for GIDC, which reflect the empirical and logical criticisms discussed in this section and in the previous one. These changes would realize two main goals: (a) to allow the clinician to make a diagnosis solely on the basis of an expanded number of discrete behavioral signs, and (b) to eliminate the distinction between the A and B criteria, which should result in fewer false negative diagnoses.

TABLE 9.4
Proposed Changes to the DSM-III-R Criteria for Gender Identity Disorder of Childhood

For boys:

1. Desire to be a girl must be expressed verbally. It should not have to be inferred from other behavioral signs.
2. The B-1 criteria in DSM-III-R should be divided into six discrete units in order to reflect more accurately the core behavioral features of the disorder: cross-dressing, cross-sex role preference, toy and activity preference, display of feminine or effeminate mannerisms, cross-sex peer preference,and phobic avoidance of rough-and-tumble play. The criteria should note that the boy prefers cross-sex behaviors and avoids same-sex behaviors (e.g., "a strong preference for female roles in fantasy play and a strong avoidance of male roles in fantasy play").
3. The distinction between the A and B criteria in DSM-III-R should be eliminated. As the alternative, the child would meet criteria if he expressed a recurrent desire to be a girl or manifests at least four of the eight possible criteria. This change would then permit a GIDC diagnosis to be applied to boys who manifest multiple signs of cross-gender-identificaiton, yet who do not specifically state the desire to be of the opposite sex.

For girls:

1. Recurrent desire to be a boy should be considered a positive sign regardless of the putative motivational basis.
2. The B-1 criteria should be expanded in a manner similar to what is proposed for boys.
3. The distinction between the A and B criteria should be eliminated, as noted for boys.

DIAGNOSTIC AND ASSESSMENT PROCEDURES

As noted in the previous section, a number of assessment techniques have been used with gender-problem children. It can be seen in Table 9.3 that the measures vary in their complexity and in the ease with which they can be implemented. This section concentrates on three procedures: first, the clinical interview with the child's parents; second, a gender identity interview with the child; and third, a brief questionnaire that covers some key gender-related behaviors and can provide the clinician with a reasonable quantitative impression about the extent of a child's cross-gender-identification.

Parent Interview

The clinical interview with the child's parents should establish whether or not the DSM-III-R criteria have been met. Table 9.5 summarizes some key areas in which clinical judgments are required. This

TABLE 9.5
Core Behavioral Features of the Gender Identity Disorder of Childhood

---

1. *Identity Statements*
   __Child frequently states the wish to be of the opposite sex or that he or she is a member of the opposite sex (e.g., "I want to be a girl, I am a girl, I want to grow up to be a Mommy, not a Daddy").
   __Child occasionally states the wish to be of the opposite sex.
   __Child rarely states the wish to be of the opposite sex.
   __Child does not state the wish to be of the opposite sex.
2. *Anatomic Dysphoria*
   __Child frequently states a dislike of his or her sexual anatomy (e.g., "I don't like my penis"; "I want a penis, not a vagina") or demonstrates this behaviorally (e.g., in a boy, sitting to urinate to simulate having female genitalia; in a girl, standing to urinate to simulate having male genitalia).
   __Child occasionally states a dislike of his or her sexual anatomy or demonstrates this behaviorally.
   __Child rarely states a dislike of his or her sexual anatomy or demonstrates this behaviorally.
   __Child never states a dislike of his or her sexual anatomy or demonstrates this behaviorally.
3. *Cross-dressing*
   __Child frequently cross-dresses (e.g., in boys, use of mother's clothes, such as dresses, high-heeled shoes, jewelry, and makeup; simulation of long hair with towels. In girls, refusal to wear culturally typical feminine clothing and use of clothing, such as boys' pants and shirts, to simulate a masculine appearance; often desire hair to be very short, in accordance with masculine convention).
   __Child occasionally cross-dresses.
   __Child rarely cross-dresses.
   __Child never cross-dresses.
4. *Toy and Role Play*
   __Child prefers to play with toys and to engage in roles stereotypically associated with the opposite sex (e.g., in boys, a preference for female dolls, such as Barbie or Gem, role play as a female, emulation of female superheroes; drawings invariably are of women. In girls, a preference for male dolls, such as GI Joe or male Transformers, role play as a male, emulation of male superheroes; drawings invariably are of men).
   __Child plays with toys and engages in roles that are both stereotypically masculine and feminine.
   __Child avoids toys and roles that are stereotypically associated with his or her sex but does not engage in toy or role play associated with the opposite sex.
   __Child prefers neutral activities (e.g., drawing, making music) and does not engage in either same-sex or cross-sex toy or role play.
   __Child prefers to play with toys and to engage in roles stereotypically associated with own sex.
5. *Peer Relations*
   __Child prefers to play with opposite-sex peers.
   __Child is a loner or is rejected.
   __Child plays with both same-sex and opposite-sex peers.
   __Child prefers to play with same-sex peers.

(*continued*)

TABLE 9.5
(continued)

6. *Mannerisms*
   __Child frequently displays motoric movements and speech characteristics that are associated with the opposite sex, either in "natural" or "exaggerated" form (e.g., in boys, this includes hand movements, hip control, elevated pitch and lisp; in girls, this includes low voice projection).
   __Child occasionally displays motoric movements and speech characteristics that are associated with the opposite sex.
   __Child rarely displays motoric movements and speech characteristics that are associated with the opposite sex.
   __Child never displays motoric movements and speech characteristics that are associated with the opposite sex.
7. *Rough-and-Tumble Play*
   __In boys, there is an aversion to rough-and-tumble play or participation in group sports, such as hockey, football, and soccer. There is often a concern regarding physical injury. In girls, there is a strong attraction to rough-and-tumble play and group sports, particularly with boys.
   __In boys, there is no interest in rough-and-tumble play or participation in group sports, but the accompanying fear is not present.
   __In boys, there is an interest in rough-and-tumble play or participation in group sports. In girls, such interests are not dependent on a male peer group, but rather, are expressed in more typical ways (e.g., mixed-sex teams, all-girls' teams).

Note. These behavioral features have been drawn from a variety of sources, including Green (1974, 1987), Rekers (1977b), Stoller (1968a,b), Zucker (1985), and Zuger (1966).

information should be sufficient to make a diagnostic decision. For the purpose of diagnosis, the interviewer should consider only the child's current behaviors, such as that displayed during the past 6 months. From a developmental perspective, however, it is also important to understand the course of these behaviors, including their onset and any changes that have occurred over time. It is not unusual, for example, to find that an older child may have had a history of expressing cross-sex wishes but that these are no longer expressed, despite the presence of other cross-gender behaviors.

Child Interview

A clinical interview with the child is also useful in establishing the extent to which children feel gender dysphoric and confused about their status as a boy or a girl. Although not required for diagnosis, such an interview also provides a qualitative impression of some of the child's conflictual issues, and thus may be helpful in planning a treat-

TABLE 9.6
Gender Identity Interview

01. Are you a boy or a girl? BOY______ GIRL______
02. Are you a (opposite of first response)? ______
03. When you grow up, will you be a Mommy or a Daddy? MOMMY______ DADDY______
04. Could you ever grow up to be a (opposite of first response)? YES______ NO______
05. Are there any good things about being a boy? YES______ NO______ If YES, say: Tell me some of the good things about being a boy. (Probe for a maximum of three responses.)
    a.
    b.
    c.
    If YES or NO, ask: Are there any things that you don't like about being a boy? YES______ NO______
    If child answers YES, say: Tell me some of the things that you don't like about being a boy. (Probe for a maximum of three responses.)
    a.
    b.
    c.
06. Do you think it is better to be a boy or a girl? BOY______ GIRL______ Why? (Probe for a maximum of three responses.)
    a.
    b.
    c.
07. In your mind, do you ever think that you would like to be a girl? YES______ NO______
    If YES, ask: Can you tell me why? (Probe for a maximum of three responses.)
    a.
    b.
    c.
08. In your mind, do you ever get mixed up and you're not really sure if you are a boy or a girl? YES______ NO______
    If Yes, say: Tell me more about that. (Probe until satisfied.)
09. Do you ever feel more like a girl than like a boy? YES______ NO______
    If YES, say: Tell me more about that. (Probe until satisfied.)
10. You know what dreams are, right? Well, when you dream at night, are you ever in the dream? If YES, ask: In your dreams, are you a boy, a girl, or sometimes a boy and sometimes a girl? BOY______ GIRL______ BOTH______
    NOT IN DREAMS______ (Probe regarding content of dreams.)
11. Do you ever think that you really are a girl? YES______ NO______
    If YES, say: Tell me more about that. (Probe until satisfied.)
12. When you were in your Mom's tummy, do you think she wanted you to be a boy or a girl? BOY______ GIRL______
13. When you were in your Mom's tummy, do you think your Dad wanted you to be a boy or a girl? BOY______ GIRL______
    (For 12 and 13, ask: What do you think about that? (Probe until satisfied.)

Note. Adapted from K. J. Zucker, "Development of a Gender Identity Interview Schedule for Children," unpublished.

ment program. Table 9.6 shows a semistructured Gender Identity Interview schedule that we currently employ in our clinical research. Control group data are not yet available, but the interview appears to have heuristic value. The following is a summary of an interview with a 12-year-old boy (IQ = 78) seen at a 3-year follow-up. At the time of his assessment, this youngster met the DSM-III criteria for GIDC and had had an extensive cross-gender history beginning with frequent cross-dressing at age 2. Since the age of 2, he had also been severely troubled in many other aspects of his life and had been in some type of treatment or under the care of child welfare authorities. Only some progress had been made in dealing with his gender identity problem.

Interviewer (I): Are you a boy or a girl?
Child (C): A boy.
I: Are you a girl?
C: Only in my dreams.
I: When you grow up, will you be a Mom or a Dad?
C: A Dad (laughs).
I: Are there any good things about being a boy?
C: Yes.
I: Tell me some of the good things about being a boy.
C: Girls don't play with their private parts, boys do . . . 'cause you don't have anything hanging. I guess playing with yourself feels a little bit good.
I: Tell me another good thing about being a boy.
C: I wanted to look at naked dolls when I was at [name of previous residential treatment facility].
I: Are there any other good things about being a boy?
C: [No reply]
I: Are there any things that you don't like about being a boy?
C: Yes.
I: Tell me some of the things that you don't like.
C: I hate playing with trucks and cars . . . I'm still glued to Barbie dolls.
I: What do you like about them?
C: Changing them and combing their hair, it's just like having a real daughter.
I: Any other things that you don't like about being a boy?
C: I don't know.

I: Do you think it is better to be a boy or a girl?

C: In my way, I like girls better.

I: Tell me why.

C: They get all these girl commercials on TV. If I had one wish, I'd be a boy and a girl or alternate each day, turn into someone different, like at recess I'd be a girl . . .

I: Any other reasons why it's better to be a girl?

C: [No further answers]

I: In your mind, do you ever think that you would like to be a girl?

C: Yes.

I: Can you tell me why?

C: I just think . . . is there such thing as changing a guy into a girl?

I: What do you think?

C: I don't know. Is there? If I was younger, I'd want to change.

I: What would be better?

C: Always having to be treated differently . . . they [i.e., girls] get treated special . . .

I: In your mind, do you ever get mixed up and you're not really sure if you are a boy or a girl?

C: Sort of, well not really, I just think I'm a boy.

I: What did you mean when you said "sort of?"

C: Sometimes when I see all girls running around, I get lonely.

I: Do you ever feel more like a girl than like a boy?

C: Sort of.

I: Tell me more about that.

C: I always act like one usually.

I: You know what dreams are, right? Well, when you dream at night, are you ever in the dream?

C: Yes.

I: In your dreams, are you a boy, a girl, or sometimes a boy and sometimes a girl?

C: Both, but mostly a girl.

I: Tell me about the dreams in which you're a girl.

C: [No reply]

I: Can you tell me about the dreams in which you're a boy?

C: Feels weird.

I: Do you ever think that you really are a girl?

C: No.

Use of Rating Scales as Screens

Some type of screening questionnaire would also facilitate a diagnostic interview. Table 9.3 summarizes some of the available questionnaires; however, these questionnaires (e.g., Bates & Bentler, 1973; Bates et al., 1973) tend to focus primarily on gender role behaviors and thus do not provide as much information as is required in making a DSM-III-R diagnostic decision. Table 9.7 shows a Gender Identity Questionnaire

TABLE 9.7
Gender Identity Questionnaire

Instructions

Please answer the following behavioral statements as they currently characterize your child's behavior. For each question, circle the response that most accurately describes your child.

01. His favorite playmates are
    a. always boys
    b. usually boys
    c. boys and girls equally
    d. usually girls
    e. always girls
    f. does not play with other children
02. He plays with girl-type dolls, such as "Barbie"
    a. as a favorite toy
    b. frequently
    c. once in a while
    d. very rarely
    e. never
03. He plays with boy-type dolls, such as "G.I. Joe" or "Ken"
    a. as a favorite toy
    b. frequently
    c. once in a while
    d. very rarely
    e. never
04. He experiments with cosmetics (makeup) and jewelry
    a. as a favorite activity
    b. frequently
    c. once in a while
    d. very rarely
    e. never
05. He imitates *female* characters seen on TV or in the movies
    a. as a favorite activity
    b. frequently
    c. once in a while
    d. very rarely
    e. never

(*continued*)

TABLE 9.7
(continued)

06. He imitates *male* characters seen on TV or in the movies
    a. as a favorite activity
    b. frequently
    c. once in a while
    d. very rarely
    e. never
07. He plays sports with boys (but not girls)
    a. as a favorite activity
    b. frequently
    c. once in a while
    d. very rarely
    e. never
08. He plays sports with girls (but not boys)
    a. as a favorite activity
    b. frequently
    c. once in a while
    d. very rarely
    e. never
09. In playing "mother/father," "house," or "school" games, he takes the role of
    a. a girl or woman at all times
    b. usually a girl or woman
    c. half the time a girl or woman and half the time a boy or man
    d. usually a boy or man
    e. a boy or man at all times
    f. does not play these games
10. He plays "girl-type" games (as compared to "boy-type" games)
    a. as a favorite activity
    b. frequently
    c. once in a while
    d. very rarely
    e. never
11. He plays "boy-type" games (as compared to "girl-type" games)
    a. as a favorite activity
    b. frequently
    c. once in a while
    d. very rarely
    e. never
12. In dress-up games, he likes to dress up
    a. in girls' or women's clothes all the time
    b. usually in girls' or women's clothes
    c. half the time in girls' or women's clothes and half the time in boys' or men's clothes
    d. usually in boys' or men's clothes
    e. in boys' or men's clothes all the time
    f. does not dress up

(continued)

TABLE 9.7
(continued)

13. He states the wish to be a girl or a woman
    a. every day
    b. frequently
    c. once in a while
    d. very rarely
    e. never
14. He states that he is a girl or a woman
    a. every day
    b. frequently
    c. once in a while
    d. very rarely
    e. never
15. He talks about *not* liking his sexual anatomy (private parts)
    a. every day
    b. frequently
    c. once in a while
    d. very rarely
    e. never

If you circled a, b, c, or d, please describe what he says:

16. He talks about *liking* his sexual anatomy (private parts)
    a. every day
    b. frequently
    c. once in a while
    d. very rarely
    e. never

If you circled a, b, c, or d, please describe what he says:

Note. Adapted from "Childhood Sex-role Behaviors: Similarities and Differences in Twins" by P. H. Elizabeth and R. Green, 1984, *Acta Geneticae Medicae et Gemellologiae, 33*, 173–179. The questionnaire may also be used with girls with pronouns appropriately changed.

TABLE 9.8
Mean Total Score on the Gender Identity Questionnaire

Group	*M*	*SD*	*Range*
Gender-referred (N=45)	2.89*	.61	1.62–4.42
Female Siblings (N=20)	3.77*	.49	2.64–4.56
Male Siblings (N=21)	4.15*	.26	3.56–4.50

Note. Absolute range, 1–5. 1 = least sex-typical response; 5 = most sex-typical response.
*$F(2,83) = 47.2$, $p < .0001$.

developed by Elizabeth and Green (1984). The original version of the questionnaire showed reasonable psychometric properties (Elizabeth, Meyer-Bahlburg, Janal, Ehrhardt, & Green, 1984; Zucker & Torkos, 1989), including internal consistency, good interparent agreement, and strong sex differences. We have added items 13–16, which focus on cross-sex desires and feelings about sexual anatomy.

Table 9.8 provides unpublished maternal report data from a sample of 45 gender-referred children (41 boys, 4 girls) and 41 siblings (21 boys, 20 girls) seen in our clinic. Each item on the questionnaire was coded such that the most sex-typical response was a 5 and the least sex-typical response was a 1. Preliminary analyses showed some sex differences among the siblings; accordingly, the data were analyzed with the sibling group divided by sex. The results showed that the gender-referred group had a significantly lower (i.e., atypical) score than both the male and female sibling controls. Only two siblings, both girls, had mean scores below the mean for the gender-referred group (i.e., more sex-atypical), whereas only two gender-referred children had mean scores above the mean of the female siblings; one of these children's mean score also exceeded the mean of the male siblings. Thus, this brief questionnaire seems to have clinical utility in differentiating gender-referred children from their siblings.

SUMMARY AND DIRECTIONS

Diagnostic and assessment procedures for children with gender identity disorder have progressed considerably since the seminal reports on this condition appeared at the beginning of the 1960s. As with many other child psychiatric problems, work has concentrated more on boys than on girls (Eme, 1979), though in recent years progress has been made in understanding the phenomenological parameters of the gender identity disorder of childhood in girls. Some of the measurement problems have become better understood as a result of recognition of the need for age-appropriate assessment tools. It is fairly clear now that the nominal approach to psychiatric diagnosis has inherent constraints and that spectrum-oriented approaches serve as a useful complement to a "yes–no" dichotomous system. The latter approach will probably facilitate a sharper understanding of the boundaries of gender identity disorder. Gender identity problems in children are relatively rare; thus standardized assessment and diagnostic techniques should facilitate cross-center collaboration with regard to various issues that are better studied with large sample sizes, such as the relative effectiveness of different forms of treatment, familial influences on genesis, and long-term follow-up.

REFERENCES

Achenbach, T. M. (1978). The Child Behavior Profile: I. Boys aged 6–11. *Journal of Consulting and Clinical Psychology, 46*, 478–488.

Achenbach, T. M. (1980). DSM-III in light of empirical research on the classification of child psychopathology. *Journal of the American Academy of Child Psychiatry, 19*, 395–412.

Achenbach, T. M. (1985). *Assessment and taxonomy of child and adolescent psychopathology*. Beverly Hills, CA: Sage Publications.

Achenbach, T. M. (1988). Integrating assessment and taxonomy. In M. Rutter, A. H. Tuma, & I. S. Lann (Eds.), *Assessment and diagnosis in child psychopathology* (pp. 300–343). New York: Guilford Press.

Achenbach, T. M., & Edelbrock, C. S. (1981). Behavioral problems and competencies reported by parents of normal and disturbed children aged four through sixteen. *Monographs of the Society for Research in Child Development, 46*(1, Serial No. 188).

Achenbach, T. M., & Edelbrock, C. (1983). *Manual for the Child Behavior Checklist and Revised Child Behavior Profile*. Burlington, VT: University Associates in Psychiatry.

American Psychiatric Association. (1952). *Diagnostic and statistical manual. Mental disorders*. Washington, DC: Author.

American Psychiatric Association. (1968). *Diagnostic and statistical manual of mental disorders* (2nd ed.). Washington, DC: Author.

American Psychiatric Association. (1980). *Diagnostic and statistical manual of mental disorders* (3rd ed). Washington, DC: Author.

American Psychiatric Association. (1987). *Diagnostic and statistical manual of mental disorders* (3rd rev. ed.). Washington, DC: Author.

Baker, R. P., & Dreger, R. M. (1973). The Preschool Behavioral Classification Project: An initial report. *Journal of Abnormal Child Psychology, 1*, 88–120.

Bakwin, H. (1960). Transvestism in children. *Journal of Pediatrics, 56*, 294–298.

Bakwin, H. (1968). Deviant gender-role behavior in children: Relation to homosexuality. *Pediatrics, 41*, 620–629.

Barbin, H. (1980). *Herculine Barbin: Being the recently discovered memoirs of a nineteenth-century French hermaphrodite* (R. McDougall, Trans.). New York: Pantheon.

Bates, J. E., & Bentler, P. M. (1973). Play activities of normal and effeminate boys. *Developmental Psychology, 9*, 20–27.

Bates, J. E., Bentler, P. M., & Thompson, S. K. (1973). Measurement of deviant gender development in boys. *Child Development, 44*, 591–598.

Bates, J. E., Bentler, P. M., & Thompson, S. K. (1979). Gender-deviant boys compared with normal and clinical control boys. *Journal of Abnormal Child Psychology, 7*, 243–259.

Bates, J. E., Skilbeck, W. M., Smith, K. V. R., & Bentler, P. M. (1974). Gender role abnormalities in boys: An analysis of clinical ratings. *Journal of Abnormal Child Psychology, 2*, 1–16.

Bem, S. L. (1981). Gender-schema theory: A cognitive account of sex typing. *Psychological Review, 88*, 354–364.

Bender, L., & Paster, S. (1941). Homosexual trends in children. *American Journal of Orthopsychiatry, 11*, 730–743.

Benjamin, H. (1954). Transsexualism and transvestism as psychosomatic somato-psychic syndromes. *American Journal of Psychotherapy, 8,* 219–230.

Bentler, P. M., Rekers, G. A., & Rosen, A. C. (1979). Congruence of childhood sex-role identity and behaviour disturbances. *Child: Care, Health and Development, 5,* 267–283.

Bradley, S. J. (1980). Female transsexualism: A child and adolescent perspective. *Child Psychiatry and Human Development, 11,* 12–18.

Bradley, S. J., & Zucker, K. J. (1984, October). *Gender-dysphoric adolescents: Presenting and developmental characteristics.* Paper presented at the meeting of the American Academy of Child Psychiatry, Toronto, Ontario.

Brown, E. V. (1979). Sexual self-identification as reflected in children's drawings when asked to "draw-a-person." *Perceptual and Motor Skills, 49,* 35–38.

Cauldwell, D. (1949). Psychopathia transsexualis. *Sexology, 16,* 274–280.

Coates, S. (1985). Extreme boyhood femininity: Overview and new research findings. In Z. DeFries, R. C. Friedman, & R. Corn (Eds.), *Sexuality: New perspectives* (pp. 101–124). Westport, CT: Greenwood Press.

Coates, S., & Person, E. S. (1985). Extreme boyhood femininity: Isolated behavior or pervasive disorder? *Journal of the American Academy of Child Psychiatry, 24,* 702–709.

Coates, S., & Zucker, K. J. (1988). Gender identity disorders in children. In C. J. Kestenbaum & D. T. Williams (Eds.), *Handbook of clinical assessment of children and adolescents* (Vol. 2, pp. 893–914). New York: New York University Press.

Cowell, R. (1954). *Roberta Cowell's story by herself.* Melbourne: Heinemann.

Cramer, P., & Hogan, K. A. (1975). Sex differences in verbal and play fantasy. *Developmental Psychology, 11,* 145–154.

Cucchiari, S. (1981). The gender revolution and the transition from bisexual horde to patrilocal band: The origins of gender hierarchy. In S. B. Ortner & H. Whitehead (Eds.), *Sexual meanings: The cultural construction of gender and sexuality* (pp. 31–79). Cambridge: Cambridge University Press.

Davenport, C. W. (1986). A follow-up study of 10 feminine boys. *Archives of Sexual Behavior, 15,* 511–517.

Deaux, K., & Major, B. (1987). Putting gender into context: An interactive model of gender-related behavior. *Psychological Review, 94,* 369–389.

Dirks, J., & Gibson, E. (1977). Infants' perception of similarity between live people and their photographs. *Child Development, 48,* 124–130.

Doering, R. W. (1981). *Parental reinforcement of gender-typed behaviors in boys with atypical gender identity.* Unpublished doctoral dissertation, University of Toronto.

Dreger, R. M. (1970). The establishment of diagnostic categories for the evaluation of specific therapies for children's emotional disorders. *Alabama Journal of Medical Sciences, 7,* 55–60.

Dreger, R. M. (1981). First-, second-, and third-order factors from the Children's Behavioral Classification Project Instrument and an attempt at rapprochement. *Journal of Abnormal Psychology, 90,* 242–260.

Edelbrock, C., & Costello, A. J. (1988). Structured psychiatric interviews for children. In M. Rutter, A. H. Tuma, & I. S. Lann (Eds.), *Assessment and diagnosis in child psychopathology* (pp. 87–112). New York: Guilford Press.

Elizabeth, P. H., & Green, R. (1984). Childhood sex-role behaviors: Similarities and differences in twins. *Acta Geneticae Medicae et Gemellologiae 33,* 173–179.

Elizabeth, P. H., Meyer-Bahlburg, H. F. L., Janal, M. N., Ehrhardt, A. A., & Green, R. (1984, September). *Do human twins show a "free-martin" like phenomenon?* Paper presented at the meeting of the International Academy of Sex Research, Cambridge, England.

Eme, R. F. (1979). Sex differences in childhood psychopathology: A review. *Psychological Bulletin, 86,* 574–595.
Erikson, E. H. (1951). Sex differences in the play configurations of preadolescents. *American Journal of Orthopsychiatry, 21,* 667–692.
Etaugh, C., Levine, D., & Mennella, A. (1984). Development of sex biases in children: 40 years later. *Sex Roles, 10,* 911–922.
Fagan, J. F., & Singer, L. T. (1979). The role of simple feature differences in infants' recognition of faces. *Infant Behavior and Development, 2,* 39–45.
Fagot, B. I., Leinbach, M. D., & Hagan, R. (1986). Gender labeling and the adoption of sex-typed behaviors. *Developmental Psychology, 22,* 440–443.
Frame, C. L., & Matson, J. L. (Eds.). (1987). *Handbook of assessment in childhood psychopathology: Applied issues in differential diagnosis and treatment evaluation.* New York: Plenum.
Freimuth, M. J., & Hornstein, G. A. (1982). A critical examination of the concept of gender. *Sex Roles, 8,* 515–532.
Freud, S. (1925). Some psychological consequences of the anatomic distinction between the sexes. In J. Strachey (Ed. and Trans.), *The standard edition of the complete psychological works of Sigmund Freud* (Vol. 19, pp. 241–260). London: Hogarth.
Friend, M. R., Schiddel, L., Klein, B., & Dunaeff, D. (1954). Observations on the development of transvestitism in boys. *American Journal of Orthopsychiatry, 24,* 563–575.
Green, R. (1968). Childhood cross-gender identification. *Journal of Nervous and Mental Disease, 147,* 500–509.
Green, R. (1970). Little boys who behave as girls. *California Medicine, 113,* 12–16.
Green, R. (1971). Diagnosis and treatment of gender identity disorders during childhood. *Archives of Sexual Behavior, 1,* 167–174.
Green, R. (1973). Twenty-five boys with atypical gender identity: A behavioral summary. In J. Zubin & J. Money (Eds.), *Contemporary sexual behavior: Critical issues in the 1970s* (pp. 351–358). Baltimore: Johns Hopkins University Press.
Green, R. (1974). *Sexual identity conflict in children and adults.* New York: Basic Books.
Green, R. (1975). The significance of feminine behavior in boys. *Journal of Child Psychology and Psychiatry, 16,* 341–344.
Green, R. (1976). One-hundred ten feminine and masculine boys: Behavioral contrasts and demographic similarities. *Archives of Sexual Behavior, 5,* 425–446.
Green, R. (1979). Childhood cross-gender behavior and subsequent sexual preference. *American Journal of Psychiatry, 136,* 106–108.
Green, R. (1980). Patterns of sexual identity development in childhood: Relationship to subsequent sexual partner preference. In J. Marmor (Ed.), *Homosexual behavior: A modern reappraisal* (pp. 255–266). New York: Basic Books.
Green, R. (1987). *The "sissy boy syndrome" and the development of homosexuality.* New Haven: Yale University Press.
Green, R., & Fuller, M. (1973). Family doll play and female identity in preadolescent males. *American Journal of Orthopsychiatry, 43,* 123–127.
Green, R., Fuller, M., & Rutley, B. (1972a). It-Scale for Children and Draw-a-Person test: 30 feminine vs. 25 masculine boys. *Journal of Personality Assessment, 36,* 349–352.
Green, R., Fuller, M., Rutley, B., & Hendler, J. (1972b). Playroom toy preferences of fifteen masculine and fifteen feminine boys. *Behavior Research and Therapy, 3,* 425–429.
Green, R., & Money, J. (1960). Incongruous gender role: Nongenital manifestations in prepubertal boys. *Journal of Nervous and Mental Disease, 131,* 160–168.

Green, R., & Money, J. (1961). Effeminacy in prepubertal boys: Summary of 11 cases. *Pediatrics, 27,* 286–291.

Green, R., Neuberg, D. S., & Finch, S. J. (1983). Sex-typed motor behaviors of "feminine" boys, conventionally masculine boys, and conventionally feminine girls. *Sex Roles, 9,* 571–579.

Green, R., Williams, K., & Harper, J. (1980). Cross-sex identity: Peer group integration and the double standard of childhood sex-typing. In J. Samson (Ed.), *Childhood and sexuality* (pp. 542–548). Montreal: Editions Etudes Vivantes.

Green, R., Williams, K., & Goodman, M. (1982). Ninety-nine "tomboys" and "non-tomboys": Behavioral contrasts and demographic similarities. *Archives of Sexual Behavior, 11,* 247–266.

Gutterman, E. M., O'Brien, J. D., & Young, J. G. (1987). Structured diagnostic interviews for children and adolescents: Current status and future directions. *Journal of the American Academy of Child and Adolescent Psychiatry, 26,* 621–630.

Hamburger, C. (1953). The desire for change of sex as shown by personal letters from 465 men and women. *Acta Endocrinologica, 14,* 361–375.

Hamburger, C., Sturup, G. K., & Dahl-Iverson, E. (1953). Transvestism. Hormonal, psychiatric, and surgical treatment. *Journal of the American Medical Association, 152,* 391–396.

Heinrich, P., & Triebe, J. K. (1972). Sex preferences in children's human figure drawings. *Journal of Personality Assessment, 36,* 263–267.

Herjanic, B., & Reich, B. (1982). Development of a structured psychiatric interview for children: Agreement between child and parent on individual symptoms. *Journal of Abnormal Child Psychology, 10,* 307–324.

Higham, E. (1976). Case management of the gender incongruity syndrome in childhood and adolescence. *Journal of Homosexuality, 2,* 49–57.

Jolles, I. (1952). A study of validity of some hypotheses for the qualitative interpretation of the H-T-P for children of elementary school age; I. Sexual identification. *Journal of Clinical Psychology, 8,* 113–118.

Klein, A. R., & Bates, J. E. (1980). Gender-typing of game choices and qualities of boys' play behavior. *Journal of Abnormal Child Psychology, 8,* 201–212.

Kosky, R. J. (1987). Gender-disordered children: Does inpatient treatment help? *Medical Journal of Australia, 146,* 565–569.

Lozinski, J. A. (1988). *Sex-typed responses in the Rorschach protocols of cross-gender-identified children.* Unpublished master's thesis, University of Toronto.

Maccoby, E. E. (1988). Gender as a social category. *Developmental Psychology, 24,* 755–765.

MacDonald, M. W. (1938). Criminally aggressive behavior in passive, effeminate boys. *American Journal of Orthopsychiatry, 8,* 70–78.

Meyer, J. K., & Dupkin, C. (1985). Gender disturbance in children: An interim clinical report. *Bulletin of the Menninger Clinic, 49,* 236–269.

Meyer-Bahlburg, H. F. L. (1985). Gender identity disorder of childhood: Introduction. *Journal of the American Academy of Child Psychiatry, 24,* 681–683.

Meyer-Bahlburg, H. F. L., Feldman, J. F., & Ehrhardt, A. A. (1985). Questionnaires for the assessment of atypical gender role behavior: A methodological study. *Journal of the American Academy of Child Psychiatry, 24,* 695–701.

Money, J. (1952). *Hermaphroditism: An inquiry into the nature of a human paradox.* Unpublished doctoral dissertation, Harvard University.

Money, J. (1973). Gender role, gender identity, core gender identity: Usage and definition of terms. *Journal of the American Academy of Psychoanalysis, 1,* 397–403.

Money, J. (1985). The conceptual neutering of gender and the criminalization of sex. *Archives of Sexual Behavior, 14,* 279–290.

Money, J., Hampson, J. G., & Hampson, J. L. (1955). Hermaphroditism: Recommendations concerning assignment of sex, change of sex, and psychologic management. *Bulletin of the Johns Hopkins Hospital, 97,* 284–300.

Money, J., Hampson, J. G., & Hampson, J. L. (1957). Imprinting and the establishment of gender role. *Archives of Neurology and Psychiatry, 77,* 333–336.

Money, J., & Russo, A. J. (1979). Homosexual outcome of discordant gender identity/role: Longitudinal follow-up. *Journal of Pediatric Psychology, 4,* 29–41.

Ollendick, T. H., & Hersen, M. (Eds.). (1983). *Handbook of child psychopathology.* New York: Plenum.

Pleak, R. R., Meyer-Bahlburg, H. F. L., O'Brien, J. D., Bowen, H. A., & Morganstein, A. (1989). Cross-gender behavior and psychopathology in boy psychiatric outpatients. *Journal of the American Academy of Child and Adolescent Psychiatry, 28,* 385–393.

Rekers, G. A. (1977a). Atypical gender development and psychosocial development. *Journal of Applied Behavior Analysis, 10,* 559–571.

Rekers, G. A. (1977b). Assessment and treatment of childhood gender problems. In B. B. Lahey & A. E. Kazdin (Eds.), *Advances in clinical child psychology* (Vol. 1, pp. 267–306). New York: Plenum.

Rekers, G. A., Bentler, P. M., Rosen, A. C., & Lovaas, O. I. (1977). Child gender disturbances: A clinical rationale for intervention. *Psychotherapy: Theory, Research, and Practice, 14,* 2–11.

Rekers, G. A., & Mead, S. (1979). Early intervention for female sexual identity disturbance: Self-monitoring of play behavior. *Journal of Abnormal Child Psychology, 7,* 405–423.

Rekers, G. A., & Mead, S. (1980). Female sex-role deviance: Early identification and developmental intervention. *Journal of Clinical Child Psychology, 9,* 199–203.

Rekers, G. A., & Milner, G. C. (1978). Sexual identity disorders in childhood and adolescence. *Journal of the Florida Medical Association, 65,* 962–964.

Rekers, G. A., & Varni, J. W. (1977). Self-monitoring and self-reinforcement in a pretranssexual boy. *Behavior Research and Therapy, 15,* 177–180.

Rekers, G. A., & Yates, C. E. (1976). Sex-typed play in feminoid boys vs. normal boys and girls. *Journal of Abnormal Child Psychology, 4,* 1–8.

Roberts, C. W., Green, R., Williams, K., & Goodman, M. (1987). Boyhood gender identity development: A statistical contrast of two family groups. *Development Psychology, 23,* 544–557.

Rosen, A. C., Rekers, G. A., & Brigham, S. L. (1982). Gender stereotypy in gender-dysphoric young boys. *Psychological Reports, 51,* 371–374.

Rosen, A. C., Rekers, G. A., & Friar, L. R. (1977). Theoretical and diagnostic issues in child gender disturbances. *Journal of Sex Research, 13,* 89–103.

Rutter, M. (1978). Diagnostic validity in child psychiatry. *Advances in Biological Psychiatry, 2,* 2–22.

Schultz, N. M. (1979). *Severe gender identity confusion in an eight-year-old boy.* Unpublished doctoral dissertation, Yeshiva University.

Serbin, L. A. (1980). Sex-role socialization: A field in transition. In B. B. Lahey & A. E. Kazdin (Eds.), *Advances in clinical child psychology* (Vol. 3, pp. 41–96). New York: Plenum.

Skilbeck, W. M., Bates, J. E., & Bentler, P. M. (1975). Human figure drawings of gender-problem and school-problem boys. *Journal of Abnormal Child Psychology, 3,* 191–199.

Slaby, R. G., & Frey, K. S. (1975). Development of gender constancy and selective attention to same-sex models. *Child Development, 46,* 849–856.

Spence, J. T. (1984). Masculinity, femininity, and gender-related traits: A conceptual analysis and critique of current research. *Progress in Experimental Personality Research, 13,* 1–97.

Spence, J. T. (1985). Gender identity and its implications for concepts of masculinity and femininity. In T. Sondregger (Ed.), *Nebraska symposium on motivation* (pp. 59–95). Lincoln: University of Nebraska Press.

Stoller, R. J. (1964). The hermaphroditic identity of hermaphrodites. *Journal of Nervous and Mental Disease, 139,* 453–457.

Stoller, R. J. (1967). "It's only a phase." Femininity in boys. *Journal of American Medical Association, 201,* 314–315.

Stoller, R. J. (1968a). *Sex and gender (Vol. 1). The development of masculinity and femininity.* New York: Jason Aronson.

Stoller, R. J. (1968b). Male childhood transsexualism. *Journal of the American Academy of Child Psychiatry, 7,* 193–209.

Stoller, R. J. (1975). *Sex and gender (Vol. 2). The transsexual experiment.* London: Hogarth.

Stoller, R. J. (1978). Boyhood gender aberrations: Treatment issues. *Journal of the American Psychoanalytic Association, 26,* 541–558.

Stoller, R. J. (1985). *Presentation of gender.* New Haven: Yale University Press.

Stoller, R. J., & Newman, L. E. (1971). The bisexual identity of transsexuals: Two case reports. *Archives of Sexual Behavior, 1,* 17–28.

Tolor, A., & Tolor, B. (1974). Children's figure drawings and changing attitudes toward sex roles. *Psychological Reports, 34,* 343–349.

Tuber, S., & Coates, S. (1985). Interpersonal phenomena in the Rorschachs of extremely feminine boys. *Psychoanalytic Psychology, 2,* 251–265.

Unger, R. K. (1979). Toward a redefinition of sex and gender. *American Psychologist, 34,* 1085–1094.

Vecchio, T. J. (1966). Predictive value of a single diagnostic test in unselected populations. *New England Journal of Medicine, 274,* 1171–1173.

Williams, K., Green, R., & Goodman, M. (1979). Patterns of sexual identity development: A preliminary report on the "tomboy." In R. Simmons (Ed.), *Research in community mental health* (Vol. 1, pp. 103–123). Greenwich, CT: JAI Press.

Williams, K., Goodman, M., & Green, R. (1985). Parent–child factors in gender role socialization in girls. *Journal of the American Academy of Child Psychiatry, 24,* 720–731.

Zucker, K. J. (1982). Childhood gender disturbance: Diagnostic issues. *Journal of the American Academy of Child Psychiatry, 21,* 274–280.

Zucker, K. J. (1985). Cross-gender-identified children. In B. W. Steiner (Ed.), *Gender dysphoria: Development, research, management* (pp. 75–174). New York: Plenum.

Zucker, K. J. (1989, March). *Girls with the gender identity disorder of childhood.* Paper presented at the meeting of the Society for Sex Therapy and Research, Tucson, AZ.

Zucker, K. J., & Bradley, S. J. (1989, January). *Gender identity and sexual orientation in cross-gender-identified children: A follow-up in adolescence.* Paper presented at the meeting of the Society for Research in Child and Adolescent Psychopathology, Miami, FL.

Zucker, K. J., Bradley, S. J., Doering, R. W., & Lozinski, J. A. (1985). Sex-typed behavior in cross-gender-identified children: Stability and change at a one-year follow-up. *Journal of the American Academy of Child Psychiatry, 24,* 710–719.

Zucker, K. J., Bradley, S. J., Corter, C. M., Doering, R. W., & Finegan, J. K. (1980). Cross-gender behavior in very young boys: A normative study. In J. Sampson (Ed.), *Childhood and sexuality* (pp. 599–622). Montreal: Editions Etudes Vivantes.

Zucker, K. J., Bradley, S. J., & Kuksis, M. (1988, August). *Gender constancy judgments in cross-gender-identified children*. Paper presented at the meeting of the International Academy of Sex Research, Minneapolis, MN.

Zucker, K. J., Doering, R. W., Bradley, S. J., & Finegan, J. K. (1982). Sex-typed play in gender-disturbed children: A comparison to sibling and psychiatric controls. *Archives of Sexual Behavior, 11*, 309–321.

Zucker, K. J., Doering, R. W., Bradley, S. J. Alon, N. & Lozinski, J. A. (1984, September). *Sex-typed fantasy play in cross-gender-identified children*. Paper presented at the meeting of the International Academy of Sex Research, Cambridge, England.

Zucker, K. J., Finegan, J. K., Doering, R. W., & Bradley, S. J. (1983). Human figure drawings of gender-problem children: A comparison to sibling, psychiatric, and normal controls. *Journal of Abnormal Child Psychology, 11*, 287–298.

Zucker, K. J., Finegan, J. K., Doering, R. W., & Bradley, S. J. (1984). Two subgroups of gender-problem children. *Archives of Sexual Behavior, 13*, 27–39.

Zucker, K. J., & Torkos, H. (1989). Assessment of androgyny in children. *Annals of Sex Research, 2*, 197–211.

Zuger, B. (1966). Effeminate behavior present in boys from early childhood I. The clinical syndrome and follow-up studies. *Journal of Pediatrics, 69*, 1098–1107.

Zuger, B. (1978). Effeminate behavior present in boys from childhood: Ten additional years of follow-up. *Comprehensive Psychiatry, 19*, 363–369.

Zuger, B. (1984). Early effeminate behavior in boys: Outcome and significance for homosexuality. *Journal of Nervous and Mental Disease, 172*, 90–97.

CHAPTER 10

The Diagnosis and Assessment of Tic Disorders

Kenneth E. Towbin
Mark A. Riddle
James F. Leckman
Donald J. Cohen
Yale University School of Medicine

The disorder manifested by multiple motor tics, phonic and verbal productions, and behavioral changes was described by and named after Georges Gilles de la Tourette a century ago (Gilles de la Tourette, 1885). Over the last 100 years, a cascade of research studies has led to new and clearer appreciation of the phenomenology, natural history, etiology, physiology, and treatment of this malady. Moreover, Tourette's syndrome, as a prototypical illness, has become like a prism through which neuropsychiatry has been able to appreciate the various contributions to the clinical picture made by genetics, perinatal and stressful life events, inner life experience, family and relationship influences, and treatment efforts. There has been uniformly unanimous consensus that the multiple chronic motor and phonic symptoms first described by Gilles de la Tourette stand at the core of the disorder—the *sine qua non* of the syndrome. But various researchers have emphasized associated features that remain objects of intensive investigation even now. The study of these associated features has provided abundant opportunities to learn more and raise questions. Perhaps the most pressing question these studies have brought forward is whether associated features represent additional symptoms arising from the same etiology as the core syndrome or they are a secondary consequence of the core—the result of a complex interplay between urges, movements, self-control, and adaptation with which a Tourette sufferer is continually, painfully, and vividly confronted. The aim of this chapter is to review and distinguish the core symptoms, identify the variety of associated features that have been related to them, and discuss several of the most common instruments and methods of evaluation currently employed.

HISTORICAL BACKGROUND

Gilles de la Tourette's original case studies included seven patients whom he described as suffering from tics, echolalia, and coprolalia. One patient in the series also described obsessional thoughts. The description offered a clear differentiation of the tics from other motor movements, such as chorea. These clear descriptions and the degree to which, in 1885, tic phenomena were already known from the detailed writings of those such as Itard (1825), Bell (1830), and Hall (1852) made the core features readily recognizable. However, for a time the severity of symptoms in Gilles de la Tourette's patients created diagnostic ambiguity and, prior to the third edition of the *Diagnostic and Statistical Manual* of the American Psychiatric Association (DSM-III), there was uncertainty over whether coprolalia or echolalia were required for the diagnosis. Gilles de la Tourette himself stated that only some of his patients suffered from coprolalia, although all the others had echolalia. He also observed that all the patients had simultaneous motor tics and verbal outbursts. By 1907 this description had been modified so that motor and phonic tics were not necessarily simultaneous (Meige & Feindel, 1907). But Meige and Feindel wrote of a mental component or urge preceding each movement or phonic production that they believed was critical. This raised the question of whether mental components or preoccupations were an additional core feature.

In the United States, early attempts to classify tic disorders were heavily influenced by the prevailing view of nosology in which there was a preference for leaving maximum latitude for clinician's judgments, grouping very different but specific syndromes together, whether their etiologies were perceived to be similar or not, and giving nonspecific designations. For example, schizophrenic reaction contained, among other subtypes, latent, childhood, and residual subtypes all in the same category. Also, disorders in which the etiology was well understood were grouped with conditions where an etiology was completely unknown. Consequently, a diagnostic label gave little information about the definition of any disorder, its etiology, or its relationship to other disorders in the same group.

In the first *Diagnostic and Statistical Manual* of the American Psychiatric Association (DSM-I; APA, 1952) tic disorders were not recognized as any separate entity, nor were they listed specifically among any of the categories. Tics were simply understood to be a part of other special symptom reactions.

The second edition (DSM-II; APA, 1968), in its handling of tic disorders, continued the tradition of juxtaposing unrelated syndromes. DSM-II identified one tic disorder, "Tic," as a subtype of Special Symptoms (Not Elsewhere Classified) Disorders that encompassed a broad range of problems including developmental disorders (e.g., developmental articulation disturbances, learning disorders), specific symptoms (e.g., enuresis, encopresis, headaches), and infantile disturbances (e.g., feeding disorders). However, the diagnostic process was complicated and confusing because the category of diagnosis would change depending on the presentation. When a patient had a single tic and then developed multiple tics, the entire diagnostic category would change from Special Symptoms (Not Elsewhere Classified) to a Musculoskeletal Psychophysiologic Disorder. Furthermore, the "rules" of DSM-II required that if two disorders were present, the clinician must decide whether the tics might not be a presentation of another primary disorder and use that label instead of an additional label of tic disorder. In this way, patients with tics arising from organic brain syndromes would be in yet another category, as would patients who exhibited tics in conjunction with childhood schizophrenia, and so on. DSM-II did not specifically acknowledge the existence of transient tics, nor did it offer definitions differentiating these from chronic tics or Tourette's syndrome. Descriptions did not identify any diagnostic relationship between these disorders; clinicians were instructed to add these labels if applicable. This was closely mirrored by the Group for Advancement of Psychiatry scheme (1966). Unusual symptom clusters or those resulting from etiologies not congruent with the categories identified by the DSM-II could not be readily brought together. Patients with tics and other disorders might not be identified as having tics at all. In addition, the questions about core features, duration, onset, and severity previously raised by various investigators were not addressed in these schemes. Specific criteria or definitions that would assist in directing clinicians in their decision about diagnosis were absent.

The DSM-III (APA, 1980) employed specific criteria that were called *operationalized* definitions. By grouping all tic disorders together and differentiating subgroups according to age of onset, tic patterns, and duration of disturbance, DSM-III first permitted clinicians and investigators to identify readily the variety of conditions in which tics arise. This was further abetted by permitting multiple diagnoses when comorbid conditions existed. DSM-III also differentiated tic syndromes from one another and left open questions of whether there were different or identical etiologies for the different subtypes.

Tic disorders encompassed four subtypes: transient tics, chronic motor tics, atypical tic disorder, and Tourette's syndrome. There was an effort to imply a diagnostic relationship between each of the subgroups. When tic disturbances were continuously present throughout a year or longer, the patient crossed a conceptual boundary between transient tics and entered the domain of the chronic tic syndromes: chronic motor tic disorder and Tourette's syndrome (TS). Tourette's syndrome was diagnosed when *vocal and motor* tics, as distinct from chronic motor tics only, were present for longer than a year. In order to remain true to the original descriptions, for TS to be diagnosed, the onset of tics was specifically designated as between 2 and 15 years of age.

The third revised edition (DSM-III-R; APA, 1987) effected three modifications to DSM-III in an effort to apply results from recent empirical research. First, the age range of onset was extended to 21. Second, it had also been reported that some individuals had chronic vocal tics *in the absence of motor tics,* so the category of chronic motor tics was expanded to include chronic motor or vocal phenomena only. Third, there was an attempt to gain greater specificity by defining a certain density of symptoms, identifying that symptoms change in severity and anatomic location, and excluding tics arising as a consequence of known central nervous system diseases such as Huntington's chorea and post-viral encephalitis.

The *International Classification of Diseases* (ICD) is entering its tenth edition, and the chapter on psychiatric disorders will undergo revisions as well. The emergence of tic disorders as a separate entity is relatively new to the *ICD* system because, as recently as the eighth edition (World Health Organization [WHO], 1969), tics were grouped with the hereditary neuromuscular disorders, in the same larger group with Duchenne's muscular dystrophy, Friedreich's spinocerebellar ataxia, and hydrocephalus. In the ninth edition (WHO, 1978), tics were differentiated and subgrouped for the first time. These subgroups included transient tics, chronic motor tics, Tourette's disorder, and unspecified tic disorder. The draft proposals to the tenth edition (WHO, 1988) suggested that the new version will offer a more expanded view and more detailed descriptions of tic disorders than its predecessors as it will contain transient tics of childhood, chronic motor or vocal tics, Tourette syndrome, and tic disorder not otherwise specified. Intrinsically, the *ICD* takes a different approach to the psychiatric diagnostic process. In contrast with its U.S. counterpart, it does not enlist operational criteria; rather, it provides concise, clear descriptions of each disorder including discussion of its borderlands with other disorders. Room for clinical judgments is implicit in this process, and the overall effect from the *ICD* is that the clinician is offered more of a picture than a blueprint for each disorder.

DEFINITION

Before entering into a detailed discussion of DSM-III-R criteria, it is important, as Gilles de la Tourette and others stress, to understand features of tics in order to differentiate them from other episodic dyskinesias. Tics are relatively quick, recurrent, stereotyped muscular contractions that have an involuntary, nonpurposeful quality. They may affect any muscle or combination of muscles in the body and so may resemble many ordinary purposeful acts. Although they may be suppressed for brief periods, they cannot be deferred indefinitely, and the person with tics is usually aware of this quality. For the purposes of discussion, both vocal and motor tics are often subdivided into complex and simple types, depending on the number of muscle groups brought into play, the duration of the movements, the number of components that may be brought together into an orchestrated bout of movements, and distinctiveness of the movement. Examples of each variety of tics are given in Table 10.1.

Tics are remarkably common childhood symptoms. As many as 12%

TABLE 10.1
Examples of Varieties of Tics

Type	*Description*
Simple motor	eyeblinks, eye darting, pursing lips or pouting, grimacing, jerking motions of the head, arm, leg, hands, feet, or stomach, snaps of the jaw, shoulder shrugs, kicks.
Complex motor	biting, making peculiar "faces" or wincing, throwing, grabbing, pinching, bending, posturing, jumping, bouncing, banging, repeated touching, copropraxia (obscene gestures).
Simple phonic	clicking, short exhalations "puh puh puh," lip "pops," grunts, sniffing, coughs, throat clearing, yelps, squeaks, spitting, initial consonants.
Complex phonic	parts of words, words, phrases, echolalia, palilalia (echoing others or self), odd prosody and inappropriate accentuation of syllables, coprolalia; examples such as: "I have to go now, now, now, now, now," "alright, alright," "here we go round the mulberry bush," or "shiiiiiit, shitttttt, shshshshshshit."

Note. See also Leckman & Cohen (1988).

to 14% of children display tics in childhood, including transient tics, chronic multiple tics, and TS (Achenbach & Edelbrock, 1981; Lapousse & Monk, 1964). The salient features of tics make them unique among involuntary movements and permit differentiation. These features include their repetitiveness, brevity, variability over time, development, situation, anatomic location, mood, their presence during sleep, their duration, and suppressibility against the background of otherwise normal development (Fahn, 1982; Fahn & Erenberg, 1988).

Unlike the athetosis of cerebral palsy or the more generalized deficits of disorders leading to myoclonus, tics occur most commonly in patients who are otherwise neurologically normal and whose motor development has been normal (Bruun, 1988). This does not mean that tics never arise in persons with other neurological disorders or with abnormal motor development, but that when this occurs it is probably in the context of comorbidity with other neurological disorders or an unusual etiology for tics (Fahn & Erenberg, 1988). When tics do arise in persons with such a history, consideration of other disorders (e.g., cerebral palsy, chorea) should be kept in mind during the complete evaluation.

Tics are episodic and brief events on the time scale of other movement disorders. Most single symptoms last less than 3 seconds, although longer bouts involving a series of movements are often seen. It should be underscored that although persons severely afflicted with tics may experience symptoms throughout the day, their movements are still quite different from the continuous movements of other disorders such as stereotypies, athetosis, or segmental myoclonus. Periods of quiescence between movements are the rule, although the examination of exceptionally severely afflicted patients may lead the clinician to question this fact. Even under these circumstances, however, patients do not experience any one particular movement nonstop, but instead display a barrage of many different movements without cessation.

Suppressibility is a relative but diagnostically important feature. Although some patients have an ability to forestall even severe symptoms for hours, others may be unable to delay even moderate symptoms for more than a few minutes. For most patients, the capacity to overpower or diminish some tics is successful many times. How long this restraint can be sustained is subject to wide variation for any particular patient. Yet, however great an ability for suppression tic sufferers experience, it stands dramatically in contrast to the inability of other movement disorder patients to delay their symptoms, such as those with chorea or myoclonus.

Variability across so many dimensions is unusual in other neurological disorders. Tics change over time, although minute to minute or week to week they usually involve the same muscle groups and look much the same. Nevertheless, the frequency, intensity, and severity of any particular tic may change throughout the day or even over an hour. Through development, the tics often undergo changes in frequency and severity, usually becoming less severe following adolescence. In persons with multiple tics, one often sees an everchanging picture derived from the combinations and permutations of the movements, each with its own variable "pacemaker," each changing in intensity.

Specific symptoms change over time, but they also appear to spread in a predictable pattern in the early phases of the disorder. From the beginning with eye blinks, mild facial twitches, or lip darting, the movements tend to progress anatomically downward to the neck, shoulders, arms, trunk, legs, and feet. Over the course of the illness most patients report a rostral to caudal spread for both TS and chronic motor tics (Jagger et al., 1982). Yet for other patients the tics may not progress beyond the face or neck, or there may be particular regions that are more severely affected.

Tics change with situations and moods. For example, some persons discover that when they are being closely observed their tics become more severe, whereas others find that this exposure diminishes their symptoms. Similarly, strong emotional arousal, pleasurable or not, may exacerbate tics. Tourette's syndrome patients commonly report increased symptoms on occasions as diverse as birthdays, final examinations, bereavement, public performance, marital arguments, or Christmas anticipation. Forceful symptoms may be obvious in the doctor's waiting room only to recede entirely when the patient enters the examining room.

Another uncommon feature of tics is their appearance during sleep. Although Gilles de la Tourette (1885) wrote that the movements disappear completely during sleep, subsequent studies confirmed that tics occur during both rapid eye movement (REM) and non-rapid-eye movement (NREM) sleep (Glaze, Frost, & Jankovic, 1983).

A clearer understanding of these features makes the logic of the DSM-III-R criteria more readily discernable. DSM-III-R defines four varieties of tic disorder: transient tics, chronic motor or vocal tics, Tourette's syndrome, and tic disorder not otherwise specified (NOS). These are listed in Table 10.2.

Leaving aside the NOS category, the tic disorders all share an onset during the developmental years, defined as prior to age 21 years, and an idiopathic etiology not attributable to any specific known toxic, infectious, or degenerative central nervous system disease. In addition, the DSM-III-R makes an attempt to define a requisite frequency (i.e., multiple times a day, nearly every day) in order to have symptoms properly

TABLE 10.2
DSM-III-R Criteria for Tic Disorders

Tourette's Disorder

A. Both multiple motor and one or more vocal tics have been present at some time during the illness, although not necessarily concurrently.
B. The tics occur many times a day (usually in bouts), nearly every day or intermittently throughout a period of more than one year.
C. The anatomic location, number, frequency, complexity, and severity of the tics change over time.
D. Onset before age 21.
E. Occurrence not exclusively during psychoactive substance intoxication, or known central nervous system disease, such as Huntington's chorea, and post-viral encephalitis.

Chronic Motor or Vocal Tic Disorder

A. Either motor or vocal tics, but not both, have been present at some time during the illness.
B. The tics occur many times a day, nearly every day, or intermittently throughout a period of more than one year.
C. Onset before age 21.
D. Occurrence not exclusively during psychoactive substance intoxication, or known central nervous system disease, such as Huntington's chorea, and post-viral encephalitis.

Transient Tic Disorder

A. Single or multiple motor and/or vocal tics.
B. The tics occur many times a day, nearly every day for at least two weeks, but for no longer than twelve consecutive months.
C. No history of Tourette's or chronic motor or vocal tic disorder.
D. Onset before age 21.
E. Occurrence not exclusively during psychoactive substance intoxication, or known central nervous system disease, such as Huntington's chorea, and post-viral encephalitis.

Tic Disorder Not Otherwise Specified

Tics that do not meet criteria for a specific tic disorder.

Note. From *Diagnostic and Statistical Manual of Mental Disorders* (3rd ed., rev.) by American Psychiatric Association, 1987, Washington, DC: Author.

termed a disorder. Once these conditions are met, the three specified disorders are differentiated by three parameters. Chronicity is defined by a duration greater than 1 year, although there is little empirical support for this specific boundary. The other two parameters are the presence of motor tics and presence of phonic tics. Diagnoses are differentiated by combining the parameters as in Table 10.3.

TABLE 10.3
Parameters Differentiating Tic Disorders

Disorder	*Symptom Duration*	*Kinds of Tics*
Transient tics	< 1 year	only motor or only phonic or motor and phonic tics
Chronic motor tics	> 1 year	motor tics only
Chronic phonic tics	> 1 year	phonic tics only
Tourette's Syndrome	> 1year	must have motor *and* phonic tics

The DSM-III-R definition of Tourette's syndrome specifically underscores that the level of complexity, number, severity, frequency, and anatomic location of tics may change constantly. It also explicitly states that motor and phonic tics need not occur simultaneously.

REVIEW OF THE LITERATURE

Tics are primarily observable or audible events and possess a subjective component that is readily understood, thus there are few controversies about their definition and the essential core of the disorders manifesting them. This can be contrasted to the conceptual ambiguity intrinsic to definitions of many other psychiatric symptoms and disorders, such as bipolar illness, schizophrenia, anxiety, and personality disorders. However, the unanimous opinions about tic symptoms do not extend to a consensus about the associated behaviors of tic disorders, differentiation between types of tic disorders, and the emotional consequences of severe tic disorders. The approach to evaluation of persons with these symptoms is heavily influenced by the clinician's understanding of these questions.

In addition, there are several questions raised by the modifications to the DSM-III when DSM-III-R was produced. These include: (a) the boundary of at least a 1-year duration of illness that separates transient tics from chronic tic disorders, (b) the age of onset being extended by 6 years to between 2 and 21 years of age, and (c) the appearance of specific exclusionary criteria. Several of these changes appear to have been established by convention or based on clinical experience, because no support for them can be found from actual studies, whereas others reflect reports from the literature. Each of these is discussed in this section.

Associated Features

Patients rarely appear with the textbook or diagnostic manual picture of a disorder. Instead, they present themselves complete with their own idiosyncratic history, relationships, symptoms, reactions, and personal interpretations about causal connections. Unraveling the "Gordian knot" created by our inability to determine whether a given symptom is a part of the same disorder, arises in reaction to the presence of a disorder, is coincidental and unrelated to a disorder, or is a part of a completely different disorder is never easy and relies heavily on the understanding of the boundaries and typical features of the primary dysfunction in question. In Tourette's syndrome, for example, questions about associated symptoms have existed for as long as investigations have been conducted and remain one of the most active foci of current research.

The history of these questions begins as early as the article introducing the disorder as Tourette's syndrome. Gilles de la Tourette's description of obsessional thoughts in one of his patients (Gilles de la Tourette, 1885) was followed by Meige and Feindel's (1907) elaboration on a mental component accompanying tics. They created an implication that Tourette's syndrome might display more symptoms than just motor and phonic tics. Other investigators, including Mahler (1944), Kelman (1965), and Fernando (1967) described increased physical restlessness, "impulsions" or impulsivity, and "hypermotility" or hyperactivity in their patients. These symptoms were commonly observed or reported early in the histories offered by patients and were considered by these investigators to be a part of the tic disorder itself. More recently, the observation of aggressive and/or sexually inappropriate behaviors (Cohen, Leckman, & Shaywitz, 1984; Shapiro, Shapiro, Wayne, & Clarkin, 1972) has been seen commonly in TS patients and has led some investigators (Comings & Comings, 1987) to also consider these symptoms as etiologically related to Tourette's syndrome as well.

However, great care must be used in evaluating the methods and findings of some of these reports. Among the most widely quoted investigators in this topic of associated symptoms, Comings and Comings (1987) conducted family studies in which they suggested that a TS gene is responsible for attention deficit disorder, conduct disorder, bipolar affective disorder, panic/anxiety disorder, phobias, and sleep disorders (Comings & Comings, 1987). As Pauls, Cohen, Kidd, and Leckman (1988) detailed, at least six critical flaws in the assembly of the subjects, design of methods and instruments, and analysis of data cast serious doubt on the sweeping conclusions Comings and Comings proposed. Current standards of family study methodology demand that research designs include safeguards (Pauls et al., 1988) to avoid biased findings: Subjects should be ascertained from a general population and not a clinic-referred one; diagnostic corroboration should be available from information provided by multiple sources; independent diagnostic and severity ratings of associated symptoms should be made by investigators blind to tic status; and interview instruments should have previously demonstrated validity and reliability in a clinical population.

It is crucial that evaluation be guided by what is currently known about morbidity and symptom phenomenology in TS. Although the answers to the questions of associated symptoms discussed earlier are not available to clinicians and investigators now, we do know that these associated symptoms may be more prevalent and, when present, can impose significant limitations in TS patients (Bruun, 1988; Towbin, 1988). This means that when patients with tics present with any of the categories of symptoms to be discussed later, their presence must have a direct bearing on the foci of evaluation, decisions about treatments, and determinations of morbidity. Whether part of the core syndrome or not, these symptoms require detailed consideration.

Attention Deficit Disorders and Tourette's Syndrome

Attention deficit-hyperactivity disorder (ADHD) is an etiologically heterogeneous group of conditions manifested by problems with concentrating on directed tasks, impulsivity, and/or increased physical restlessness. Several investigators have observed that problems with these symptoms are seen early in the history of patients who later go on to develop Tourette's syndrome (TS) (Jagger et al. 1982; Moldofsky, Tullis, Lamon, 1974; Shapiro, Shapiro, Bruun, & Sweet, 1978). It is not surprising that there would be some confusion over whether the increased activity seen in young children who later go on to exhibit Tourette's syndrome is an early manifestation of that same disorder; both problems are involved with efforts to overcome bodily activity and impulsivity. On the one hand, it is easy to understand that children with Tourette's syndrome would exhibit difficulties with control of their bodies and exhibit symptoms as a consequence of these struggles that would include distractibility, impulsivity, and restlessness. On the other, not every child with Tourette's syndrome has had or currently exhibits these difficulties.

It is not known whether symptoms of ADHD in TS patients are part of the TS etiology or whether these symptoms are the expression of a separate disorder. Evidence from carefully constructed family studies of probands with both TS and ADHD suggests that the phenomena sort independently in their families (Pauls et al., 1986). Pauls and co-workers (1986) explained the increased prevalence of ADHD symptoms in patients referred for evaluation of Tourette's syndrome on the premise of Berkson's (1946) bias in which the probability of seeking medical attention for a disorder is increased when two disorders are present. Support for this hypothesis can be found in the epidemiologic survey in Monroe County, New York, by Caine and co-workers (1988) in which 100% of the 11 subjects with TS plus ADHD had been previously evaluated by physicians, whereas only 10 of the remaining 30 (33%) with Tourette's syndrome only (without ADHD) had been clinically evaluated—a threefold difference. This difference between the rates of referral in patients with TS only compared to those with TS plus ADHD is also seen in the retrospective review of patients seen in the extensive experience of Shapiro and Shapiro (Shapiro, Shapiro, Young, & Feinberg, 1988).

However, caution must be exercised before rushing to dismiss the other side of the question. The evidence from epidemiologic studies (Caine et al., 1988; Jagger et al., 1982) suggests a prevalence of ADHD of roughly 24% to 25% in TS patients, and this remains strikingly elevated from the general child population prevalence of roughly 9% in recent studies (Offord et al., 1987). This would imply some relationship greater than chance in the expression of these symptoms in this population. It need not be that either ADHD is part of TS or that they are entirely independent; the possibility of yet a more complex interaction between ADHD and TS also exists. For example, ADHD and TS could sort independently, whereas TS might increase the severity or decrease the threshold for expression of an ADHD disorder. A great deal has yet to be understood about the relationship between these two syndromes.

Disorders of Inhibition

Violent and increased sexual behavior have also been described among TS patients. Stefl's (1983) survey of persons with Tourette's syndrome in Ohio claimed that 25% to 30% suffered from episodes of aggressive outbursts, whereas Jagger and co-workers (1982) discovered that 36% of persons in their survey exhibited sexualized touching of themselves or others. The figure for self-abusive behavior resembles that for aggressive outbursts and has been reported in clinical investigations of referred patients with values ranging from a low of 7% to a high of 40% (Brunn, 1988; Comings & Comings, 1985; Nee, Caine, Polinsky, Eldridge, & Ebert, 1980; Shapiro et al., 1972). Viewed on a spectrum of difficulties with bodily control and impulsivity, it might be said of these symptoms, as of ADHD, that it is difficult to draw a tidy boundary between the core symptoms and the associated behaviors. Certainly, any surveys of patients referred for Tourette's syndrome showing violent or inappropriate sexual behavior will suffer from referral bias, because the morbidity from symptoms like these is so high and the threshold for seeking treatment so much lower than when these symptoms are absent. Until more rigorous studies are completed, it will not be possible to determine whether these symptoms are an offshoot consequence of Tourette's syndrome or in what way they may be directly related to it, if at all. For the purposes of evaluation, it can only be underscored that the expression of these symptoms is more frequent in Tourette's syndrome sufferers than in the general population, and such symptoms demand specific inclusion in any survey or review of symptoms undertaken by the clinician.

Obsessions and Compulsions

Obsessions are involuntary thoughts, images, urges, doubts, or worries that invade patients' awareness and which they usually understand as unnecessary and arising from their own mental life. Classically, compulsions are stereotyped behavioral acts performed in reaction to obsessions, either as a substitute to ward them off or in response to their demands. Compulsions are highly diverse and run a gamut of complexity and duration from relatively brief simple movements to endlessly intricate rituals. Examples of typical obsessions and compulsions are given in Table 10.4.

Descriptions of obsessions and compulsions associated with tics and with Tourette's syndrome in particular have been noted since the initial designation of TS and have appeared consistently in both the classic literature and modern research into tic phenomenology and natural history (Gilles de la Tourette, 1885; Caine et al., 1988; Grad, Pelcovitz, Olson, Matthews, & Grad, 1987; Jagger et al., 1982; Miege & Feindel, 1907; Shapiro et al., 1988; Towbin, 1988). Although in general it appears that most persons develop these symptoms late in the course of their illness, this is not a universal finding. Most studies discover that symptoms arise after 5 to 10 years from the onset of the first simple motor movements (Bruun, 1988). This relationship to the duration of the illness may explain the wide range of prevalence figures that have been proposed for obsessions and compulsions in Tourette's syndrome patients. When older samples are queried, the rates may be as high as 90% (Nee, Polinsky, & Ebert, 1982), whereas younger samples have given rates as low as 25% (Frankel et al., 1986; Grad et al., 1987). Taken altogether, the findings probably support a general prevalence statistic of 50% to 60% of all TS patients exhibiting obsessive-compulsive (OC) symptoms. This is to be compared to the general population prevalence

TABLE 10.4
Examples of Obsessions and Compulsions

Symptom Type	*Examples*
"Classic" Obsessions	Thoughts, images, words, doubts. Prayers, scenes of violence or sex, difficulties making choices about minor purchases, trying to remember every word of a conversation, thinking words backwards, thinking in "pig-latin"
"Classic" Compulsions	Washing/cleaning, checking, counting. Washing hands 20 or 30 times a day; scrubbing floors and dusting 20 or 30 times each day; repeatedly checking doors, windows, locks, lights, one's own body for signs of cancer; repeatedly checking the streets for dead animals, checking for false alarms; counting tiles, floor boards, spots.
"Tic-related" obsessions	Thinking about tics. Constant incapacitating worrying when the next tic will occur; mentally counting tics; endless wondering whether people saw or heard a tic; thoughts that intrude just before a tic, such as an sexual or violent image.
"Tic-related" compulsions	Actions employed to "block" a tic, such as blurting out a cough instead of saying an obscene word, hitting one's leg instead of touching someone's genitals; actions that preceed a tic such as tapping before a complex tic, or repeatedly asking about whether anyone saw a tic.

from the Epidemiologic Catchment Area surveys (Robins et al., 1984) which, using similar methods of determination, arrived at a figure of 2.5% of the population.

There are no clinically distinctive characteristics of the compulsive behaviors that might distinguish persons with OC in TS from those with obsessions and compulsions; the full range of obsessions and compulsions usually associated with obsessive-compulsive disorder (OCD) may be also seen in Tourette's syndrome patients. It does appear that the OC symptoms most common in OCD patients are not the most common OC symptoms in persons with TS (Frankel et al., 1986, Grad et al., 1987; Rasmussen & Tsuang, 1986). Despite this, the variety of symptoms remains quite broad and cannot be distinguished from the symptoms found in OCD. This has relevance for determining what instruments might be useful in evaluating the OC symptoms of Tourette's syndrome sufferers. Also, it should be emphasized that the distinction between complex tics and compulsions is often difficult to make in patients with moderate to severe TS (Towbin, 1988). This confusion, which cannot be readily clarified by medication response alone, is a continuing focus of investigation.

In contrast to the contradictory or weak evidence for a direct relationship between the symptoms of attention deficits or disinhibition of aggression and Tourette's syndrome, there is strong evidence supporting a view that, in the presence of TS, obsessions and compulsions share the same etiology as the one producing TS. The evidence comes from family-genetic studies (Nee et al., 1980; Pauls, Cohen, Heimbuch, Detlor, & Kidd, 1981; Pauls & Leckman, 1986) and from findings of a greatly increased prevalence of OC symptoms in TS patients, as previously noted. Preliminary results of ongoing work suggest that some first-degree family members of TS probands have only obsessions or compulsions without any history or current expression of any tics (Pauls, Towbin, Leckman, Zahner, & Cohen, 1986). Whereas this result might be expected if the OC symptoms were transmitted genetically as a separate comorbid condition, the evidence for OCD presenting as an alternative expression of the same etiology as TS was strongly supported by three findings: (a) OCD was discovered among first-degree relatives of TS probands at greatly increased rates compared to even the highest general population figures (12% to 13% in relatives of TS probands, compared to population prevalence of 2.0%) (Robins et al., 1984), (b) "OCD-only" was discovered in first-degree relatives of TS probands when the probands themselves did not have histories or display OC symptoms, and (c) rates of "OCD-only" among first-degree relatives of TS probands with histories of OC symptoms were equal to rates in first-degree relatives of those TS probands for whom there was no such history (Pauls et al., 1986). This suggests a high probability that some obsessions and compulsions share the same specific genetic etiology with Tourette's syndrome (Pauls & Leckman, 1986).

The relationship between OCD and TS has also been implicated from clinical surveys of OCD patients. In one study where subjects were carefully interviewed for lifetime histories of tics, roughly 40% produced histories of tics either in childhood, which were absent at the time of the study, or mildly present but not readily observed at the time of the study (Green & Pittman, 1986). If the results of the family-genetic studies are true, in time it may be demonstrated that some obsessions and compulsions *in the absence of current or past history of tics* are a consequence of the same etiology as the one leading to TS (Towbin, 1988).

Questions of Diagnostic Modifications

As described in a previous section, DSM-III-R made modifications in DSM-III in order to decrease the time between new findings and clinical application. Although the modifications were supposed to be based on results from empirical research, this was not possible in all cases, and the clinical experience of the committee was substituted. In the tic disorders, three modifications were imposed: The age range was extended, a new diagnostic subtype emerged for chronic vocal tics, and specificity was given to the chronic tic disorders. For TS specifically, DSM-III-R created two additional changes. One was applying exclusionary criteria in recognition of known organic conditions that give rise to tics and require some nosologic clarification, and the other was a change in the number of chronic vocal tics required in order for a diagnosis of TS to be made.

Age of Onset

In DSM-III there was some inconsistency in the specification of the age of onset. Although there was some logic as to why transient tics and Tourette's syndrome specifically required a childhood onset, there were no obvious reasons provided to explain why chronic multiple tics did not require such an age of onset. When DSM-III-R was produced, the age range of onset was extended from the 2 to 15 years in DSM-III to 2 to 21 years of age. This was a response to Abuzzahab and Anderson's (1976) report of 15 patients in their registry who developed symptoms after age 20, several case reports (Areneta, Magen, Musci, Singer, & Vahn, et al., 1979; Marneros, 1984), and the observations of those with extensive clinical experience (Brunn, 1988; Shapiro et al., 1988).

New Diagnostic Subtypes

It had been reported that some individuals exhibited chronic vocal tics in the absence of motor tics, although rarely. For this reason, the category of chronic motor tics was expanded to include chronic motor or vocal phenomena only (Leckman & Cohen, 1988). No studies have specifically addressed the population that shows only vocal phenomena so that the natural history, relationship to other tic disorders, and etiology remain unclear. The validity of equating chronic vocal with chronic motor tics has not been established. It has been suggested that the movements of the throat made during vocal tics may not be rare but occur commonly in normal individuals (Shapiro et al., 1988). This hypothesis holds that, in their pathological form, vocal tics are exaggerations of movements that never reach expression normally, but in the disoder reach high levels of intensity and frequency.

Increased Specificity of the Designation

DSM-III-R made an attempt to gain greater specificity by defining a certain density of symptoms, identifying that symptoms change in severity and anatomic location, and excluding tics arising as a consequence of known central nervous system diseases such as intoxication, Huntington's chorea, and postviral encephalitis. This change represents a departure from a purely descriptive method of identifying and studying tic disorders and highlights the prevailing view that TS is a separate disease entity (i.e., it is not an alternative expression of any other known disorder). It also was an attempt to underscore that these were symptoms with a level of expression or morbidity warranting designation as a disorder.

Changes in the Number of Vocal Tics

Although it may seem trivial, the number of vocal tics required to make a diagnosis of TS was changed from "multiple vocal tics" in DSM-III to "one or more" in DSM-III-R. This change extended the population of patients who would warrant the diagnosis in the newer scheme because clinical experience suggests that many patients do have only one vocal tic. Evidence is not available on what percentage of TS patients have one versus more than one vocal tic, but the intent was clarified in DSM-III-R. There is no evidence to support a prognostic or etiologic difference on the basis of one or more than one vocal tic, although research data is lacking.

Additional Questions

At least two questions remain to be studied further in order to clarify arbitrary demarcations in the current diagnostic scheme. First, there have been no satisfactory studies to justify the 1-year duration separating transient tics from chronic tics. In fact, some investigators have argued that the disorders may not be so readily differentiated by any evaluation at a single point in time (Shapiro et al., 1988). The suggestion of separating these disorders and the 1-year duration has been based on clinical experience but, to date, no natural history study of transient tics has indicated whether 12 months yields a more valid dividing line than, for example, 6 or 18 months.

Furthermore, because the genetic risks of developing Tourette's syndrome are the same for first-degree relatives of those having chronic multiple tics as for relatives of probands with Tourette's syndrome itself, there may be legitimate questions about whether these are separate disorders (Pauls, Kruger, Leckman, Cohen, & Kidd, 1984; Pauls & Leckman, 1986). Evidence that both disorders yield the same vulnerability to first-degree relatives for a similar outcome argues for their identity and may finally lead to a single diagnostic label.

Questions of Placement in a Psychiatric Nosology

Some investigators have suggested that because Tourette's syndrome is a genetic disorder of the central nervous system, analogous to Huntington's chorea, it should be classified as a neurological illness and is not appropriate in a psychiatric classification. Although the lines dividing neurological illnesses and psychiatric conditions are notoriously vague, there are other illnesses in the psychiatric classification that have a neurological basis, such as autism, mental retardation, specific developmental learning disorders, and organic mental disorders. This does not even begin to consider the burgeoning knowledge of the genetics and neurology of traditional psychiatric disorders such as schizophrenia and bipolar illness. Obviously, a psychiatric disorder does not have to be ipso facto idiopathic or without biological features. In a broader way the suggestion to move TS to a neurological category proposes that classification should be based solely on etiology. But because classification schemes are constructed and designed for specific reasons, different schemes will reflect different purposes. It is quite valid to base a classification on etiology, but it is just as appropriate to consider where patients with various conditions go for care, what professional groups see the most patients, the age of onset, and the treatment approaches employed. Tourette's syndrome has traditionally been treated by mental health professionals using a variety of modalities and has been considered under the broad rubric of psychiatric conditions, thus its placement in psychiatric nosology is equally valid.

DIAGNOSTIC AND ASSESSMENT PROCEDURES

Tic disorders arise during development and therefore demand that clinicians assess not only patients' current state, but also where patients are in their development and how the disorder threatens to dislodge them from the optimal developmental path. The procedures employed in the assessment of a person seeking diagnosis and treatment for a tic disorder should reflect our most complete understanding of both the features that contribute to the day-to-day severity of symptoms and the factors that, in the face of a potentially chronic illness, affect development and subsequent emotional adjustment. This can be best secured by a knowledge and thorough application of the modalities and the instruments that are available.

Modalities

In order to gain this kind of comprehensive understanding of individuals and their illness, the evaluator must include an assessment of who patients are in their family, at work, and to themselves. One must also include assessment of general health and the symptoms currently exhibited. In order to accomplish this, three modalities are employed: direct interviews, videotaping, and laboratory/physical examinations.

Direct Interviews

Interviews of patients separately and with their family stand at the center of the evaluation of tic disorders. There are four main goals of the interviews with patients: (a) to obtain accurate historical and descriptive information; (b) to gain a clear understanding of patients' strengths and defenses, the meaning of the symptoms to patients, and their impact on patients; (c) to convey accurate information about the disorder; and (d) to establish the context of a relationship that will optimally promote subsequent treatment and observation. Patients usually come to clinical attention because they exhibit symptoms that disrupt their lives at home and school or work; thus, the severity of their distress and immediacy of their demands may lead the clinician to adopt too narrow a scope—that is, focusing only on the tics. A clinician may be too readily drawn to the symptoms as the sole problem requiring attention. Clinicians may neglect the vital elements of the patient's premorbid adjustment and development, current thoughts, anxieties and frustrations, the disruption of social and occupational or academic adjustment, and the impact of their dysfunction on their families.

Seen in this way, the interviews become more than a means of gathering the medical history. Usually the interview is the primary means of obtaining the patient's personal history and learning about activities that aggravate or diminish symptoms. But when conducted in a warm, caring, unhurried, unassuming way, the interview is a therapeutic intervention in and of itself. It is the only opportunity a patient may have to reflect on the various internal effects of symptoms and their interpersonal consequences, to receive accurate information about prognosis and to raise embarrassing questions. Patients learn to observe themselves without the need to "attack" the symptoms impulsively and vigorously and can gradually come to understand how the symptoms affect their inner life in such areas as self-esteem, aspirations, and coping strategies. The clinician may assist in reducing the patient's anxiety, improve the ability to observe specific symptoms and defensive reactions, and discover new ways to contend with the consequences of the illness. This cannot be accomplished in one or several interviews but becomes an ongoing endeavor as the patient and the clinician work together over months or years. When one recalls that symptoms may wax and wane, the foundation in this relationship becomes important from the initial contact with the patient, even when symptoms may be quite mild. In more severe cases, the relationship between clinician and patient assumes an even more crucial role in treatment and care. In these situations the frustration about unresponsiveness, social impairment, and academic/occupational disability loom even larger. Patients may feel quite hopeless and helpless, become quite depressed, and require assistance in obtaining even basic living needs. The clinician may shift from being a collaborator to an advocate, which may include contacts with other important adults in the patient's life.

The role of the interview with the patient and family is equally crucial. As is discussed later, the parents in particular are vital for providing history, assisting in making assessments of severity, and in rating progress. Particularly for children, the earliest entry into their illness is through the family. But in addition, clinicians are required to appreciate the multiple ways in which Tourette's syndrome is also a familial disorder. It is a disorder that runs through families and affects families directly and indirectly.

Tourette's syndrome is a chronic illness in which children may be severely affected and that may have a profound social effect on parents and siblings (Cohen, Ort, Leckman, Riddle, & Hardin, 1988). This can be as simple as the immediate feelings aroused in any parent who sees their child with a chronic, potentially disabling malady. The parents may experience anger, shame, a sense of failure, and grief. Similarly, siblings may experience guilt or jealousy, sadness, frustration, and anger as their brother or sister demands increasing amounts of the family's resources, or causes the sibling embarrassment in his or her peer group. Sometimes the symptoms themselves may be the cause of conflict. As noises and tics lead to disruption of family routines or intimate times, or as compulsive rituals become elaborate and time consuming, the entire family can feel burdened. Occasionally, aggressive behaviors may surface, and family members may become targets of verbal or physical assaults or threats. The patient may become generally irritable or dispirited and increasingly isolated from the family, consequently causing or evoking anger.

But beyond its immediate impact on the family, Tourette's syndrome is also a familial genetic disorder. This has several other ramifications. The genetic etiology means that multiple family members are affected, and patients have at least one parent with whom they have a special genetic as well as emotional connection relative to their disability. They may also have siblings who are affected to greater or lesser degrees of severity. The special emotional relationship contains all those features previously identified, as with any chronic illness, but also contains components of the parent's past history and coping strategies with the same kinds of problems. As has been emphasized by Cohen and coworkers (Cohen, Ort, Leckman, Riddle, & Hardin, 1988), this emotional connection to the parent's past can be strongly positive or negative. Sometimes the special connection with a parent can work in a patient's favor, providing reassurance and compassion, and reinforcing self-esteem. Conversely, children may find that their symptoms force the afflicted parent to contend with conflicts and questions of self-esteem that were never resolved, and, subsequently, these symptoms rearouse or continue to arouse self-disdain and derogation in their parents. As children struggle to come to terms with their own symptoms and illness, they bring into the process a parent or grandparent who now must embark on a similar journey, often for the first time. Just as children must come to understand their own responsibilities and conflicts about the symptoms, so the parents are often faced with reassessing difficulties in academic/occupational achievement, interpersonal relationships, and their self-concepts. Frustrations about their bodies and lives may represent the recrudescence of internal conflicts that have never been successfully resolved. The parent may attempt to apply the same vigorous efforts to control affects and behaviors with their own children as they used to control their own symptoms. The child may come to personify unconsciously the parent's negative introjects and place the parent into direct conflict with the child for reasons neither one can understand. The judicious use of family interviews can diminish these struggles and, in a way similar to the individual interview, provide an arena for examining the fears, frustrations, disappointments, and reactivated self-disdain that the symptoms may create. The family interviews form the foundation for determining whether further intensive specific family therapy may be needed and what strengths can be enjoined from within the family to assist in treatment.

Another adult in the child's constellation of relationships with whom direct contact can be essential is the teacher. This contact also has elements of assessment and treatment. In general, narrative information from teachers can assist in the evaluation of any childhood disturbance that brings a child to attention. Particularly in Tourette's syndrome, when symptoms may be much less evident during the class day than at home, the impact on peers may be more evident, and an objective rating of frequency and severity can be essential. Here, the teachers' information and role are critical. But when a teacher is uninformed and misinformed about the symptoms, their etiology, morphology, and ability to be controlled, the child can face intense stress and, as a result, symptoms may be worsened. An informed teacher can adjust expectations to meet the child's emotional and educational needs optimally. The observations of these interventions allow the clinician to assess how stress-responsive a particular patient's symptoms may be and also help to understand whether stress makes a significant contribution to the patient's severity. This kind of consultative contact alone can diminish symptoms in the classroom and improve a child's standing in the group.

Videotape

The next major modality that has been used to assess initial severity and monitor progress is videotape material. This can be as informal as conducting portions of the initial clinical interview on videotape or having the patient sit "quietly" for a videotaped segment, or as formalized as the protocol employed by Tanner, Goetz, and Klawans (1982). Videotapes are valuable because symptoms, especially complex prolonged ones, can be accurately recorded and the patient's overall physical response to intervention can be assessed in a similar way over time. However, videotaped segments may not be reliable measures of severity. The stress of being videotaped may lead many patients to have greater or fewer symptoms, the symptoms themselves may be changed by the procedure, and patients may refuse. High-quality equipment can also be expensive. Nevertheless, work by at least two research groups suggests that videotaped material can be a reliable reflection of actual severity (Shapiro & Shapiro, 1984; Tanner et al., 1982).

Physical Examination and Laboratory Investigation

The last major modalities of assessment are physical examination and laboratory investigations. The need for a complete physical examination goes without question. Although no established procedure of laboratory assessment exists, the usual investigation includes complete blood count, blood chemistries, and can include radiographic examinations, as indicated in Table 10.5.

There is little support for a general requirement of electroencephalograms (EEG) in patients evaluated for Tourette's syndrome despite reports of increased rates of nonspecific findings such as slow wave and posterior spiking (Krumholtz, Singer, Neidermeyer, Burnite,

TABLE 10.5
Laboratory Studies Suggested for Evaluation of Tourette's Syndrome

Urinalysis		
Complete blood count with differential		
Blood chemistries:		
Glucose	SGOT	Ceruloplasmin*
BUN	SGPT	Serum copper*
Creatinine	Alk. Phos.	
Sodium	LDH	
Potassium	CPK	
Chloride	Calcium	
HCO_3	Phosphorous	
Electrocardiogram		
Radiographic studies:		
Computerized Axial Tomography*		
Karyotype*		
Slit Lamp Examination for Kayser–Fleischer rings*		

*These studies may be ordered as the presentation and history warrant specific investigation.

& Harris, 1983; Shapiro et al., 1988; Volkmar et al., 1984). There is a general feeling that EEG findings do not contribute any prognostic, therapeutic, or etiologic significance. A similar statement might be made of Computerized Tomographic (CT) Scans, although the literature has not established this as firmly (Volkmar et al., 1984). When the presentation raises serious questions about possible Huntington's disease or Hallervorden-Spatz disease, a CT scan can be useful (Shapiro et al., 1988). However, investigations of CT scans in Tourette syndrome suggest that patients generally have normal CT scans when, except for tics, other focal neurological findings are absent (Caparulo et al., 1981; Harcherick et al., 1985).

Instruments and Assessment

In order to obtain reliable assessments using formal instruments, it is vital to understand the limitations, problems, and function of the instrument employed. The functions are fully discussed later, but several limitations and problems can be generalized for all the instruments.

The same features that define tics make their assessment and measurement a challenge. They change over short spans of time in a way that jeopardizes the reliability of short periods of assessment. A child may display constant tics at home or school, and then present in an appointment without so much as even a mild symptom picture. Conversely, the patient may exhibit much more severe symptoms in the assessment than are exhibited elsewhere. Generally, the movements or sounds cannot be suppressed completely, but severity can vary dramatically across settings.

An instrument must encompass the entire range of severity from the mildest tic symptoms to the most severe TS or chronic multiple tics in a way that permits meaningful comparisons. As one understands the range of tic illnesses more completely, severity becomes a more elusive concept. What comparison can be made between the severity of multiple very mild simple tics and one constant but very obvious complex tic? What comparison can be made between very severe symptoms confined to an hour or two of the day in the privacy of home and a more evenly distributed set of symptoms of moderate severity that is obvious all day long in every setting? Should very obvious vocal tics be equated with more discreet but equally forceful motor movements?

The appropriate standard against which symptoms are to be rated is a third problem. If three different parties (the patient, the parent, and the clinician) make different observations about the severity of symptoms, which one should determine the "actual severity"? For the patient, there may be no acknowledgment that the symptoms are disruptive, while the mother may see these symptoms as the worst to date and "very severe." At the same time, clinicians may see moderate symptoms relative to the population with which they are most familiar (i.e., the very impaired persons who are referred for treatment). Each one may be accurate in their perception, but which severity rating should be the basis for intervention and gauging improvement?

A final problem is that the morphology of complex tics may make distinguishing the number of movements impossible. When is a series of simple movements that always occur in succession and always in the same way one complex tic and when is it a series of simple tics? When patients have nonstop movements, how are these to be divided into identifiable components?

In order to achieve the most reliable responses, it is important to take the time to review the instrument, explain terms, and define time frames carefully with the parents and patient. When this is not done, the reliability of the responses cannot be trusted. Clinical decisions based on unreliable responses may affect subsequent ratings of improvement, the relationship with the clinician, and the outcome of treatment.

Tic Ratings

Tic ratings can be divided into three varieties: self- or parent-assessed historical data bases, self- or parent-assessed ratings of tic frequency and severity, and clinician ratings of severity. Self-ratings have been routinely employed by researchers for ascertainment of symptoms that are not observable in the office. In addition, a self-assessed historical data base has been employed to obtain information about onset, severity, course, and developmental milestones and progress (Jagger et al., 1982; Stefl, 1983). Gradually, both of these have been incorporated into general clinical practice. A historical data base, called the Tourette's Syndrome Questionnaire (TSQ), has become increasingly useful as a screening device prior to the initial session in order to provide a superficial overview of the patient's past history (Cohen, Leckman, & Shaywitz, 1984). The lists assist patients, their families, and the clinician in identifying progress or deterioration and in arriving at a complete picture of symptoms that otherwise may be overlooked. One of the most commonly employed lists was devised by the Yale group and called the Tourette's Syndrome Symptom List (TSSL) (Cohen et al., 1984). The list surveys a 7-day period, asking the respondent to identify the general frequency of each listed tic for each day. Associated behaviors, such as irritability and low frustration tolerance, are also included. The scoring yields five summary frequency scores and "number of symptoms" scores, one for each of the four groupings of simple and complex motor and phonic tics, and one for the group of associated behaviors.

Anecdotal reports and open clinical trials led to new medications capable of reducing tics or associated behaviors. With the need to confirm the efficacy of these agents came a pressing demand for standardized measures to assess severity of tics and Tourette's syndrome. Each of the two scales that were first developed reflected different concepts of severity. The Shapiro Tourette's Syndrome Severity Scale (Shapiro et al., 1988) views severity as based on five factors: whether tics are noticeable to others, whether they elicit comments or curiosity, whether others consider the person odd or bizarre, whether they interfere with functioning, and whether the patient is incapacitated, homebound, or hospitalized because of tics. Each of these factors is scored on its own scale, each with a different ceiling ranging from 1 to 3, and each with a floor of 0 when the factor is absent. Reliability and validity studies have been published and indicate acceptable levels for both (Shapiro et al., 1988). The scales are not straightforward, and the scatter of ranges can be cumbersome.

The Tourette's Syndrome Global Scale (TSGS) (Cohen et al., 1984) takes a view of Tourette's syndrome severity as arising from two domains: tics and social functioning. In the tic domain, each of the four subtypes of tics (simple and complex, motor and vocal) are rated separately on frequency and disruption of symptoms using a scale of 0 to 5. The score for each subtype is derived from the product of frequency and disruption. The social domain also consists of four subelements (i.e., behavior, school problems, occupational problems, and motor restlessness), each assessed according to a global 0- to 25-point scale resembling the Global Assessment of Functioning (GAF), on the V Axis in DSM-III-R. Published reliability and validity suggest acceptable levels (Harcherick, Leckman, Detlor, & Cohen, 1984; Leckman, Towbin, Ort, & Cohen, 1988). Difficulties with the metric of the TSGS result in an increased emphasis on the social domain compared with the tic domain, and the frequency-by-disruption product weights infrequent tics more heavily than may be appropriate (Leckman et al., 1989).

A third clinician-rated scale, the Yale Global Tic Severity Scale (YGTSS), has now been added (Leckman et al., 1988; Leckman et al., 1989). The YGTSS was derived from an appreciation of portions of information provided by both the TSGS and Shapiro scales and the additional merit of clinician-rated symptom checklists. The scale was created in an effort to bring together the strong features of each. Recent experience with the YGTSS suggests that it is both reliable and valid as a measure of tic severity (Leckman et al., 1989). It is an attempt to measure clearly defined components of frequency, intensity, complexity, interference, and impairment for each of the symptoms identified by the patient. The additive summary score purportedly suggests that each of these domains contributes equally to the concept of severity, and high scores in any one domain suggest significant severity. It also contains a metric for quantifying overall impairment, much like the Global Assessment Scales for Adults and Children (Endicott, Spitzer, Fleiss, & Cohen, 1976; Shaffer et al., 1983), which permits the rater to identify total impairment from TS, taking stock of elements of associated behaviors and intrapsychic, academic, and familial effects, in addition to tics. It includes a checklist section in order to supply a cross-sectional narrative picture of the current tics exhibited by the patient.

Attention Deficit Disorder/Hyperkinesis Ratings

The inclusion of measures for rating severity of attention deficit-hyperactivity disorder (ADHD) or hyperkinesis in a discussion of evaluation of TS patients implies a closer relationship between the two than the literature is currently capable of supporting. Until the nature of impulsivity, attentional deficit, and hyperactivity in TS patients is better understood, it should be made clear that the convention of rating severity of ADHD symptoms is recommended, both because symptoms of ADHD are surprisingly common in this population and because so many TS patients are impaired by them. However, it bears repeating that it would be premature to conclude that symptoms of inattention, impulsivity, or hyperactivity in TS patients are either completely separate from TS or a core part of the tic disorder.

Attention Deficit-Hyperactivity Disorder (ADHD) remains an elusive entity to measure despite a long history of investigation. At this time there are no reliable self-rated measures of severity and impairment. This is not surprising in view of the general difficulties patients with moderate to severe degrees of dysfunction have in appreciating their high levels of activity and the impact their behaviors have on others.

Several different methods of gaining objective information about impulsivity, inattention, and hyperactivity have arisen, although none have offered a proven standard. The need for sampling multiple sources for their observations is as critical in ADHD as in TS itself; in the clinician's office the patient may appear quiet, appropriate, and even subdued despite having severe symptoms virtually everywhere else. Standard practice would favor using the Connors Parent and Teacher Rating Scales because of their widespread use, ready comparison to a variety of studies of attention deficit disorder with hyperactivity (ADD+H) and ADHD, ease of administration, and good reliability in the hands of trained lay persons (Goyette, Connors, & Ulrich, 1978). Studies of children with TS have traditionally employed either the Connors scales or global impression scales.

Another measure that has been applied for ADD+H patients but also has the advantage of screening for other symptoms and difficulties, is the Achenbach Child Behavior Checklist (CBCL; Achenbach & Edelbrock, 1981). One of the major advantages of the CBCL is its extensive application across a wide range of disorders, cultures, and populations. This has permitted highly reliable figures for norms and ranges. In addition to the hyperactivity subscale, the CBCL also yields scores for externalizing behaviors, social competence, and behavior problems without hyperactivity.

An additional alternative for assessing patients with suspected ADD+H are subscales of standardized neuropsychological tests, including the Weschler Intelligence Scale for Children-Revised (WISC-R). In particular, the Trailmaking Test parts A and B, Underlining test, digit symbol modalities test (Smith, 1973), and vocabulary and coding subtest of the WISC-R may be useful. The Tourette's Syndrome Association[1] is currently making an effort to develop a unified Tic Rating Scale that would recommend or suggest tests for the assessment of these and other TS-related symptoms.

As the technology for employing microcomputer-based continuous performance tests (Halperin et al., 1988; Rosvold, Mirsky, Sarason, Bransome, & Beck, 1956) proliferates, these may be added to the clinician's repertoire for the assessment of distractibility or impulsivity.

[1]Tourette's Syndrome Association, 42–40 Bell Boulevard, Bayside, New York, 11361, (718) 224–2999.

Continuous performance tests show great promise as a laboratory measure of these cognitive dysfunctions, and therefore as an objective measure related to attention deficit disorder with hyperactivity. The greatest problem with them remains the question of what cognitive process is being assessed, impulsivity (O'Dougherty, Neuchterlein, & Drew, 1984) or inattention (Halperin et al., 1988). As currently constructed, these tests may assist a clinician in gaining additional information about errors of commission, but questions of which dimension of cognition results in these errors cannot be answered yet.

Another tool that may be useful in the future is the motion actometer (Porrino et al., 1983). These devices, usually a solid state motion sensor strapped to a subject's arm or leg, can reliably assess features of fidgetiness and restlessness by quantitative counts of movements. The reliability of actometer measures in patients with TS has not been established, and these remain primarily a research tool. Nevertheless, the possibility of their application as yet another laboratory measure for tic frequency is intriguing.

Obsessions and Compulsions (OC)

Self-rating instruments for persons with OC symptoms are becoming more acceptable. In general, no pencil-and-paper task can reliably make the diagnosis of OC Disorder without a corresponding clinical determination so that these instruments remain almost exclusively research devices for assessment of severity. The most commonly used instruments are the Leyton Obsessional Inventory (LOI) (Cooper, 1970) and the Yale-Brown Obsessive Compulsive Scale (Y–BOCS) (Price, Goodman, Charney, Rassmussen, & Heninger, 1987). Both have child versions, and the children's LOI has received formal assessment for reliability and validity (Berg, Rapoport, & Flament, 1986). These instruments may be useful for determining the degree to which OC symptoms cause impairment and interfere with day-to-day function. The LOI is a pencil-and-paper task that can be presented to the subject at any time during the assessment, whereas the Y-BOCS is a semistructured interview that requires trained administrators in order to obtain reliable information. Although neither instrument is valid for making diagnoses of OC without a clinical interview and careful investigation, the child LOI has been pared down for use as a screening device for epidemiologic investigation (Flament et al., 1988).

When employing these instruments routinely, the greatest problem arises because most patients are quite secretive about their symptoms and may not begin to reveal them until the clinical relationship is firmly established. Unlike the tics themselves, these symptoms may exist only in the patient's thoughts or be carried out in the seclusion of their bathrooms or bedrooms. Many patients are quite embarrassed about uncontrollable habits or thoughts that have sexual or scatological content and about the silliness of the actions they take knowing they have no foundation. For children, in particular, these symptoms can be a subject that arouses great personal distress and avoidance. In addition, children may not appreciate the degree of disruption these habits create for those they live with and may underestimate their impact.

For these reasons, objective assessments of interference and disruption are equally important. There are, as yet, no observer-based structured instruments for the assessment of OC symptoms by teachers or family members. It is vital to conduct a clinical interview with the parents and teachers of children presenting with symptoms, because this remains an indispensable tool in determining the actual level of preoccupation, paralysis, or action. Careful explanation of these symptoms is essential and often assists parents and teachers in becoming better observers of the patient.

Other Psychopathology

There are several reasons to conduct a complete examination for the presence of other general psychopathology in patients suffering from TS or chronic tics. Comorbid disorders may have an impact on the patient's ability to make the best use of other health care providers or teachers, or to enter into successful employment. Some comorbid conditions (e.g., major depression, social phobias, serious personality disorders) may effect patients' abilities to form healthy, supportive relationships and leave them alone without emotional resources when their symptoms are severe (Towbin, Riddle, Leckman, et. al., 1988). Reciprocally, comorbid conditions may become intensified by the movement disorder, especially as tic symptoms become worse. There is good reason to believe that the overall prognosis and general adjustment to the movement disorder may be adversely influenced by comorbid conditions. Serious substance abuse, depression, or severe personality disorder may influence the way in which the patient copes with tic disorder and may diminish the patient's capacity to contend with fluctuations in symptoms. Clinicians may find the need to treat two disorders simultaneously if they intend to intervene. In addition, the relationship between the tic disorder and comorbid conditions may be relevant for treatment. If, for example, the comorbid condition is a consequence of an upsurge in tic symptoms, this must be taken into account and monitored as treatment progresses. Treating the tics may decrease depression, social isolation, and low self-esteem. Alternatively, the comorbid condition may have a life of its own and remain prominent even when tics diminish. Separate treatments may be needed for these symptoms and consequently affect the severity or treatments for the movement disorder itself.

SUMMARY AND FUTURE DIRECTIONS

The future of assessment of tic disorders mirrors the anticipated changes in neuropsychiatry. The development of molecular biological techniques, sophisticated metabolic imaging and physiologic probe techniques, the mapping of the human genome, and increasing knowledge of the disorders themselves will substantially change methods of diagnosis and assessment in the next decade.

As molecular biological techniques are increasingly applied to TS, it may be possible to discover the specific autosomal genes responsible for the vulnerability to TS. Once discovered, biological markers that would permit early identification may become available. As we now recognize that environmental contributions to the clinical picture are large, preventative measures may be instituted for vulnerable individuals. Imaging and physiologic probe techniques may reveal the relationships between genetic vulnerability and clinical expression. We may see identification of the common pathways and neurohumoral substances that activate and moderate symptoms. New treatments based on these findings may become available. As the expression of the disorder and natural history are better described, more complete family and personal histories may be obtained, and an ever clearer understanding of the essential core symptoms of the syndrome will become available.

However, even without these optimistic predictions, the reachable advances in understanding natural history and risk or protective factors will mean better care for patients with tics. From the perception that TS was a rare eccentricity of nature at the turn of the century, we have moved to appreciate a now common, frequently mild disorder compatible with a full, rewarding life. More effective treatments are currently available than ever before. There now are more clinicians who are better informed about this disorder than ever, and this has resulted in patients receiving more compassionate, informed, thorough, and comprehensive assessment and intervention than at any time in the history of TS.

REFERENCES

Abuzzahab, F. S., & Anderson, F. O. (1976). *Gilles de la Tourette's syndrome, International registry* (Vol. 1). St. Paul, MN: Mason.

Achenbach, T. M., & Edelbrock, C. S. (1981). Behavioral problems and competencies reported by parents of normal and disturbed children aged 4 through 16. *Monographs of the Society of Research in Child Development, 46*(188).

American Psychiatric Association. (1952). *Diagnostic and statistical manual of mental disorders* (1st ed.). Washington, DC: Author.

American Psychiatric Association. (1968). *Diagnostic and statistical manual of mental disorders* (2nd ed.). Washington, DC: Author.

American Psychiatric Association. (1980). *Diagnostic and statistical manual of mental disorders* (3rd ed.). Washington, DC: Author.

American Psychiatric Association. (1987). *Diagnostic and statistical manual of mental disorders* (3rd ed., rev.). Washington, DC: Author.

Areneta, E., Magen, J., Musci, M. N., Jr., Singer, P., & Vann, C. R. (1979). Tourette's syndrome symptom onset at age thirty-five. *International Journal Social Psychiatry, 25*, 4–9.

Bell, C. (1830). *The nervous system and the human body.* London: Longman, Rees, Orme, Brown, & Green.

Berg, C. J., Rapoport, J. L., & Flament, M. (1986). The Leyton Obsessional Inventory-Child Version. *Journal of the American Academy of Child Psychiatry, 25*, 84–91.

Berkson, J. (1946). Limitations of the application of a fourfold table analysis to hospital data. *Biometric Bulletin, 2*, 47–53.

Bruun, R. D. (1988). The natural history of Tourette's syndrome. In D. J. Cohen, R. D. Bruun, & J. F. Leckman, *Tourette's syndrome and tic disorders: Clinical understanding and treatment* (pp. 21–40). New York: Wiley.

Caine, E. D., McBride, M. C., Chiverton, P., Bamford, K. A., Redliess, S., & Shiao, J. (1988). Tourette's syndrome in Monroe County school children. *Neurology, 38*, 472–475.

Caparulo, B. K., Cohen, D. J., Rothman, S. L., Young, J. G., Katz, J. D., Shaywitz, S. E., & Shaywitz, B. A. (1981). Computed Tomographic Brain Scanning in children with developmental neuropsychiatric disorders. *Journal of the American Academy of Child Psychiatry, 20*, 338–357.

Cohen, D. J., Detlor, J., Young, J. G., & Shaywitz, B. A. (1980). Clonidine ameliorates Gilles de la Tourette syndrome. *Archives of General Psychiatry, 37*, 1350–1357.

Cohen, D. J., Leckman, J. F., & Shaywitz, B. A. (1984). The Tourette syndrome and other tics: In D. Shaffer, A. A. Ehrhardt, & L. Greenhill (eds.), *The clinical guide to child psychiatry* (pp. 3–28). New York: Free Press.

Cohen, D. J., Ort, S. I., Leckman, J. F., Riddle, M. A., & Hardin, M. T. (1988). Family functioning in Tourette syndrome. In D. J. Cohen, R. D. Bruun, & J. F. Leckman, *Tourette's syndrome and tic disorders: Clinical understanding and treatment* (pp. 179–197). New York: Wiley.

Comings, D. E., & Comings, B. G. (1985). Tourette syndrome: Clinical and psychological aspects of 250 cases. *American Journal of Human Genetics, 37*, 435–450.

Comings, D. E., & Comings, B. G. (1987). A controlled study of Tourette syndrome: I-VI. *American Journal of Human Genetics, 44*, 701–838.

Cooper, J. (1970). The Leyton Obsessional Inventory. *Psychological Medicine, 1*, 48–64.

Endicott, J., Spitzer, R. L., Fleiss, J. L., Cohen, J. (1976). The Clinical Global Scale: A procedure for measuring overall severity of psychiatric disturbance. *Archives of General Psychiatry, 33*, 766–771.

Fahn, S. (1982). The clinical spectrum of motor tics. In T. N. Chase, & A. J. Friedhoff (Eds.), *Gilles de la Tourette syndrome. Advances in Neurology, 35*, 341–345. New York: Raven Press.

Fahn, S., & Erenberg, G. (1988). Differential diagnosis of tic phenomena: A neurologic perspective. In D. J. Cohen, R. D. Bruun, & J. F. Leckman, (Eds.), *Tourette's syndrome and tic disorders: Clinical understanding and treatment* (pp. 41–55). New York: Wiley.

Fernando, S. J. M. (1967). Gilles de la Tourette syndrome. *British Journal of Psychiatry, 113*, 607–617.

Flament, M., Whitaker, A., Rapoport, J. L., Davies, M., Berg, C., Kalikow, K., Sceery, W., & Shaffer, D. (1988). Obsessive compulsive disorder in adolescence: An epidemiological study. *Journal of the American Academy of Child and Adolescent Psychiatry, 27*, 764–772.

Frankel, M., Cummings, J. L., Robertson, M. M., Trimble, M. R., Hill, M. A., & Benson, D. F. (1986). Obsessions and compulsions in Gilles de la Tourette syndrome. *Neurology, 36*, 378–382.

Gilles de la Tourette, G. (1885). Etude sur une affection nerveuse caracterisee par de l'incoordination motrice accompagnee d'echolalie et de coprolalie. *Archives de Neurologie, 9*, 19–42, 158–200.

Glaze, D. G., Frost, J. D., & Jankovic, J. (1983). Gilles de la Tourette syndrome: Disorder of arousal. *Neurology, 33*, 586–592.

Goyette, C. H., Connors, C. K., & Ulrich, R. F. (1978). Normative data on revised Connors Parent and Teacher Rating Scales. *Journal of Abnormal Child Psychology, 6*, 221–236.

Grad, L. R., Pelcovitz, D., Olson, M., Matthews, M., & Grad, G. (1987). Obsessive-compulsive symptomotology in children with Tourette syndrome. *Journal of the American Academy of Child Psychiatry, 26*(1), 69–74.

Green, R. C., & Pittman, R. K. (1986). Tourette syndrome and Obsessive-Compulsive Disorder. In M. Jenike, L. Baer, & W. F. Minichiello, (Eds.), *Obsessive-compulsive disorder: Theory and management*. Littleton, MA: PSG Publishers.

Group for Advancement of Psychiatry. (1966). *Psychopathological disorders in childhood theoretical considerations and a proposed classification*. Report No. 62. New York: Group for Advancement of Psychiatry.

Hall, M. (1852). On muscular tic. *Lancet, 2*, 510.

Halperin, J., Wolf, L., Pascualvaca, D., Newcorn, J., Healey, J., O'Brien, J., Moragansein, A., & Young, J. G. (1988). Differential assessment of attention and impulsivity in children. *Journal of the American Academy of Child and Adolescent Psychiatry, 27*(3), 326–329.

Harcherick, D. F., Cohen, D. J., Ort, S. I., Paul, R., Shaywitz, B. A., Volkmar, F. R., Rothman, S. L. J., & Leckman, J. F. (1985). Computed tomographic brain scanning in 4 neuropsychiatric disorders of childhood. *American Journal of Psychiatry, 142*, 731–734.

Harcherick, D. F., Leckman, J. F., Detlor, J., & Cohen, D. J. (1984). A new instrument for clinical studies of Tourettes syndrome. *Journal of the American Academy of Child Psychiatry, 23*(2), 153–160.

Itard, J. M. G. (1825). Memoire sur Quelques Fonctions Involontaires des Appareils de la Locomotion de la Prehension et de la Voix. *Archives Generales de Medicine, 8*, 385–407.

Jagger, J., Proshoff, B. A., Cohen, D. J., Kidd, K. K., Carbonari, C. M., & John,

K. (1982). The epidemiology of Tourette syndrome: A pilot study. *Schizophrenia Bulletin, 8*(2), 267–279.

Kelman, D. H. (1965). Gilles de la Tourette's disease in children: A review of the literature. *Journal Child Psychology and Psychiatry, 6,* 219–226.

Krumholtz, A., Singer, H. S., Neidermeyer, E., Burnite, R., & Harris, K. (1983). Electrophysiological studies in Tourette's syndrome. *Annals Neurology, 14,* 638–641.

Lapouse, R., & Monk, M. (1964). Behavior deviations in a representative sample of children; Variations by sex, age, race, social class, and family size. *American Journal Orthopsychiatry, 34,* 436–446.

Leckman, J. F., & Cohen, D. J. (1988). Descriptive and diagnostic classification of tic disorders. In D. J. Cohen, R. D. Bruun, & J. F. Leckman, (Eds.), *Tourette's syndrome and tic disorders: Clinical understanding and treatment* (pp. 3–21). New York: Wiley.

Leckman, J. F., Riddle, M. A., Hardin, M. T., Ort, S. I., Swartz, K. L., Stevenson, J., & Cohen, D. J. (1989). The Yale Global Tic Severity Scale (YGTSS): Initial testing of a clinician rated scale of tic severity. *Journal of the American Academy of Child and Adolescent Psychiatry, 28*(4), 566–574.

Leckman, J. F., Towbin, K. E., Ort, S. I., & Cohen, D. J. (1988). Clinical assessment of tic disorder severity. In D. J. Cohen, R. D. Bruun, & J. F. Leckman, (Eds.), *Tourette's syndrome and tic disorders: Clinical understanding and treatment* (pp. 55–79). New York: Wiley.

Mahler, M. J. (1944). Tics and impulsions in children: A study of motility. *Psychoanalytic Quarterly, 13*(4), 430–444.

Marneros, A. (1984). Gilles de la Tourette syndrome. *Fortschreift Neurologie und Psychiatrie, 52,* 250–257.

Meige, H., & Feindel, E. (1907). *Tics and their treatment.* (A. K. Wilson, Ed. and Trans.). New York: William Wood.

Moldofsky, H., Tullis, C., & Lamon, R. (1974). Multiple Tic Syndrome (Gilles de la Tourette Syndrome): Clinical, biological and psychological variables and their influence with haloperidol. *Journal of Nervous and Mental Diseases, 159,* 282–292.

Nee, L. E., Caine, E. D., Polinsky, R. J., Eldridge, R., & Ebert, M. H. (1980). Gilles de la Tourette Syndrome: Clinical and family study of 50 cases. *Annals of Neurology, 7,* 41–49.

Nee, L. E., Polinsky, R. J., & Ebert, M. H. (1982). Tourette syndrome: Clinical and family studies. In T. N. Chase, & A. J. Friedhoff, (Eds.), *Gilles de la Tourette syndrome. Advances in Neurology, 35,* 291–295. New York: Raven Press.

O'Dougherty, M., Neuchterlein, K. H., & Drew, B. (1984). Hyperactive and Hypoxic Children: Signal detection, sustained attention, and behavior. *Journal Abnormal Psychology, 92,* 4–28.

Offord, D. R., Boyle, M. H., Szatmari, P., Rae-Grant, N. I., Links, P. S., Cadman, D. T., Byles, J. A., Crawford, J. W., Blum, H. M., Byrne, C., Thomas, H., & Woodward, C. A. (1987). Six-month prevalence of disorders and rates of service utilization. *Archives of General Psychiatry, 44*(9), 832–836.

Pauls, D. L., Cohen, D. J., Heimbuch, R., Detlor, J., & Kidd, K. K. (1981). Familial pattern and transmission of Gilles de la Tourette syndrome and multiple tics. *Archives of General Psychiatry, 38,* 1091–1093.

Pauls, D. L., Cohen, D. J., Kidd, K. K., & Leckman, J. F. (1988). Tourette syndrome and neuropsychiatric disorders: Is there a genetic relationship? *American Journal of Human Genetics, 42,* 206–209.

Pauls, D. L., Hurst, C. R., Kruger, S. D., Leckman, J. F., Kidd, K. K., & Cohen, D. J. (1986). Evidence against a genetic relationship between Tourette syndrome and Attention Deficit Disorder. *Archives of General Psychiatry, 43,* 1177–1179.

Pauls, D. L., Kruger, S. D., Leckman, J. F., Cohen, D. J., & Kidd, K. K. (1984). The risk of Tourette's syndrome and multiple tics among relatives of Tourette syndrome patients obtained by direct interview. *Journal of the American Academy of Child Psychiatry, 23,* 134–137.

Pauls, D. L., & Leckman, J. F. (1986). The inheritance of Gilles de la Tourette syndrome and associated behaviors: Evidence for an autosomal dominant transmission. *New England Journal of Medicine, 315,* 993–997.

Pauls, D. L., Towbin, K. E., Leckman, J. F., Zahner, G. E. P., & Cohen, D. J. (1986). Gilles de la Tourette syndrome and obsessive-compulsive disorder. *Archives of General Psychiatry, 43,* 1180–1182.

Porrino, L., Rapoport, J., Behar, D., Sceery, W., Ismond, D. R., & Bunney, W. E. (1983). A naturalistic assessment of the motor activity of hyperactive boys I: Comparison with normal controls. *Archives of General Psychiatry, 40*(6), 681–688.

Price, L. H., Goodman, W. K., Charney, D. S., Rassmussen, S. A., & Heninger, G. R. (1987). Treatment of severe obsessive compulsive disorder with Fluvoxamine. *American Journal of Psychiatry, 144*(8), 1059–1061.

Rasmussen, S. A., & Tsuang, M. T. (1986). Clinical characteristics and family history in DSM-III OCD. *American Journal Psychiatry, 143,* 317–322.

Robins, L. N., Helzer, J. E., Weissman, M. M., Orvaschel, H., Gruenberg, E., Burke, J. D., Jr., & Regier, D. A. (1984). Lifetime prevalence of specific psychiatric disorders in three sites. *Archives of General Psychiatry, 41*(10), 949–959.

Rosvold, H. E., Mirsky, A. F., Sarason, I., Bransome, E. D., & Beck, L. H. (1956). A continuous performance test of brain damage. *Journal of Consulting Psychology, 20,* 343–350.

Shaffer, D. L., Gould, M. S., Brasic, J., Ambrosini, P., Fisher, P., Bird, H., & Aluwahalia, S. (1983). A children's Global Assessment Scale. *Archives of General Psychiatry, 40,* 1228–1231.

Shapiro, A. K., & Shapiro, E. S. (1984). Controlled study of Pimozide vs. Placebo in Tourette's syndrome. *Journal of the American Academy of Child Psychiatry, 23*(2), 161–173.

Shapiro, A. K., Shapiro, E. S., Bruun, R. D., & Sweet, R. D. (1978). *Gilles de la Tourette syndrome.* New York: Raven Press.

Shapiro, A. K., Shapiro, E. S., Wayne, H. L., & Clarkin, J. (1972). The psychopathology of Gilles de la Tourette syndrome. *American Journal of Psychiatry, 129,* 427–434.

Shapiro, A. K., Shapiro, E. S., Young, J. G., & Feinberg, T. E. (1988). *Gilles de la Tourette syndrome* (2nd ed.). New York: Raven Press.

Smith, A. (1973). *Symbol Digit Modalities Test.* Los Angeles, California: Western Psychological Services.

Stefl, M. E. (1983). *The Ohio Tourette's Study.* Cincinnati: School of Planning, University of Cincinnati.

Tanner, C. M., Goetz, G. G., & Klawans, H. L. (1982). Chloinergic mechanisms in Tourette syndrome. *Neurology, 32,* 1315–1317.

Towbin, K. E. (1988). Obsessive-compulsive symptoms in Tourette's syndrome. In D. J. Cohen, R. D. Bruun, & J. F. Leckman, (Eds.), *Tourette's syndrome and tic disorders: Clinical understanding and treatment* (pp. 137–151). New York: Wiley.

Towbin, K. E., Riddle, M. A., Leckman, J. F., Bruun, R. D., & Cohen, D. J. (1988). The clinical care of individuals with Tourette's syndrome. In D. J. Cohen, R. D. Bruun, & J. F. Leckman, (Eds.), *Tourette's syndrome and tic disorders: Clinical understanding and treatment* (pp. 329–353). New York: Wiley.

Volkmar, F. R., Leckman, J. F., Detlor, J., Harcherick, D. F., Pritchard, J. W., Shaywtiz, B. A.,

& Cohen, D. J. (1984). EEG abnormalities in Tourette syndrome. *Journal of the American Academy of Child Psychiatry, 23,* 352–353.

World Health Organization. (1969). *Manual of the international statistical classification of diseases, injuries and causes of death* (8th ed.). Geneva: World Health Organization.

World Health Organization. (1978). *Mental disorders: Glossary and guide to their classification in accordance with the ninth revision of the International Classification of diseases.* Geneva: World Health Organization.

World Health Organization. (1988). *Manual of the international statistical classification of diseases, injuries and causes of death (10th ed.). Draft of Chapter V. Mental, Behavioral, and Developmental Disorders: Clinical descriptions and diagnostic guidelines.* Geneva: World Health Organization.

CHAPTER 11

Elimination Disorders

William E. MacLean, Jr.
George Peabody College of Vanderbilt University

Robert M. Brayden
Vanderbilt University School of Medicine

The developmental milestones of early childhood herald the continuing maturation of the child. Most parents readily recall their child's first steps, first words, and the like. Many of these developmental phenomena are biobehavioral in nature given the dynamic system created by the child's physiological readiness and responsiveness of the environment. The development of bowel and bladder control is no exception. Despite the wishes of parents and caregivers, a basic level of physical readiness must be achieved and instruction provided before toilet training can be fully accomplished (Christophersen & Rapoff, 1983; MacKeith, Meadow, & Turner, 1973).

The failure to obtain an age-appropriate level of continence represents a widely accepted form of behavioral disturbance (Walker, 1978). Whether the disorder is characterized by continued incontinence (primary) or a period of continence followed by a reoccurrence (secondary), the topographies of the disorders remain the same. Unlike other forms of childhood psychopathology, where there has been controversy over the nature of the disorder, there has been little difficulty agreeing on the basic aspects of elimination disorders. Simply stated, the passage of waste materials represents a discrete observable event. Furthermore, passage of waste into inappropriate places, as determined by cultural standards, is easily detected by parents, teachers, and other children.

Given the widespread agreement that there is a basis for such diagnoses, efforts have been directed toward determining under what circumstances a diagnosis is appropriate. Consequently, there has been considerable elaboration of the diagnostic criteria for elimination disorders since 1952 when the first *Diagnostic and Statistical Manual* was published by the American Psychiatric Association (APA).

HISTORICAL BACKGROUND

In DSM-I (APA, 1952), enuresis was included as a special symptom reaction. This group of disorders was distinguished from the remainder of DSM-I in that a specific symptom was the "single outstanding expression of psychopathology." A diagnosis of enuresis was not appropriate if the symptom was associated with, or was secondary to, organic illness or physiological defect, or some other psychiatric disorder. Although diagnosticians were provided with these exclusionary criteria, they were not given other guidelines for making the diagnosis, such as the age at which diagnosis would be appropriate or an objective definition of enuresis. It is noteworthy that encopresis was not included as a diagnostic category in DSM-I. Doleys (1989) made the case that the relative underattention that encopresis has received, as contrasted with the burgeoning literature on enuresis, may be due to its greater association with medical-organic factors (such as fecal incontinence) and Anthony's (1957) observation that many professionals find encopresis to be particularly offensive to treat or write about.

Both enuresis and encopresis were included in a category called Special Symptoms Not Elsewhere Classified in DSM-II (APA, 1968). As in DSM-I, there was no further delineation of defining criteria for the diagnoses, although it remained that these diagnoses were not appropriate if there was an organic basis for the disorder or if the behavior was associated with another DSM-II diagnostic category.

In DSM-III, functional encopresis and functional enuresis were included in a diagnostic subclass labeled Mental Disorders With Physical Manifestations (APA, 1980). In contrast to the previous two editions, objective behavioral definitions (e.g., voiding of urine or passing of feces into places not appropriate for that purpose) were provided for each disorder. Further, there was specification of the age at which diagnosis would be appropriate and the frequency of these events that would be considered psychopathological. Moreover, the addition of the term *functional* to the diagnoses emphasized the already recognized need to exclude those children whose elimination disorder was due to known organic etiology.

Table 11.1 provides a comparative analysis of the criteria for functional encopresis and enuresis through the four editions of the *Diagnostic and Statistical Manual.* This comparison highlights the considerable elaboration of diagnostic criteria that occurred in the third edition and further refinement of the criteria in DSM-III-R (APA, 1987). The most obvious change in the criteria as presented in DSM-III-R is the subtyping into primary or secondary categories and, for functional enuresis, whether the disorder occurs on a diurnal and/or nocturnal basis. Although specification of these subtypes has the potential to provide identification of discrete subgroups, there is some question as to whether such distinctions will be helpful. For example, Levine (1982) argued that children with encopresis present for care with a spectrum of clinical symptoms that includes partial bowel training, and classifications of primary and secondary subgroups may be misleading. Nevertheless, classification systems that take into account more factors than the chronological age of the child will enhance the diagnostic specificity of elimination disorders. Whether such precision has relevance, for example, in specifying optimal intervention approaches remains to be determined.

Another change from DSM-III to DSM-III-R, evident for both forms of elimination disorders, was the addition of mental age as a further criterion in establishing the appropriateness of the diagnosis for a given child. In DSM-III, no further specification of age was provided. However, the DSM-III-R criteria made separate references to chronologic and mental age. Children whose overall development is delayed with respect to their chronologic age must have attained a mental age of at least 4 years for these diagnoses to be appropriate. This further refinement emphasizes the already recognized developmental gradient that underlies the attainment of bowel and bladder control. This gradient has two separate but interrelated components: (a) the neuromaturation necessary for sphincter control and (b) the cognitive level necessary to engage in independent toileting behavior.

Additional changes in the DSM-III-R criteria are also apparent in the definitions of each disorder. With respect to functional encopresis, both the reference to the "individual's own sociocultural setting" in determining whether the child is eliminating appropriately and specification of "normal or near-normal consistency" feces were deleted. Although not explicitly stated, it would appear that such deletions were made because these phrases were not deemed essential to the disorder. In the United States, the sociocultural expectations for managing human waste do not vary from one part of the country to another, nor do they vary from one ethnic or cultural subgroup to the next. Similarly, fecal matter in any form that is placed in any location not appropriate for its sanitary management is deemed sufficient for diagnosis. Professionals who regularly treat children with functional encopresis

TABLE 11.1
Comparative Aspects of *Diagnostic and Statistical Manual* Criteria for Functional Encopresis and Enuresis

Edition	*Definition*	*Frequency*	*Age Considerations*	*Differential Diagnosis*	*Subtypes*
Functional Encopresis					
DSM-I	—	—	—	—	—
DSM-II	No specific criteria	—	—	—	—
DSM-III	Repeated voluntary or involuntary passage of feces of normal or near-normal consistency into places not appropriate for that purpose in the individual's own sociocultural setting	At least one event a month	After the age of 4 years	Not due to a physical disorder such as aganglionic megacolon	—
DSM-III-R	Repeated passage of feces into places not appropriate for that purpose (e.g., clothing, floor), whether involuntary or intentional (The	At least one event each month for at least 6 months	Chronologic and mental age, at least 4 years	Not due to a physical disorder such as aganglionic megacolon	Primary or secondary

	disorder may be over-flow incontinence secondary to functional fecal retention)				
Functional Enuresis					
DSM-I	No specific criteria	—	—	—	—
DSM-II	No specific criteria	—	—	—	—
DSM-III	Repeated involuntary voiding of urine by day or night	At least two such events per month for children between the ages of 5 and 6, and at least one event per month for older children	After the age of 5 years	Not due to a physical disorder, such as diabetes or a seizure disorder	—
DSM-III-R	Repeated voiding of urine during the day or night into bed or clothes, whether involuntary or intentional	At least two such events per month for children between the ages of 5 and 6, and at least one event per month for older children	Chronologic age at least 5, mental age at least 4	Not due to a physical disorder, such as diabetes, urinary tract infection, or a seizure disorder	Primary or secondary Nocturnal, diurnal, or both

point out that, given the defecation dynamics involved in children with megacolon, the fecal matter can vary considerably in consistency (Levine, 1975). In DSM-III-R, the definition of functional enuresis was elaborated to include repeated voiding of urine during the day or night into bed or clothes, whether involuntary or intentional. Specification of an inappropriate location for elimination serves to clarify the nature of the disorder, and the inclusion of the phrase "whether involuntary or intentional" removes the need to establish intentionality in making the diagnosis.

Specific definitional issues pertaining to the diagnosis of elimination disorders, as set out in DSM-III-R, are discussed in turn.

DEFINITIONAL ISSUES

Functional Encopresis

Definition

There is little question regarding the presence of stool given its distinct physical and olfactory characteristics. The specific physiology responsible for rectal evacuation is well understood (Roy, Silverman, & Cozzetto, 1975). However, the contributory processes leading to inappropriate defecation are more complex. Previous typologies have distinguished between those children who withhold defecation (retentive) from children who evacuate and place their feces in inappropriate places (Gavanski, 1971; Levine, 1975, 1982; Walker, 1978).

Retentive-type encopresis generally follows constipation of longstanding duration (Roy et al., 1975). The retained fecal mass, termed an *impaction*, distends and eventually dilates the rectum. The size of the impacted stool results in painful defecation; dilation of the anal canal may also lead to anal fissure, additionally causing painful defecation (Levine, 1982; Wrenn, 1989). Unless passed from the body, fecal matter continues to collect and involves the colon. The dilated colon, known as megacolon, may allow some soft or liquid fecal matter to pass around its edges. This manner of excretion, termed *paradoxical diarrhea* or *overflow incontinence*, is considered to be mostly out of the control of the child (Bellman, 1966; Levine, 1975). Retentive encopresis may have behavioral antecedents, such as toilet phobia described by Doleys (1978) or pot refusal syndrome (Berg & Jones, 1964), and/or a physiologic basis such as low fiber intake, dehydration secondary to febrile illness, or a side effect of medication.

The nonretentive type is less frequent in occurrence, less noted in the literature, and the subject of considerable speculation (Gavanski, 1971; Walker, 1978). Some of the discussion has focused on whether the bowel movements came about through involuntary or intentional processes. In cases where it appears that the encopresis is related to incomplete toilet training (accidents), the distinction appears less useful. Conversely, manipulative soiling or intentional placement of feces in inappropriate places is probably linked to antisocial processes (Walker, 1978) that may warrant an additional DSM-III-R diagnosis.

Frequency

During the first 4 years of life—that is, the years before a diagnosis of encopresis would be made—the frequency of bowel movements decreases from more than four per day in the first week of life to an average of 1.2 per day at 4 years of age (Weaver & Steiner, 1984). Children generally develop a pattern or routine of defecation that facilitates toilet training. For most children, elimination occurs following mealtime, such as breakfast or dinner, in response to the gastrocolic reflex, and toilet training for bowel control is rapidly accomplished (Christopherson & Rapoff, 1983).

Beyond 4 years of age, one event per month over a 6-month period has been determined sufficient frequency to warrant a diagnosis of functional encopresis. Recent literature suggests that retentive encopretic children have soiling (overflow) episodes much more frequently than once per month. For example, Loening-Baucke, Cruikshank, and Savage (1987) found that 38 encopretic children (mean age 8.8 years, range 6 to 11 years) experienced infrequent and incomplete bowel movements; however, they experienced overflow soiling a minimum of 3.0 times per week. Friman, Mathews, Finney, Christophersen, and Leibowitz (1988) found that 39 retentive and 11 nonretentive encopretics (mean age 6.7, range 4 to 12 years) averaged 14.8 episodes of soiling per week, and Gabel found a mean of 11 soiling episodes per week in 38 encopretic boys (Gabel, Chandra, & Shindledecker, 1988). These data suggest that the current frequency criterion, at least once per month for a period of 6 months, would be highly sensitive to the clinical population.

Age Considerations

At about 1 year of age, a baby begins to appreciate aversive attributions to feces by caretakers (Fleisher, 1976). Gradually, the toddler becomes aware of the stimulation of receptors signaling the need to defecate and starts to make toileting needs known by age 18 to 24 months (Behrman & Vaughn, 1987). Most parents initiate behaviors to

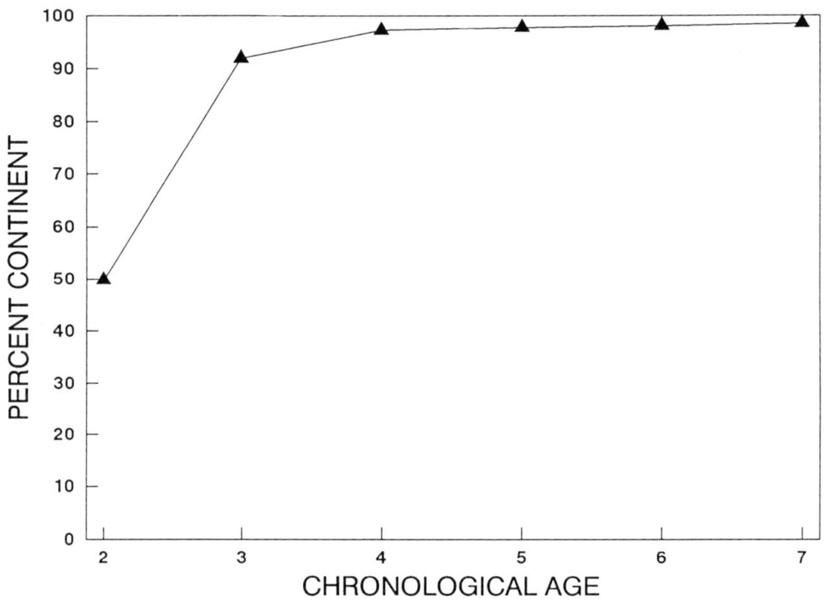

FIG. 11.1. Percentage of children, ages 2–7 years, who achieved bowel continence (defined as a frequency of less than once per month for greater than 3 months) in a sample from Sweden reported by Bellman (1966).

encourage the passage of waste into toilets at this time. Cross-sectional longitudinal studies of young children reveal that by the age of 4 years, developmentally and chronologically, most children have achieved full bowel control (Bellman, 1966; Stein & Susser, 1967). Figure 11.1 provides a graphic representation of the data presented in Bellman (1966). According to this cross-sectional study, half of the children had achieved bowel continence by their second birthday. By 3 years of age, upwards of 90% of the children exhibited bowel control by day and night. Although no statistical test was conducted, the authors concluded that girls acquire bowel control at somewhat younger ages than boys (Bellman, 1966).

Although bowel movements vary in frequency, volume, and consistency during infancy, the finding of true constipation in infancy is uncommon (Rappaport & Levine, 1986). In infants and toddlers, Levine (1982) cited multiple factors that may prompt withholding of stool. Among the factors Levine included are "early colonic inertia," voluntarily withholding of defecation, negative interactions with caretakers, and painful experiences such as passing bowel movements while one has anal fissures or perianal irritation. As children become older, stresses coinciding with toilet training and initiation of school may influence defecation patterns (Levine, 1982).

Differential Diagnosis

A thorough physical examination is necessary to rule out physical conditions that may result in fecal incontinence. Table 11.2 presents a listing of representative medical diagnoses that should be considered when evaluating these children.

A careful medical history can assist in diagnosing organic causes of elimination disorders. Medications and toxins may have constipating effects, thus promoting fecal retention that then leads to fecal soiling. Narcotics and their derivatives, phenothiazines, tricyclic antidepressants, some antihypertensive medications, diuretics, iron, and bulk-

TABLE 11.2
Conditions that Have Encopresis and Enuresis as Associated Features

Encopresis	*Enuresis*
Retentive	Endocrinological disorders
Anorectal anomalies	Diabetes mellitus
Hirschprung's disease	Diabetes insipidis
Anal narrowing	Urinary tract infection
Anterior displacement of the anus	Genitourinary disorders
Anal fistula	Genitourinary malformations
Anal fissures	Chronic renal failure
Pelvic mass	Small functional bladder capacity
Medications	Uninhibited bladder contractions
Narcotics	Neurological disorders
Phenothiazines	Convulsive disorder
Tricyclic antidepressants	Central nervous system tumor
Iron	Meningomyelocele
Endocrinological/physiological anomalies	Sleep and arousal immaturity
Hypothyroidism	Cerebral palsy
Hypercalcemia	Constitutional delay in neuromaturity
Neurological abnormalities	
Meningomyelocele	
Cerebral palsy	
Nonretentive	
Gastrointestinal abnormalities	
Inflammatory bowel disease (Crohn's disease, ulcerative colitis)	
Lactose intolerance	
Pancreatic insufficiency	

forming laxatives with insufficient water intake are among reported drugs causing fecal impaction (Wrenn, 1989). A history of significant immobility, rarely found in normally developing children, is important because exercise enhances colonic motility (Read & Timms, 1986).

Physical examination of encopretic children should include assessment of the metabolic, endocrine, gastrointestinal, and neurological systems. Constipation is commonly present in hypothyroidism; however, cessation of growth, sleepiness, and lethargy are also usually present (Behrman & Vaughn, 1987). Disorders of calcium resulting in hypercalcemia can cause constipation. Gastrointestinal tract abnormalities leading to diarrhea and soiling include inflammatory bowel diseases (ulcerative colitis and Crohn's disease), surgical shortening of the bowel, and prolonged recovery from bowel infection. Lactose intolerance and pancreatic insufficiency due to cystic fibrosis are examples of absorption disorders resulting in diarrhea. One manifestation of these disorders could be soiling. Anomalies of the anus and rectum such as narrowing, anterior displacement, fistulas, and severe fissuring may also contribute to constipation, particularly in its early presentation (Levine, 1982). Abnormalities resulting in a pelvic mass may also cause the impaction of fecal material (Schmitt, 1984a). Diseases of the cerebral cortex, spinal cord, or peripheral nervous system may cause colonic motility abnormalities (Behrman & Vaughn, 1987; Fleisher, 1976).

Numerous chronic conditions may affect elimination, resulting in fecal retention and, in some cases, soiling. These include myelomeningocele, "Prune belly" syndrome, and cerebral palsy (Fleisher, 1976; Fitzgerald, 1987). Defects of closure of the neural tube, especially those that do not involve the skin, such as spina bifida occulta, may present or be complicated by both enuresis and encopresis.

Lack of fecal bulk may be associated with constipation (Wrenn, 1989). Undernutrition or a diet high in carbohydrates or proteins and low in dietary fiber may lead to chronic constipation (Fitzgerald, 1987).

Encopresis has been recognized in a few reports as a presenting and/or accompanying sign of anal sexual abuse (Brayden & Altemeier, 1989). The prevalence of this symptom is nearly the same as the rate in the general population.

Type

The duration of continence determines whether the encopresis is classified as primary or secondary. Continence over a 12-month period is deemed sufficient proof of bowel control. Regression following this period is unusual and evidence that a maturational delay alone cannot explain the development of the symptoms. Thus, in secondary disorders, investigation should focus on organic processes or psychosocial determinants of recent onset.

Functional Enuresis

Definition

Given the explicit nature of the disorder, there has been no disagreement regarding the definition of the behavioral act. Whatever the clinician's perspective on etiology, the repeated voiding of urine into the bed or clothing is the crucial aspect of the disorder. In DSM-III-R this criterion was expanded to include intentional as well as involuntary voiding.

Some authors (Fielding & Doleys, 1988) advocate use of the size of the wet spot as an additional measure of each enuretic episode. Such information appears to have greater relevance for determining progress of treatment (such as dry bed training) than in making the diagnosis per se.

Frequency

According to DSM-III-R, a diagnosis of functional enuresis requires that there be at least two events per month in children ages 5 to 6 years. For older children, one event per month (presumably over a period of several consecutive months) is sufficient. In a large population-based study, Foxman, Valdez, and Brook (1986) found that of 1,753 children aged 5 to 13 years, 14% had at least one enuretic episode in the previous 3 months. Children who were reported to wet their beds tended to be younger (age 5 to 8 years) and male. The frequency of wetting among these children was described as sporadic, with 15% of the enuretic children at each age group wetting nightly and 40% wetting one to five times per week. However, these frequencies are well within the criteria necessary for a diagnosis of functional enuresis as presented in DSM-III-R.

Age Considerations

This criterion acknowledges the underlying developmental acquisition of bladder control. During infancy, distention of the bladder causes the spinal cord to reflexively stimulate the muscle in the bladder wall, the detrusor, to contract. The physiological process that results in urination is termed *micturition*. As the child grows, the total bladder capacity increases proportionately more rapidly than the total growth of the child (Goellner, Ziegler, & Fomon, 1981). Concomitantly, the volume of urine the child produces per body weight decreases (Goellner et al., 1981; Koff, 1983). Control over urination begins when a child learns to control the voluntary sphincter muscles around the outlet tract for urine. Continence develops with the integration of voluntary inhibition of urination with the spinal reflexes of micturition.

Acquisition of dryness tends to be gradual, and influenced both by maturation of the organism and the effect of its environment. Figure 11.2 provides a cross-sectional longitudinal comparison of day and night bladder control acquisition from 1 to 12 years of age (Oppel, Harper, & Rider, 1968). The data are presented here as the percentage of children who have achieved a totally dry state at each age. Children attain daytime control at much earlier ages than they achieve nighttime control. Inspection of Fig. 11.2 reveals that, by age 3, 84% of children are dry during the day, and 64% are dry at night. By age 12, the prevalence rates become 99% and 92% for daytime and nighttime, respec-

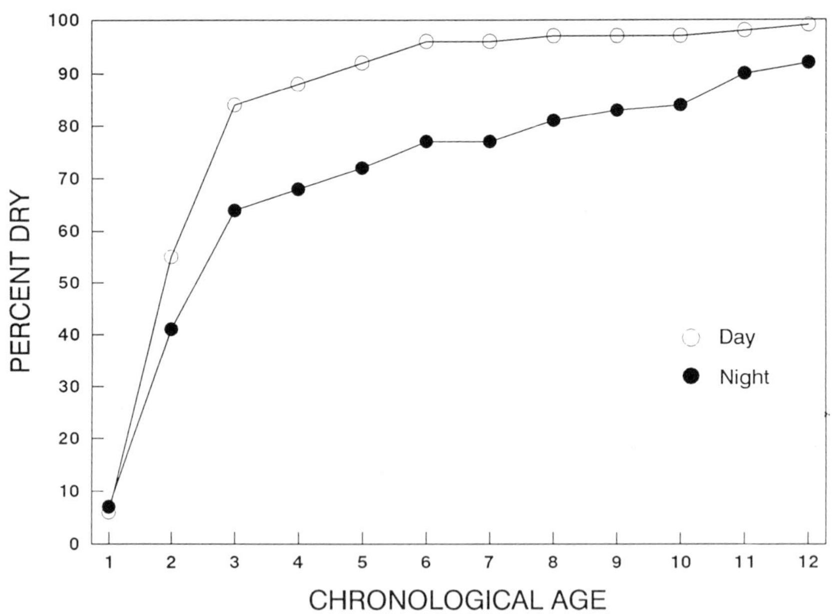

FIG. 11.2. Percentage of children, ages 1–12 years, who achieved bladder continence (defined as a frequency of less than once per month for at least 1 month) by day and night in a sample from Baltimore, Maryland, reported by Oppel et al. (1968).

tively. Although the data presented would suggest that over 20% of children have not achieved a totally dry state by 6 years of age, these prevalence rates are based on even one wet episode in a month period, a more rigorous frequency criterion than is presently in use.

Differential Diagnosis

In some children, enuresis may be a primary manifestation of a physical disorder. Representative conditions are presented in Table 11.2. Children occasionally have infections, malformations, or disease processes that may predispose them to this symptom.

Urinary tract infections are cited as a cause of enuresis, particularly when the enuresis is both diurnal and nocturnal (Behrman & Vaughn, 1987). Stansfeld (1973) found that between 5% and 10% of girls with bedwetting and 1% of boys had urinary tract infections. Wetting resolved, however, in less than 50% of these children when the infection was treated with antibiotics.

Anatomical malformations are found in less than 1% of children with enuresis (Forsythe & Redmond, 1974). Clinical indicators of malformation include an abnormal urinary stream, persistent dampness, or recurrent urinary tract infections. Abnormalities of the bones of the lumbar region of the spinal cord may also influence continence. Myelomeningocele and spina bifida occulta are among the disorders with difficulties in maintaining urinary continence due to abnormal development of neural control mechanisms (McLorie & Husmann, 1987).

Bedwetting may be one of the presenting symptoms of diseases such as diabetes and chronic renal failure that result in the formation of large amounts of urine (Meadow, 1987). Enuresis may also be associated with neurological disease. Seizure disorders, some of which tend to occur during sleep, may have presenting symptoms of loss of continence. Pituitary gland tumors or injuries may cause urine volumes to markedly increase by destruction of cells responsible for the production of antidiuretic hormone (ADH) (Behrman & Vaughn, 1987). Dysregulation of the pituitary function of antidiuresis could also affect the volume of urine formed (Birkasova, Birkas, Flynn, & Cort, 1978). Birkasova and colleagues found that some enuretics produce paradoxically large volumes of dilute urine at night and suggested that a physiological variation in the control of antidiuresis could be the cause. The role of abnormal neural control over urine volume formation remains uncertain and requires further investigation (Terho & Kekomaki, 1984).

Quite aside from these disease processes, there is evidence that functional differences may be responsible for the observed enuresis. For example, physiological differences in bladder function have been theorized to contribute to the symptom of enuresis. Several studies have found that enuretic children have smaller functional bladder capacities; that is, the children tend to report the need to void with smaller volumes of urine (Esperenca & Gerrard, 1969; Starfield, 1967). In a study conducted under general anesthesia, enuretic children have been found, however, to have total bladder capacities no different from those of nonenuretic children (Troup & Hodgson, 1971). The role of smaller functional bladders as a cause of enuresis awaits further study.

Some authors have found that sudden strong contractions of the bladder are more common in enuretic children, both during the day and the night (Mahony, Laferte, & Blais, 1981). The role of uninhibited contractions of the bladder, also called *detrusor instability,* in enuresis is uncertain, because many nonenuretic children also have these contractions (Koff & Murtagh, 1983). Response to anticholinergic medications, which should decrease uninhibited contractions, has had equivocal results.

Sleeping and arousal patterns have been studied in enuretic children. Evidence suggests that enuresis occurs randomly throughout sleep (Norgaard et al., 1989), and patterns of sleep are no different when enuretics are compared to age-matched control children (Inoue et al., 1987). Inoue found that electroencephalographic (EEG) patterns of rhythmic slow wave episodes preceded enuretic episodes; age-related decreases in this pattern compared to controls were slower to occur in enuretic children than control children, suggesting an immaturity of sleep patterns. There is no current consensus on whether the rate at which one changes from sleep to conscious alertness differs between enuretic children and nonenuretic children (Fielding & Doleys, 1988).

There is evidence that enuresis may have a familial basis (Bakwin, 1973). Studies of twins show that enuresis in one child places the twin at risk of developing the problem (Bakwin, 1971). These findings suggest a genetic predisposition, presumably determined by multiple genes, to be causal in this process. Theoretically, however, environmental determinants in settings where interactions around the symptom have occurred could wholly account for these findings. Most likely, both genetic and environmental factors are operative.

Type

The differentiation of type (primary or secondary) is dependent on the length of time that a child has sustained bladder control. One year represents an arbitrary, but significant, time period. The distinction presumably has importance for intervention (Fielding & Doleys, 1988).

The time of day in which the passage of urine occurs is an important distinction. Less than 10% of children with the symptom of enuresis will have daytime (diurnal) enuresis (Schmitt, 1984b). Evidence suggests that the mechanisms believed responsible for diurnal enuresis are different from those responsible for nocturnal enuresis. Diurnal wetting may be related to reflux of urine into the vagina, involuntary emptying of the bladder associated with laughter (giggle or stress incontinence), and uninhibited bladder contractions (Schmitt, 1982). Diurnal-nocturnal enuretics are more resistant to treatment, drop out of treatment more frequently, and exhibit greater behavioral deviance (Fielding, 1982). They are less likely to report familial nocturnal enuresis than nocturnal-only enuretics (Berg, 1979).

Reliability of Current Diagnostic Criteria

Pursuant to the development of DSM-III, extensive field trials were conducted to determine coefficients of agreement for the proposed diagnostic categories (Spitzer & Forman, 1979; Spitzer, Forman, & Lee, 1979). The results were reported separately for adults and youth (ages 18 years and younger). In each report, the data were grouped with the category Other Disorders With Physical Manifestations, in which functional encopresis and enuresis were only two possible diagnoses. For adults, the reported kappa was 1.00 for 0.6% of the sample of 331 patients ($N = 2$), as compared with an overall kappa of .72 across all categories. In contrast, a kappa of .48 for 5.5% of the 55 children and adolescents studied ($N = 3$) was reported, as compared with an overall kappa of .52. It is difficult to interpret these results because it is not possible to determine whether the disagreement evident among the child and youth data corresponded to the diagnoses of interest in this discussion. Similar analyses were not undertaken during the development of DSM-III-R. It remains an open question whether the current criteria for functional encopresis and enuresis would result in high rates of interobserver agreement among diagnosticians who have little experience with children and youth.

SELECTIVE REVIEW OF THE LITERATURE

Developmental Aspects of Elimination Behavior

A developmental gradient underlies the expression of the symptomatology of both functional enuresis and encopresis. As evidence of this biobehavioral phenomenon, the attainment of bowel and bladder control follows a predictable developmental sequence for most children. The sequence was determined from a short-term longitudinal study of 356 boys and 316 girls, ages 18 months to 54 months, attending day nurseries and 648 children, 54 boys and 54 girls at each age from $2\frac{1}{2}$ to 5 years in 6-month intervals, visited regularly by home health visitors. In both groups, the parents and/or nursery personnel kept home charts of soiling and wetting over at least 4 days and nights. Nocturnal bowel control was achieved first, followed by daytime bowel, daytime bladder, and finally nocturnal bladder control (Stein & Susser, 1967). The sequence was the same for boys and girls and was also evident among children whose overall rate of sphincter control was delayed relative to their same-age peers (Stein & Susser, 1967). Although the sequence is very stable within particular samples, Stein and Susser (1967) reported some differences between children raised in the United States and children from the United Kingdom, thus attesting to the malleability of early childhood through social and cultural factors. However, the biological limits as set by maturation of organs and the nervous system must be acknowledged.

Both disorders represent behaviors that are developmentally appropriate for a period of time. What distinguishes the pathology from the developmentally appropriate behavior is how long it persists beyond a particular developmental age. This boundary represents an age at which the majority of children have attained bowel and bladder control and have acquired the skills necessary to eliminate in socially appropriate ways.

Cross-sectional longitudinal data available at the time of the third revision of the *Diagnostic and Statistical Manual* indicated that most children achieve bowel control by the age of 4 and bladder control by 5 years of age (Bellman, 1966; Oppel et al., 1968; Stein & Susser, 1967). Acquisition data vary somewhat based on the criteria used to define control. Some reports are based on the age at which the child first demonstrated control, a fairly liberal index, whereas others report the age at which the child had control with no further relapse (accidents), a much more stringent criterion. Generally, the time between incontinent episodes (or frequency per month) is used as an index of the attainment of continence. As the time period between incontinent episodes approaches 1 year, there is general agreement that continence has been attained (APA, 1980). Although previous studies reported some difference among boys and girls in the ages at which control is achieved, the differences were minimized by the authors (Bellman, 1966; Oppel et al., 1968).

Therefore, a major factor in determining a diagnosis of functional encopresis or functional enuresis is the developmental and chronological age of the child. Against these limits are placed the frequency of encopretic or enuretic episodes each month. There has been little discussion of the age and frequency criteria for functional encopresis. In contrast, there has been some question about the age criterion for a diagnosis of functional enuresis. At present, a chronological age of 5 years and a mental age of at least 4 years represent a commonly agreed on point when bladder control, either diurnal or nocturnal, should be achieved (APA, 1980, 1987). Such limits place as many as 20% of children, depending on the particular epidemiological study and its defining criteria, potentially eligible for a diagnosis of functional enuresis (DeJonge, 1973). What is the rate of spontaneous "cure" among children who meet the criteria for a diagnosis of functional enuresis? In a long-term follow-up study of 1,129 children with enuresis who were not treated with an electric alarm, there was an annual spontaneous cure rate of 14% between 5 and 9 years, 16% between 10 and 14 years, and 16% between 15 and 19 years of age for children with primary nocturnal and diurnal enuresis (Forsythe & Redmond, 1974). Such data underscore the individual variability in the rate of development of bladder control, and that maturation alone may be as successful as some intervention approaches in bringing about cessation of nocturnal and diurnal enuresis.

Since the publication of DSM-III, there has been some consideration of the epidemiology of functional enuresis based on the age criterion. In an interesting study conducted by Verhulst and colleagues (1985), there were significant declines in the prevalence of bedwetting with increasing age and differential rates of decline between boys and girls. In particular, the girls' decline was four-and-a-half times faster than the boys (71% vs. 16%) over the period of 4 to 6 years of age. Previous epidemiological studies had not made much of the apparent gender differences (Bellman, 1966; Oppel et al., 1968). Verhulst and associates proposed that future DSM criteria should reflect gender as well as age considerations. Following from the data reported by Verhulst and associates, a diagnosis of functional enuresis would be made for girls age 5 and older and for boys age 8 and older.

Elimination Disorders: Mental, Behavioral, or Developmental?

With the advent of the multiaxial classification system in DSM-III, a distinction was made between clinical syndromes (Axis I) and specific developmental disorders (Axis II). The distinction has to do with providing a mechanism for describing aspects of the person's adaptation (Axis II) that have not been traditionally included in taxonomies of mental disorder. The case could be made that functional enuresis and functional encopresis are primarily developmental disorders and should be recorded on Axis II. One basis of this argument would be the individual differences apparent in the acquisition of continence reviewed earlier. Although there are many factors that may play a role in these individual differences, the influence of genetically programmed neuromaturation must be acknowledged, given its prepotent influence. At the same time, parents must develop the expectation that children will attain bowel and bladder continence if the potential made available by neuromaturational processes is to be realized. It would be tempting to assume that all parents would derive measurable relief from their children's attainment of independent elimination behavior, but the rate and skill with which parents develop their resolve to engage in training varies considerably from parent to parent. Given the need for two developmental processes to become manifest, one could make the case that the *primary types* of either disorder really represent developmental disorders and should therefore be recorded on Axis II. The rationale for such a change is reinforced when a developmental delay (relative to other children) in acquiring bowel or bladder continence (primary type) is contrasted with the situation in which a child has demonstrated continence for a 12-month period and then regresses. Acquisition of continence for a period of 1 year establishes that the developmental underpinnings, neuromaturation, and parental expectations have been achieved and that some pathological process, either physical and/or psychological in nature, has interrupted these developmental milestones. It follows then that the *secondary types* of both diagnoses represent acquired mental disorders and fit best with Axis I (Rapoport & Ismond, 1984).

The differentiation of functional encopresis into retentive and nonretentive subtypes has been considered previously (Walker, 1978) given the marked difference in the manifestation of the presenting problem. On the one hand, clinicians find themselves confronted with children who retain their feces to the point that impaction and megacolon may result, whereas on the other hand children excrete normal feces but place their excrement in inappropriate places.

Differentiating functional encopresis into retentive or nonretentive subtypes would also assist in discriminating between developmental and mental/behavioral components of disorder. Retentive encopresis typically has physiological components (e.g., composition of the diet, the rate of bowel motility and water intake) and behavioral components (e.g., parent–child interactional issues) (Fleischer, 1976; Houts, Mellon, & Whelan, 1988; Schmitt, 1984a). Moreover, fecal retention to the degree that impaction results is a highly abnormal state during childhood (Behrman & Vaughn, 1987). Despite a paucity of case-control literature supportive of a behavioral component of fecal retention, case report evidence supporting behavioral treatment is plentiful (Friman & Christophersen, 1986).

However, among nonretentive children, there is considerable difference between children who are incompletely toilet trained and those children who have achieved continence for significant periods of time (12 months) and then regress. Nonretentive encopretic children who do not have a physical disorder and who have had a preceding period of 1 year of fecal continence are likely to also meet the diagnostic criteria for some other Axis I disorder. In cases where children are incompletely toilet trained, a diagnosis on Axis II is appropriate. Although such considerations appear justified on a conceptual basis, there has been almost no empirical study of functional encopresis. It is hoped that such discussion will foster further investigation.

It is clear that a perfect classification system is elusive (Levine, 1982). Pediatricians often approach this disorder with dietary and cathartic interventions, information about toilet habits and training, and parental support designed to decrease anxiety, blaming, and coercion. This level of intervention is often sufficient to resolve the elimination disorder. Unknown is whether other problems arising from parental anxiety and coercion are also diminished or whether they tend to become manifest in other aspects of family interactions. Primary care providers should be trained in the identification of mental or behavioral components of elimination disorders, even in those that appear to respond solely to physiological interventions.

Proposed Changes in Diagnostic Criteria

Tables 11.3 and 11.4 present alternative classification criteria for functional encopresis and functional enuresis. For functional encopresis, these changes include a differentiation between retentive and nonretentive subtypes and rules for determining whether the disorder should be placed on Axis I or Axis II. The distinction between retentive and nonretentive subtypes requires that the child is withholding feces such that constipation, impaction, or megacolon is present. Such a determination would be readily achieved in consultation with the child's primary health provider. Cases meeting the criteria would be recorded on Axis I. Children presenting without evidence of retention or impaction would receive further consideration. A diagnosis would be made on Axis II if the child had never been completely toilet trained (primary)

TABLE 11.3
Proposed Diagnostic Criteria for Functional Encopresis

Retentive type—Axis I

A. Repeated passage of feces into places not appropriate for that purpose (e.g., clothing), whether involuntary or intentional in a child with evidence of fecal retention.
B. At least one such event a month for at least 6 months.
C. Chronologic and mental age, at least 4 years.
D. Not due to a physical disorder, such as aganglionic megacolon.

Nonretentive type (Primary-Axis II; Secondary-Axis I)

A. Repeated passage of feces into places inappropriate for that purpose without evidence of fecal retention.
B. At least one soiling event a month for at least 6 months.
C. Chronologic and mental age at least 4 years.
D. Primary type—the disturbance was not preceded by a period of fecal continence lasting at least 1 year (Axis II).
   Secondary type—the disturbance was preceded by a period of fecal continence lasting at least 1 year (Axis I).
E. Not due to a physical disorder, such as neurological abnormalities of the anal sphincter or chronic diarrhea due to infections or inflammatory causes.

and on Axis I if there was a regression following 1 year of continence (secondary).

For functional enuresis, the changes follow from the observed gender differences in the acquisition of urinary continence for boys (especially nocturnal type) and the discussion of classification on Axis I for secondary functional enuresis and Axis II for primary functional enuresis.

TABLE 11.4
Proposed Diagnostic Criteria for Functional Enuresis

A. Repeated voiding of urine during the day or night into bed or clothes, whether involuntary or intentional.
B. At least two such events per month for children between the ages of 5 and 6, and at least one event per month for older children.
C. Females: Chronological age at least 5, and mental age at least 4.
   Males: Chronologic age at least 8 and mental age at least 7.
D. Not due to a physical disorder, such as diabetes, urinary tract infection, or a seizure disorder.
E. Specify primary or secondary type.
   Axis I Primary type: The disturbance was not preceded by a period of urinary continence lasting at least 1 year.
   Axis II Secondary type: The disturbance was preceded by a period of urinary continence lasting at least 1 year.
F. Specify nocturnal only, diurnal only, or nocturnal and diurnal.

PROPOSED DIAGNOSTIC AND ASSESSMENT PROCEDURES

Given the similarity in the data required for a diagnosis of either functional encopresis or enuresis, a general model is presented with references made to particular aspects of the diagnoses. The general assessment scheme includes pediatric screening, developmental screening, clinical interviews, and behavioral record keeping.

Pediatric Screening

Presentation of symptoms suggestive of functional encopresis and enuresis should prompt assessment by the child's primary care physician. In cases where there is no primary medical care provider, referral can be made to a regional medical center that offers a pediatric service. The purpose of the physical examination is to determine whether there is an identifiable organic basis for the symptoms.

In encopresis, the next diagnostic decision, assuming physical conditions—as described earlier in this chapter—have been ruled out, is to determine whether or not rectal impaction is present (Schmitt, 1984a). Evidence of impaction is supported by a history of leakage of liquid fecal matter with occasional large, hard, painful bowel movements. Physical evidence corroborating impaction includes palpable fecal matter on abdominal examination, rectal distention with feces, and the presence of fecal matter on abdominal X ray.

Impacted feces should be treated to remove the impaction and insure that bowel movements become soft and formed in consistency (Levine, 1982). If retentive encopresis and enuresis are present in the same child, treatment of the fecal impaction should be the initial aim of medical intervention (Fielding & Doleys, 1988). A variety of methods of treating bowel impaction are available (Fitzgerald, 1987). Although some practitioners express hesitation in forcing children to take medicine for constipation or disimpaction (Fleisher, 1976), Fleisher advocates that the child should be told how laxatives will help the constipation and given control of when and how long laxatives will be administered.

Increases in water and dietary fiber may be helpful in treatment. Parents and children should be warned that until the stretched intestine (megacolon) is allowed time to resume its smaller size, laxatives may cause an increase in the number of soiling episodes (Fleisher, 1976).

In the evaluation of enuresis the primary health provider also must be principally concerned with diagnosing organic diseases causing the symptom of enuresis. The important possible organic diseases causing enuresis have been discussed earlier in this chapter. Children with organic etiologies, such as urinary tract infections, anomalies of the urinary tract, and diabetes should have appropriate treatment for the primary problem. On follow-up, the symptom of enuresis should be evaluated. Generally, in slightly less than half, the symptom will be resolved (Meadow, 1987). Persistence of what is thought to be organically medicated enuresis may indicate insufficient treatment, incorrect diagnosis, or confounding psychosocial facilitators that were present before or developed with the organic process. A synthetic peptide called DDAVP, which has similar biological effects as ADH in reducing the urine volume, has been empirically used and has demonstrated efficacy in the treatment of childhood enuresis (Terho & Kekomaki, 1984). The safety of DDAVP has been documented in a small number of patients over the age of 10 years when it is used over long periods of time (Rew & Rundle, 1989); however, reversal of nocturnal dryness after discontinuation of DDAVP is immediate (Terho & Kekomaki, 1984).

Children for whom an organic basis for enuresis is not established should be distinguished by the time pattern of the enuresis. Those with diurnal wetting, with or without nocturnal enuresis, may benefit from evaluation and treatment of uninhibited bladder contractions (Schmitt, 1984b). Schmitt stated these children present with histories of urgency incontinence; functionally strengthening the urethral sphincter by stream interruption exercises may help these children to develop continence by allowing them to effectively resist elevated bladder pressure.

Assessing whether the elimination symptom is primary or secondary, as described in Table 11.1, is important diagnostically only in as much as it indicates that the processes resulting in the symptom are more likely of recent onset. Primary or secondary elimination disorders may be either organic or nonorganic in their etiology. In secondary elimination disorders, the investigation is directed toward physical and mental conditions that are of recent onset; both psychosocial factors and undetected organic diseases should be considered. Primary elimination disorders suggest that neuromaturational factors are more likely to be operative, although primary disorders do not rule out psychosocial determinants.

Developmental Screening

Both diagnoses require that a child have a developmental level of at least 4 years. Gross delays in development may be readily apparent to the diagnostician, whereas milder degrees may be more difficult to discern without formal assessment. In either case, if delay is suspected, then a thorough evaluation is warranted to determine the child's developmental level. The developmental assessment of young children is a highly specialized process that requires considerable knowledge of child development, familiarity with a variety of assessment instruments, and sophistication in child behavior management (Stagg, 1988). Individual clinicians will have to judge for themselves whether they have sufficient competence to carry out such an evaluation. Referral to a developmental evaluation center may be both prudent and advisable in many instances. Should developmental delay be detected as a result of these efforts, the evaluation would also provide data necessary for a referral for early intervention.

Clinical Interview

Most practitioners advocate for clinical interviews of the immediate caregivers (parents and daycare providers) as well as the child. Doleys (1981) proposed that the interview consist of a history and description of the problem, family and medical history, assessment of other problems, assessment of home and family environment, and a review of previous intervention attempts. For the purposes of establishing a diagnosis, the interview should reveal the degree to which bowel or bladder control has been achieved and show that the child does not manifest some other form of psychological disturbance. In consideration of this latter possibility, the interview may be supplemented with a formal psychological assessment using a variety of objective and projective methods.

Diagnosticians must rely on the parent's recall in determining the longest period of continence. Although there are always concerns about bias and error in such recall, the 12-month period necessary for a diagnosis of the secondary type for each disorder would facilitate recall. In cases meeting the requirements for secondary type, assessment should include some consideration of the events that may have contributed to the observed regression.

Some authors suggest that the parent interview also include a thorough description of the antecedent and consequent events, previous attempts to intervene, the parents' tolerance for the elimination disorder, the parents' attitude toward the problem, and the like (Fielding & Doleys, 1988). Although such information does assist intervention planning, these data are not necessary for the diagnosis.

Behavioral Record Keeping

Parents or caregivers should be asked to provide a diary of toileting accidents. Such information is generally recorded on a form provided by the diagnostician. The forms are usually tailored to either functional

EVENING	CHILD'S BEDTIME	TIME OF EVENING CHECK (IMMEDIATELY BEFORE YOUR BEDTIME)	WAS THE BED WET (PUT 'W') OR DRY (PUT 'D')	SIZE OF WET PATCH PUT 'S' for small (0-10cm) 'M' for medium (10-20cm) 'L' for large (more than 20 cm)	MORNING	TIME OF MORNING CHECK (WHEN CHILD WAKES)	WAS THE BED WET (PUT 'W') OR DRY (PUT 'D')	SIZE OF WET PATCH PUT 'S' for small (0-10cm) 'M' for medium (10-20cm) 'L' for large (more than 20 cm)	DID THE CHILD WAKE TO USE THE TOILET BY HIM/HERSELF DURING THE NIGHT	ANY COMMENTS
Example	7.30pm	11.15pm	D			6.30am	W	L	YES AT 11.30pm	Away from home at Grandma's
SATURDAY					SUNDAY					
SUNDAY					MONDAY					
MONDAY					TUESDAY					
TUESDAY					WEDNESDAY					
WEDNESDAY					THURSDAY					
THURSDAY					FRIDAY					
FRIDAY					SATURDAY					

FIG. 11.3. Representative pretreatment assessment chart for nocturnal enuresis, reprinted from Fielding and Doleys (1988).

encopresis or enuresis, given the inherent differences in the disorders. For functional encopresis, the record form usually reports whether the child had a bowel movement in the toilet on a given day (Christopherson & Rainey, 1976). The record form for functional enuresis has been substantially more elaborate. For example, a sample record sheet taken from Fielding and Doleys (1988) is presented in Fig. 11.3. The diary has a column for the day of the week, time that wetting or soiling was first noted, whether the children awakened to use the toilet by themselves during the night, and any extenuating circumstances that may have occurred. The frequency and pattern of these accidents can then be determined. Such data yield important diagnostic information and also represent a baseline from which to judge the efficacy of later intervention. These records are completed by an informant, usually the child's parents, and are returned weekly.

With regard to functional enuresis, some investigators propose that parents measure the size of the wet spot (Fielding & Doleys, 1988). Such data may be extremely useful in determining the outcome of an intervention, but this information is not necessary to make a diagnosis. For DSM-III-R, voiding is voiding, no matter how much.

SUMMARY AND FUTURE DIRECTIONS

Acquisition of control of eliminatory functions requires the confluence of biological and social factors. Without the necessary integrity and maturity of the physiological underpinnings, there is little chance of attaining full control. Likewise, without a nurturant, supportive environment, the need to attain control is not present. The interplay of biological and environmental factors represents a complex biobehavioral phenomenon where change over time, from incontinence to continence, represents growth, adaptation, and maturity. The continued presence of the behavior, or some change in intensity or frequency, beyond a period of time when they are considered typical or normal has been defined as psychological disorder.

There is little disagreement with the current criteria for the diagnosis of functional enuresis. The most salient question was raised by Verhulst and colleagues (1985) with regard to the influence of gender on the acquisition of nocturnal bladder control. Should we have the same developmental criteria for a diagnosis of functional enuresis for boys as for girls? Given the data presented by Verhulst and colleagues and our knowledge that maturity proceeds more quickly in girls than in boys, it seems reasonable to alter the diagnostic criteria in this regard.

A further consideration follows from the inclusion of functional enuresis and functional encopresis on Axis I (Clinical Disorders) in the current DSM (APA, 1987). We have questioned the logic behind this listing and agree with Rapoport and Ismond (1984) that a strong case could be made for the transfer of these disorders to Axis II, considering their developmental underpinnings. In recommending changes in the diagnoses of functional encopresis and functional enuresis, we have proposed that the primary types of each disorder should be recorded on Axis II, whereas cases of regression following a 12-month period of demonstrated continence represent Axis I disorders.

With regard to functional encopresis, we have proposed a differentiation between retentive and nonretentive types. This distinction is based primarily on the extent to which the presenting problem involves constipation and/or impaction. We have argued that such a distinction is warranted because of the fundamental difference in the nature of the problem, the likelihood that dietary factors play a role in fecal retention, and that the subtypes would suggest different treatment approaches. Further research will be helpful in determining whether there are other aspects of the DSM-III-R criteria that warrant modification.

ACKNOWLEDGMENTS

Preparation of this chapter was supported by an institutional training grant award from the National Institute of Child Health and Human Development (HD 07285).

REFERENCES

American Psychiatric Association. (1952). *Diagnostic and statistical manual of mental disorders*. Washington, DC: Author.

American Psychiatric Association. (1968). *Diagnostic and statistical manual of mental disorders* (2nd ed.). Washington, DC: Author.

American Psychiatric Association. (1980). *Diagnostic and statistical manual of mental disorders* (3rd ed.). Washington, DC: Author.

American Psychiatric Association. (1987). *Diagnostic and statistical manual of mental disorders* (3rd ed., rev.). Washington, DC: Author.

Anthony, E. G. (1957). An experimental approach to the psychopathology of childhood encopresis. *British Journal of Medical Psychology, 30*, 146–175.

Bakwin, H. (1971). Enuresis in twins. *American Journal of Diseases of Children, 121*, 222–225.

Bakwin, H. (1973). The genetics of enuresis. In I. Kolvin, R. C. MacKeith, & S. R. Meadow, (Eds.), *Bladder control and enuresis* (pp. 73–77). London: W. Heinemann Medical Books.

Behrman, R. E., & Vaughn, V. C. (1987). *Nelson textbook of pediatrics* (13th ed.). Philadelphia: Saunders.

Bellman, M. (1966). Studies on encopresis. *Acta Paediatrica Scandinavica, 170*(Suppl), 1–151.

Berg, I. B. (1979). Day wetting in children. *Journal of Child Psychology and Psychiatry, 20*, 167–173.

Berg, I. B., & Jones, K. V. (1964). Functional fecal incontinence in children. *Archives of Disease in Childhood, 39*, 465–472.

Birkasova, M., Birkas, D., Flynn, M. J., & Cort, J. H. (1978). Desmopressin in the management of nocturnal enuresis in children: A double-blind study. *Pediatrics, 62*, 970–974.

Brayden, R. M., & Altemeier, W. A. (1989). Encopresis and child sexual abuse. *Journal American Medical Association, 262*, 2446.

Christophersen, E. R., & Rainey, S. K. (1976). Management of encopresis through a pediatric outpatient clinic. *Journal of Pediatric Psychology, 1*, 38–41.

Christophersen, E. R., & Rapoff, M. A. (1983). Toileting problems of children. In C. E. Walker & M. C. Roberts (Eds.), *Handbook of clinical child psychology* (pp. 593–615). New York: Wiley.

Doleys, D. M. (1978). Assessment and treatment of enuresis and encopresis in children. In M. Hersen, R. Eisler, & P. Miller (Eds.), *Progress in behavior modification* (Vol. 6, pp. 85–123). New York: Academic Press.

Doleys, D. M. (1981). Elimination problems: Enuresis and encopresis. In E. J. Mash & L. G. Terdal (Eds.), *Behavioral assessment of childhood disorders* (pp. 679–710). New York: Guilford Press.

Doleys, D. M. (1989). Functional enuresis and encopresis. In C. G. Last & M. Hersen (Eds.), *Handbook of child psychiatric diagnosis* (pp. 427–442). New York: Wiley.

DeJonge, G. A. (1973). Epidemiology of enuresis: A survey of the literature. In I. Kolvin, R. C. MacKeith, & S. R. Meadow (Eds.), *Bladder control and enuresis:* No. 48/49. Clinics in developmental medicine (pp. 39–47). Philadelphia: Lippincott.

Esperenca, M., & Gerrard, J. W. (1969). Nocturnal enuresis: Studies in bladder function in normal children and enuretics. *Canadian Medical Association Journal, 101*, 324–327.

Fielding, D. M. (1982). An analysis of the behaviour of day and night wetting children: Towards a model of micturition control. *Behaviour Research and Therapy, 20*, 49–60.

Fielding, D. M., & Doleys, D. M. (1988). Elimination problems: Enuresis and encopresis. In E. J. Mash & L. G. Terdal (Eds.), *Behavioral assessment of childhood disorders*, (2nd ed., pp. 586–623). New York: Guilford Press.

Fitzgerald, J. F. (1987). Constipation in children. *Pediatrics in Review, 8*, 299–302.

Fleisher, D. R. (1976). Diagnosis and treatment of disorders of defecation in children. *Pediatric Annals, 5*, 700–722.

Forsythe, W. I., & Redmond, A. (1974). Enuresis and spontaneous cure rate: Study of 1129 enuretics. *Archives of Disease in Childhood, 49*, 259–263.

Foxman, B., Valdez, R. B., & Brook, R. H. (1986). Childhood enuresis: Prevalence, perceived impact, and prescribed treatments. *Pediatrics, 77*, 482–487.

Friman, P. C., & Christophersen, E. R. (1986). Biobehavioral prevention in primary care. In N. A. Krasnegor, J. D. Arasteh, & M. F. Cataldo (Eds.), *Child health behavior: A behavioral pediatrics perspective* (pp. 254–280). New York: Wiley.

Friman, P. C., Mathews, J. R., Finney, J. W., Christophersen, E. R., & Leibowitz, J.

M. (1988). Do encopretic children have clinically significant behavior problems? *Pediatrics, 82*, 407–409.

Gabel, S., Chandra, R., & Shindledecker, R. (1988). Behavior ratings and outcome of medical treatment for encopresis. *Journal of Developmental and Behavioral Pediatrics, 9*, 129–133.

Gavanski, M. (1971). Treatment of non-retentive secondary encopresis with imipramine and psychotherapy. *Canadian Medical Association Journal, 104*, 227–231.

Goellner, M. H., Ziegler, E. E., & Fomon, S. J. (1981). Urination during the first three years of life. *Nephron, 28*, 174–178.

Houts, A. C., Mellon, M. W., & Whelan, J. P. (1988). Use of dietary fiber and stimulus control to treat retentive encopresis: A multiple baseline investigation. *Journal of Pediatric Psychology, 13*, 435–445.

Inoue, M., Shimojima, H., Chiba, H., Tsukahara, N., Tajika, Y., & Taka, K. (1987). Rhythmic slow wave observed on nocturnal sleep encephalogram in children with idiopathic nocturnal enuresis. *Sleep, 10*, 570–579.

Koff, S. A. (1983). Estimating bladder capacity in children. *Urology, 21*, 248.

Koff, S. A., & Murtagh, D. S. (1983). The uninhibited bladder in children: Effect of treatment on recurrence of urinary infection and on vesicoureteral reflux resolution. *Journal of Urology, 130*, 1138–1141.

Levine, M. D. (1975). Children with encopresis: A descriptive analysis. *Pediatrics, 56*, 412–416.

Levine, M. D. (1982). Encopresis: Its potentiation, evaluation, and treatment. *Pediatric Clinics of North America, 29*, 315–330.

Loening-Baucke, V., Cruikshank, B., & Savage, C. (1987). Defecation dynamics and behavior profiles in encopretic children. *Pediatrics, 80*, 672–679.

MacKeith, R., Meadow, S. R., & Turner, R. K. (1973). How children become dry. In I. Kolvin, R. C. MacKeith, & S. R. Meadow (Eds.), *Bladder control and enuresis:* No. 48/49. Clinics in developmental medicine (pp. 3–21). Philadelphia: Lippincott.

Mahony, D. T., Laferte, R. O., & Blais, D. J. (1981). Studies on enuresis. IX. Evidence of a mild form of compensated detrusor hyperreflexia in enuretic children. *Journal of Urology, 126*, 520–523.

McLorie, G. A., & Husmann, D. A. (1987). Incontinence and enuresis. *Pediatric Clinics of North America 34*(5), 1159–1174.

Meadow, S. R. (1987). Enuresis. In M. A. Holliday, T. M. Barratt, & R. L. Vernier (Eds.), *Pediatric nephrology* (2nd ed., pp. 696–699). Baltimore: Williams & Wilkins.

Norgaard, J. P., Hansen, J. H., Wildschiotz, G., Sorensen, S, Rittig, S., & Djurhuus, J. C. (1989). Sleep cystometries in children with nocturnal enuresis. *Journal of Urology, 141*, 1156–1159.

Oppel, W. C., Harper, P. A., & Rider, R. V. (1968). The age of attaining bladder control. *Pediatrics, 42*, 614–626.

Rapoport, J. L., & Ismond, D. R. (1984). DSM-III *training guide for diagnosis of childhood disorders*. New York: Brunner/Mazel.

Rappaport, L. A., & Levine, M. D. (1986). The prevention of constipation and encopresis: A developmental model and approach. *Pediatric Clinics of North America, 33*, 859–869.

Read, N. W., & Timms, J. M. (1986). Defecation and the pathophysiology of constipation. *Clinical Gastroenterology, 15*, 937–965.

Rew, D. A., & Rundle, J. S. (1989). Assessment of the safety of regular DDAVP therapy in primary nocturnal enuresis. *British Journal of Urology, 63*, 352–353.

Roy, C. C., Silverman, A., & Cozzetto, F. J. (1975). Constipation, fecal incontinence and proctologic conditions. In *Pediatric clinical gastroenterology* (2nd ed., pp. 320–341). St. Louis: Mosby.

Schmitt, B. D. (1982). Daytime wetting (diurnal enuresis). *Pediatric Clinics of North America, 29,* 9–20.

Schmitt, B. D. (1984a). Encopresis or soiling. In S. Berman (Ed.), *Pediatric decision making* (pp. 196–197). Philadelphia: B. C. Decker.

Schmitt, B. D. (1984b). Enuresis. In S. Berman (Ed.), *Pediatric decision making* (pp. 198–199). Philadelphia: B. C. Decker.

Spitzer, R. L., Forman, J. B. W., & Lee, J. (1979). DSM-III field trials: I. Initial interrater diagnostic reliability. *American Journal of Psychiatry, 136,* 815–817.

Spitzer, R. L., & Forman, J. B. W. (1979). DSM-III field trials: II. Initial experience with the multi axial system. *American Journal of Psychiatry, 136,* 818–820.

Stagg, V. (1988). Clinical considerations in the assessment of young handicapped children. In T. D. Wachs & R. Sheehan (Eds.), *Assessment of young developmentally disabled children* (pp. 61–73). New York: Plenum.

Stansfeld, J. M. (1973). Enuresis and urinary tract infection. In I. Kolvin, R. C. MacKeith, & S. R. Meadow (Eds.), *Bladder control and enuresis:* No. 48/49. Clinics in developmental medicine (p. 102). Philadelphia: Lippincott.

Starfield, B. (1967). Functional bladder capacity in enuretic and non-enuretic children. *Journal of Pediatrics, 70,* 777–781.

Stein, Z., & Susser, M. (1967). Social factors in the development of sphincter control. *Developmental Medicine and Child Neurology, 9,* 692–706.

Terho, P., & Kekomaki, M. (1984). Management of nocturnal enuresis with a vasopressin analogue. *Journal of Urology, 131,* 925–927.

Troup, C. W., & Hodgson, N. B. (1971). Nocturnal functional bladder capacity in enuretic children. *Journal of Urology, 105,* 129–132.

Verhulst, F. C., van der Lee, J. H., Akkerhuis, G. W., Sanders-Woudstra, J. A. R., Timmer, F. C., & Donkhorst, I. D. (1985). The prevalence of nocturnal enuresis: Do DSM-III criteria need to be changed? A brief research report. *Journal of Child Psychology and Psychiatry, 26,* 989–993.

Walker, C. E. (1978). Toilet training, enuresis, and encopresis. In P. Magrab (Ed.), *Psychological management of pediatric problems* (Vol. 1, pp. 129–189). Baltimore: University Park Press.

Weaver, L. T., & Steiner, H. (1984). The bowel habit of young children. *Archives of Disease in Childhood, 59,* 649–652.

Wrenn, K. (1989). Fecal impaction. *New England Journal of Medicine, 321,* 658–662.

CHAPTER 12

Elective Mutism

Stephen R. Hooper
University of North Carolina School of Medicine

Thomas D. Linz
Marshall University School of Medicine

Mutism is the inability or the unwillingness to speak. Although communicative intent may be present, the individual typically is devoid of any vocal utterances. Given this basic premise, there would appear to be several different kinds of mutism in children. One form of mutism might be mediated by neurological or biological factors, such as the mutism seen in children with profound hearing loss and deafness, profound mental retardation, and severe neuromuscular involvement. Another form of mutism involves more psychologically based factors in which the child refuses to speak, despite being quite capable of verbalizations. Although this form of mutism includes hysterical forms of mutism, which theoretically might arise from a traumatic emotional experience, these cases in children and adolescents tend to be extremely rare and directly tied to a specific traumatic event (Kolvin & Fundudis, 1981). Another type of mutism with a psychological basis is elective mutism. Children who are electively mute are typically quite capable of verbalizing, but they choose to talk only in circumscribed situations and/or with particular individuals.

In contrast to most of the other psychiatric diagnoses available to practitioners, the diagnosis of elective mutism has existed for many years without significant questioning, scrutiny, or debate. Consequently, the diagnostic criteria and assessment strategies have not changed radically over the last century. This chapter addresses this need to review and critique the available literature pertaining to elective mutism. A particular emphasis is directed toward examining the specific criteria used to diagnose this disorder in children and adolescents. Suggestions for future directions are offered.

DEFINITIONAL ISSUES

Stories describing individuals with elective mutism go back 1,500 years (Goll, 1979). However, Tramer (1934) typically is credited with coining the term *elective mutism*. According to Tramer's study of several cases, elective mutism referred to a group of verbally intact children who exhibited no speech in selected situations, but who would talk relatively normally to certain peers and family members. Although the child typically is mute in the school setting, there have been reports of children who were mute primarily in the home setting (Wilkins, 1985). Prior to Tramer, many other investigators had described a similar syndrome in children. Probably the first investigator to describe such a clinical phenomenon was Kussmaul (1877) who, in describing three cases, used the term *aphasia voluntaria* to refer to persons who forced themselves into mutism for purposes they refused to disclose. Since that time, a variety of other terms have been used to describe this behavioral presentation. These terms include *speech inhibition* (Truper, 1897), *speech shyness* (Nadoleczng, 1926; Rothe, 1928; Spieler, 1941), *thymogenic mutism* (Waterink & Vedder, 1936), *functional mutism* (Amman, 1958), *speech phobia* (Mora, DeVault, & Schopler, 1962), *learned mutism* (Reed, 1963), *speech avoidance* (Lerea & Ward, 1965), and *selective mutism* (Hesselman, 1983; Kass, Gillman, Mattis, Klugman, & Jacobson, 1967; Williamson, Sewell, Sanders, Haney, & White, 1977).

Although the operational criteria used by these various investigators have varied to a great degree (e.g., low frequency vs. zero frequency speech; elective vs. progressive mutism), and although the debate over these operational criteria continues without clear resolution (e.g., Labbe & Williamson, 1984; Paniagua & Saeed, 1988; Piersel & Kratochwill, 1981), it is clear that children showing such behavioral patterns do represent an interesting and distinct psychiatric phenomenon. Despite the apparent clarity of this phenomenon, only within the last 10 to 15 years have psychiatric nosologies established a separate diagnostic category for elective mutism.

The World Health Organization (WHO) was perhaps the first professional group to include elective mutism into its classification of mental disorders. The ninth revision of the *International Classification of Diseases* (ICD-9; WHO, 1978) and its clinical modification for the United States (ICD-9-CM; Commission on Professional and Hospital Activities, 1978) were the first classification systems to include elective mutism as a separate diagnostic category. Specifically, these classifications included the diagnosis of elective mutism as one of several disorders of "sensitivity, shyness, and social withdrawal," which was included under the broader clinical domain of Disturbance of Emotions Specific to Childhood and Adolescence. Elective mutism was to be distinguished from similar behaviors that were secondary to an adjustment reaction and from developmental speech and language disorders.

At about the time that the ICD-9 and the ICD-9-CM were published, the *Diagnostic and Statistical Manual of Mental Disorders* was undergoing its third revision (DSM-III, American Psychiatric Association, 1980). Similar to the ICD, the DSM-I (American Psychiatric Association, 1952) and DSM-II (American Psychiatric Association, 1968) did not include a separate diagnostic category for elective mutism, but the DSM-III did. Specifically, the DSM-III included this diagnosis as a separate diagnostic entity under the general category of other disorders of infancy, childhood, or adolescence. The DSM-III stated that the primary feature of this disorder was the "continuous refusal to speak in almost all social situations, including at school, despite ability to comprehend spoken language and to speak. These children may communicate via gestures, by nodding or shaking the head, or, in some cases, by monosyllabic or short, monotone utterances" (American Psychiatric Association, 1980, p. 62). Although the DSM-III acknowledged that some of these children could present with speech and language delays, it noted that these children typically exhibited normal development in these domains. A variety of associated features were also reported: excessive shyness, social isolation, social withdrawal, clinging, school refusal, functional encopresis and enuresis, compulsive traits, negativism, and temper tantrums. Specifically, the three diagnostic criteria included: "(a) continuous refusal to talk in almost all social situations, including at school; (b) ability to comprehend spoken language and to speak; and (c) not due to another mental or physical disorder" (American Psychiatric Association, 1980, p. 63).

Although the revision of the DSM-III was largely unchanged in terms of its description of elective mutism and its associated features, the DSM-III-R (American Psychiatric Association, 1987) did make two rather significant modifications to this diagnostic category. First, the

DSM-III-R modified the essential diagnostic feature by stating the need for "persistent refusal to talk in one or more major social situations" (American Psychiatric Association, 1987, p. 88) as opposed to "nearly all social situations" as described in DSM-III. In addition, DSM-III-R removed the DSM-III criterion of "not due to another mental or physical disorder," perhaps in an effort to acknowledge the comorbidity of other associated disorders that may mediate or actually cause elective mutism. This latter modification, however, increases the range of conditions that could be contributing to the mutism and indirectly underscores the need for a thorough diagnostic evaluation. Currently, the DSM-III-R diagnostic criteria include: (a) persistent refusal to talk in one or more major social situations (including at school); and (b) ability to comprehend spoken language and to speak (American Psychiatric Association, 1987, p. 89). It is unclear, however, what data contributed to these changes in criteria. It is clear from the behavioral literature, however, that exact definitional criteria for elective mutism may have direct linkages to particular treatment strategies (Kratochwill, Brody, & Piersel, 1979; Labbe & Williamson, 1984), and the specificity of these definitional criteria need to be detailed further. In addition, the DSM-III-R continues to view elective mutism as a separate and distinct disorder of childhood and adolescence, whereas the ICD-9 has conceptualized it as one kind of disturbance under a broader clinical domain.

As can be seen, there are several areas of debate surrounding the diagnosis of elective mutism. Is it one manifestation of a broader group of emotional disorders, or is it a separate and distinct form of emotional disturbance? How much or how little speech is required for a diagnosis of elective mutism? With respect to this latter question, some investigators have stated that the diagnosis of elective mutism should be reserved only for children and adolescents showing *zero* speech in selected situations (Kratochwill et al., 1979), and it should not be confused with reluctant speech (Blake & Moss, 1967). Other investigators (e.g., Williamson et al., 1977), given the relative rarity of this disorder, have advocated that reluctant speech and elective mutism are the same diagnostic entity in an attempt to extend the boundaries of this disorder for scientific study. Furthermore, some investigators have suggested that it should be important to distinguish between "pure" elective mutism and that which might arise as a behavioral manifestation secondary to other problems, such as hysteria, schizophrenia (Laybourne, 1979; Tramer, 1934), or speech difficulties (Rutter, 1977). These definitional issues have contributed to the paucity of the research on elective mutism.

SELECTED REVIEW OF THE LITERATURE

Since Kussmaul (1877) first described this disorder over 100 years ago, there has been ongoing interest, with this phenomenon being described cross-culturally (i.e., in Germany, Great Britain, Switzerland, the United States) and relatively consistently over the years (e.g., Adams & Glasner, 1954; Tramer, 1934; Weber, 1950). In general, two global trends appear in this literature. One trend has been largely descriptive and has attempted to define selected features of elective mutism. The other has been directed toward detailing specific intervention plans for children with elective mutism. Taken together, these trends have contributed to a long-standing history of research on elective mutism; however, nearly all of the literature to the present has employed case study methodology in presenting elements of this disorder. Although many of the case presentations are wonderfully rich in detail, with more recent cases attempting to speculate about etiological factors (e.g., Goll, 1979), the problems with the case study approach are widely known (e.g., idiosyncratic methods of assessment; difficulty with generalization of findings) and likely have slowed our scientific understanding of this disorder. Nonetheless, several reviews of this topic have been undertaken (Rutter, 1977; von Misch, 1952), although most have been devoted to reviewing the treatment literature with respect to elective mutism (Cunningham, Cataldo, Mallion, & Keyes, 1983; Kratochwill, 1981; Kratochwill et al., 1979; Labbe & Williamson, 1984). The literary summary of Hesselman (1983) likely provides the most extensive review of this topic available to date.

This section provides a selective review of the past and present literature with respect to elective mutism. A description of this disorder is provided by discussing the important aspects of any diagnostic entity. These include the topography of the disorder, epidemiology, etiological issues, prognosis, and response to treatment. Given the relatively rare prevalence of this disorder and the subsequent dependence on case study methodology, a review of the cases published in the literature since 1980 is presented in Table 12.1. This time period was selected for two reasons. First, it provides a minimal overlap between the relatively thorough review by Hesselman (1983), which included cases published in the literature through 1981. Second, it roughly coincides with the inclusion of the formal diagnosis of elective mutism into the ICD-9 and DSM-III, and this contributed to more consistency in the types of cases described across studies. The cases listed in Table 12.1 are not only important from a descriptive perspective, but they also

TABLE 12.1
Case Studies of Elective Mutism in Children and Adolescents (1980–1989)

Study	*N*	*Subject Description*	*Diagnostic Procedures*	*Findings*
Lipton (1980)	1	6-year-old White female; older of two children; kindergarten	Case history from home and school; school observations	No speech for 2 years in the school setting except for occasional laughter; did not talk to friends or relatives; normal speech reported in immediate family; above-average intelligence
Heimlich (1981)	1	9-year-old female	Child interview; undefined case history	Shallow affect; looked depressed; answered questions by whispering or nodding her head; talked freely to family; communicated with teacher and students via toy telephone
Hesse (1981)	1	4-year-old female; special education kindergarten	Teacher observations; undefined case history; ruled-out organic causes, autism, and psychosis	Disturbances in her interpersonal relationships; did not speak at all; deemed a refusal to communication rather than an inability to relate; normal voice functions

Croghan & Craven (1982)	1	8-year-old-female; third grade	Case history from home and school; standardized group achievement scores	Speech reluctance noted at age 2 years coinciding with birth of brother; speech declined and by age 4 years would only speak to her family; did not speak to anyone at school; above-average school achievement
Kupietz & Schwartz (1982)	3	4-year-old White male; oldest of three children; nursery school	Case history from home and school; pediatric neurodevelopmental assessment and Draw-A-Person at age 5	Spoke to mother at home, but not at school; never spoke at school and virtually to nobody outside the home; shy; timid; adjusted poorly to new surroundings; impulsive, overactive, distractible, and disobedient at home; inhibited behavior with limited participation at school
		14-year, 10-month-old White male; oldest of 4 children; school for emotionally disturbed	Case history from home and school; physical exam; neurological exam; Bender; Leiter International Performance Scale	Spoke freely at home, although speech was described by parents as high-pitched and immature; responded to teachers via gestures; early behavior was noncommunicative and withdrawn; shy and insecure as young child; IQ = 52; visual-motor delays; mild tremor; walked with limp

(continued)

TABLE 12.1
(continued)

Study	*N*	*Subject Description*	*Diagnostic Procedures*	*Findings*
		9 year, 5-month-old White male; learning adjustment class	Case history from home and school; physical exam; skull series; CAT scan; electrocardiogram	Related well to siblings; mother described him as sensitive, quiet, and afraid of failure; did not speak to family members until age 4 years; no school participation; taunted by peers to which he responded with aggression; bilateral enlargement of posterior ventricles (L>R); hypotonia
Morin, Ladouceur, & Cloutier (1982)	1	6-year-old male; middle to low SES; fifth of 6 children; kindergarten	Case history from school	Isolated rural family with few social contacts; spoke fluently at home; no verbalizations and minimal eye contact with strangers; refused to speak to teachers or peers; rarely participated in school activities, but performed in-class projects at home
Subak, West, & Carlin (1982)	1	15-year-old female	Interview attempted with child; case history from family; school information; prior medical history	Refusal to leave house; school absenteeism; responded nonverbally to questions; previous hospital admission revealed a silent

					withdrawn person who refused to eat with others or participate in activities; no in-class participation; did not talk to students or teachers; described as manipulative with monosyllabic speech and temper tantrums at home; mother was chronically depressed, fearful, and mistrustful; overprotective of children; minimal family interactions by father
Cunningham, Cataldo, Mallion, & Keyes (1983)	2	$3\frac{1}{2}$-year-old male		Case history from home and school; direct observations	Delays in expressive langauge development; normal comprehension and nonverbal abilities; spoke freely at home and to his mother outside the home; if someone entered the room, his speech would lessen as person came closer; did not speak to peers, relatives, friends of family, or strangers; experienced early hospitalizations; both parents described themselves as shy and socially inactive; paternal history of refusing to speak to strangers until age 4–5

(continued)

TABLE 12.1
(continued)

Study	*N*	*Subject Description*	*Diagnostic Procedures*	*Findings*
		15-year-old male; low SES; sixth grade	Case history from home and school; cognitive and achievement information	Spoke comfortably to family members; refusal to speak at age 5 with school entry; communicated to teachers and students via gestures or writing; IQ = Borderline to Mildly Retarded; academic performance at third to fourth grade level
Lazarus, Gavilo, & Moore (1983)	2	6-year-old female; oldest of six children; repeating kindergarten	Classroom observations; nonverbal assessment, including Leiter International Performance Scale, Bender, VMI, PPVT, and Draw-A-Person	Verbal at home, but no communication with teachers and peers; poor school attendance; bed wetting, thumb sucking, noncompliance, and stubborn; results of nonverbal assessment not reported
		7-year-old female; parents divorced	Psychological evaluation (tasks not specified); undefined case history	Did not speak to teachers and spoke infrequently to classmates; history of mutism since age 3 when she started preschool; poor peer relations, need for control, and overdependence on mother

Sluzki (1983)	2	9-year-old female; only child; Mexican-American family; bilingual; reconstituted family	Case history from school and family; family interview	Progressively ceased talking at school over 6 to 8 months; she spoke English primarily at home, although a mixture of Spanish and English was spoken; decrease in verbal output also seen at home, with mother using dolls/puppets to prompt speech
		9-year-old female; both parents were Salvadorian; youngest of three children	Case history from school and family; family interview	Did not speak at school, but spoke at home; written school work was satisfactory; primary language at home was Spanish, but mother and daughter would speak English; parents denied problem
Bozigar & Hansen (1984)	4	Undifferentiated sample of females, ages 6 to 9 years; three Hispanic, one Black; three were receiving speech therapy	Psychoeducational evaluations (tasks not specified); physical exams; undefined case history	None had spoken in school despite normal developmental milestones for speech; in 2 of 3 Hispanic families the parents were monolingual for Spanish; children speaking normally in home; the youngest child experienced a neck laceration at 26 months of age that required hospitalization

(*continued*)

TABLE 12.1
(continued)

Study	*N*	*Subject Description*	*Diagnostic Procedures*	*Findings*
Elder, Bleich, Apter, & Tyano (1985)	1	16-year-old female of Bulgarian-Jewish descent; high SES; oldest of three sisters	Undefined case history; EEG; CT scan; behavioral observation	Refused to speak on entrance to kindergarten, although spoke at home in age-appropriate manner; shy and experienced difficulty making friends; enuretic until age 12; manifested schizophrenic symptoms at approximately age 14; EEG showed nonspecific abnormalities; normal CT scan
Hill & Scull (1985)	1	$9\frac{1}{2}$-year-old male; third of four children; rural school	Behavioral observations in residential treatment facility; medical history	Rarely spoke in school except to comment on events in class, but followed simple directions; socially isolated and did not participate in school activities; inadequate self-help skills; enuresis and encopresis present; when pressured to speak he would show head and hand tremors, although these appeared when other demands were placed on him as well; had meningitis at 6 weeks of age and

				developed hydrocephalus, which required shunting; mother noted a history of speech delay
Lachenmeyer & Gibbs (1985)	1	$4\frac{1}{2}$-year-old male; middle of three children; nursery school	School observation; family interview; school history	Did not speak to teachers or students in $1\frac{1}{2}$ years in nursery school; spoke only to members of his immediate family; family was socially isolated; cognitive functioning above age level; history of otitis media and delayed speech onset
Wilkins (1985)	3	13-year-old male; middle of three children	Hospital case notes	Spoke normally at school and in neighborhood, but he was mute toward family for 7 months prior to referral; described as shy; average intelligence; dominant mother
		$14\frac{1}{2}$-year-old male; youngest of three children	Hospital case notes	Mutism began 8 months prior to referral and occurred about the time of maternal hospitalization; spoke normally at school and to friends, but not to any family member; described as shy, sulking, unhappy, and manipulative; marital problems between parents; paternal alcoholism; average intelligence

(continued)

TABLE 12.1
(continued)

Study	*N*	*Subject Description*	*Diagnostic Procedures*	*Findings*
		10-year, 2-month-old male; oldest of four children	Hospital case notes	Mutism began 10 months prior to referral and coincided with severe parental argument; spoke normally at school and in neighborhood, but not to family members; marital discord between parents; always described as shy, timid, but somewhat manipulative; overprotective mother and distant aggressive father
Wright, Miller, Cook, & Littmann (1985)	3	4-year, 4-month-old female; younger of two children	Case history from mother; speech therapy history	Child never spoke to strangers, but would speak spontaneously to brother; whispered and gestured in the presence of extended family and church members; described as a shy, but happy child; moderate articulation problem
		4-year, 11-month-old male; only child of divorced parents	Undefined case history	Never spoke to anyone outside of immediate family since age 2 years; 1 month premature with initial feeding problems;

				lived with maternal grandmother from age 14 to 20 months, then returned to mother where he was talkative to mother, but quiet and withdrawn around others
		5-year, 7-month-old male; older of two children; father in military and visited bimonthly; kindergarten	Case history from mother	Never spoke to teachers or peers; minimal participation; temper tantrums at home and school; spoke freely at home; meningitis at 4 weeks of age and hospitalized for 6 weeks; experienced a urethral dilation requiring second hospitalization; overprotective mother; speech and language delays with occasional stuttering; shy around strangers, but provocative and destructive
Barlow, Strother, & Landreth (1986)	1	5-year-old female; middle of three children; special education transition class	Case history from mother and school	Refused to talk outside of home; no social skills; teacher described her as passive, resistant, and occasionally hostile; also described as compulsive, controlling, and emotionally unexpressive; enuretic

(continued)

TABLE 12.1
(continued)

Study	*N*	*Subject Description*	*Diagnostic Procedures*	*Findings*
Hoffman & Laub (1986)	1	$4\frac{1}{2}$-year-old female; younger of two children; kindergarten	Undefined case history	Refused to speak to adults with the exception of her parents and grandparents; spoke to her friends at school but used her best friend as an intermediary in communication with teacher; hospitalized at age 2 with severe case of ataxia; average intelligence; long history of anxiety when approached by adults
Lesser-Katz (1986)	15	Black; low SES; Headstart preschoolers from inner city	Case history from teacher; classroom observations	All of the children were communicating verbally at home in age-appropriate manner, but were mute in school setting; two subtypes were described, compliant and noncompliant; the compliant children were described as timid, passive, immature, and dependent on their mothers; the noncompliant children were described as aggressively avoidant

Beck & Hubbard (1987)	1	7-year-old female; multilingual family; missionary family	Case history from parents	Spoke in high, squeaky voice in school; spoke normally only to her immediate family; excelled in school; extreme distress in verbal interaction situations; emotionally sophisticated with strong social skills; no marital discord or major cross-cultural adjustment problems; no family pathology
Louden (1987)	1	6-year-old Jamaican male; living with uncle	Case history from guardian; attempted clinical interview; WISC-R	Totally mute for about 4 months following his uncle's marriage; rejected on numerous occasions by his parents since age 4 months; emotionally withdrawn; poor academic skills; frequent crying and temper tantrums
Pigott & Gonzales (1987)	1	9-year-old Black male; third grade	Case history from parents; playroom observations in clinic; school report; classroom observations during a reading group	Mute in school for over 4 years; did not speak even when directly addressed; engaged with others in the presence of family members; talked quietly and infrequently to 1 selected peer; described as extremely shy, socially withdrawn, and sad/depressed; above-average academic achievement; severe psychomotor retardation

(*continued*)

TABLE 12.1
(continued)

Study	*N*	*Subject Description*	*Diagnostic Procedures*	*Findings*
Lesser-Katz (1988)	2	4-year-old Black male; middle of three children; intact family; low SES	Case history from mother; school observation	Did not communicate verbally or nonverbally to anyone in school; played and communicated verbally with siblings; described as a quiet infant, but later as manipulative and demanding; paternal history of reluctant speech
		3-year-old Black female; middle of three children; low SES	Case history from mother and teachers	Refused to communicate at school and frequently withdrew or isolated herself; active, talkative, playful but oppositional at home; congenital anomaly of eye muscle; chaotic homelife with helpless mother and no father

Carr & Afnan (1989)	1	$6\frac{1}{2}$-year-old female; middle of three children; intact family	Case history from parents; CBCL; McMaster Family Assessment Device	Four-year history of mutism whose onset coincided with birth of younger brother; mutism confined to play-school environment; CBCL Internalized $T = 59$; Externalized $T = 67$; a large number of conduct problems were reported; no evidence of marital discord or serious family pathology; enmeshed mother–child dyad

Note. CAT = Computer Axial Tomography; CBCL = Child Behavior Checklist; EEG = Electroencephalogram; IQ = Intelligence Quotient; L>R = Left greater than Right; PPVT = Peabody Picture Vocabulary Test; SES = Socioeconomic Status; VMI = Developmental Test of Visual-Motor Integration; WISC-R = Wechsler Intelligence Scale for Children-Revised.

serve to advance our understanding of the assessment and diagnostic procedures used currently for children and adolescents showing these diagnostic characteristics. Much of the information in this chapter has been extracted from these more recent case presentations, especially the specific subject descriptions and diagnostic procedures.

Topography

In comparison to many other psychiatric disorders, elective mutism is an unusually distinct syndrome in which the primary defining feature is the reluctance to speak in selected situations. As such, the topography of this disorder would appear to be reasonably straightforward. There is some debate, however, as to the straightforwardness of this primary defining feature. Should the diagnosis be reserved only for individuals showing zero speech in selected situations (Kratochwill et al., 1979), or should it be applied in some fashion to individuals who show an extremely low frequency of speech (e.g., one word utterances) or odd speech (e.g., unnecessary whispering) in certain situations (Williamson et al., 1977)? Labbe and Williamson (1984) noted that the latter behavioral presentation could be viewed as a less severe form of elective mutism. Systematically broadening the topography of elective mutism to include children with these behavioral manifestations would serve to increase the potential number of subjects for scientific study.

In addition to the refusal or reluctance to talk in selected situations, the topography of elective mutism typically includes a host of other distinguishing individual, demographic, and familial characteristics. The DSM-III-R notes that specific speech (e.g., developmental articulation disorder, dysarthria) and/or language (e.g., developmental receptive language disorder) deficits may be present. Many anxiety features such as excessive shyness, social isolation, social withdrawal, clinging to parents, school refusal, and compulsive traits may also be present. The DSM-III-R also noted that children with elective mutism can manifest frequent temper tantrums and oppositional tendencies.

Rutter (1977) noted that most individuals with elective mutism show specific temperamental features characterized by timidity, heightened anxiety, fearfulness, and withdrawn behaviors. Clear and significant emotional disturbance was present in many of the cases. Wergeland (1979) also noted these associated features of anxiety in children diagnosed with elective mutism and reported that many of these children also show depressive tendencies and emotional immaturity. In addition to these anxious features, some investigators have reported behavioral difficulties in these children (Kolvin & Fundudis, 1981; Wright, 1968; Wright, Miller, Cook, & Littmann, 1985), with bowel and bladder control and overactivity being the most common.

Multidimensionality

This variability in personality features has led some investigators to hypothesize a multidimensional conceptualization of elective mutism. For example, over 50 years ago Waterink and Vedder (1936) classified mutism into six types. The first type was described as *hysterical mutism* and was typically seen in adults. The second type, *elective mutism*, was seen in children only under selected circumstances and/or with particular people. The third type, *Heinzian mutism*, arose from the case descriptions of Heinze (1932) and referred to overly sensitive children showing a severe reaction to environmental changes. The fourth and fifth types were both anxiety-based: *neurotic mutism* was an expression of an anxiety neurosis, while *thymogenic mutism* was an acute reaction to trauma but without other accompanying hysterical features. The final type of mutism, *ideogenic mutism*, pertained to individuals who believed there was something wrong with their speech mechanism.

Another multidimensional conceptualization was espoused by Reed (1963) in an early review of the literature. Reed divided elective mutism into two subgroups based on behavioral theory. One subgroup learned to be electively mute as an evasive behavioral strategy and as an appeal for attention, while the other subgroup learned to be mute as a fear-reduction mechanism. Similarly, Friedman and Karagan (1973) and Lesser-Katz (1988) suggested that there appears to be two subgroups of children with elective mutism. One group tends to be more oppositional in their personality styles in an attempt to manipulate their environments. The second group has significantly heightened anxiety, particularly around speech demands.

More recently, Hayden (1980) classified 68 children with elective mutism into four subgroups. The largest subgroup, *symbiotic mutism*, was described as having a strong symbiotic relationship with a caretaker. Hayden noted that in about 84% of the cases this relationship was with the mother. The child with this type of mutism showed a shy, overly sensitive, and inhibited behavioral style, but was not withdrawn. In fact, these children were described as highly manipulative and negative with peers and adults. In contrast, *speech phobic mutism* represented the least common type of elective mutism. These children showed an active fear of hearing their own voices, possibly because of the fear of revealing family secrets. Hayden noted that nearly all of these children evidenced accompanying ritualistic and obsessive-compulsive tendencies. *Reactive mutism* was clustered clinically by the findings that a single traumatic event or series of events precipitated this mutism (e.g., rape, a significant loss or death in the family, mouth injuries). Hayden noted that these events typically occur during formative years, and may even go unnoticed by their caregivers. These children appear depressed and socially withdrawn, and they may lack age-appropriate social skills. Children showing the last type of elective mutism, *passive-aggressive mutism,* use their silence as a weapon. Their refusal to speak is an oppositional feature that is an expression of anger and hostility. These children typically were characterized as the family scapegoat, but they were also described as strong-willed and capable of manipulating their disorganized environment.

Neurocognitive Abilities

Variability in the neurocognitive abilities of children diagnosed with elective mutism also has been reported. For example, speech difficulties have been reported to co-occur in children with elective mutism; however, rates have varied considerably. Kolvin and Fundudis (1981) found speech immaturities or deficits in 50% of their clinic sample, whereas Wright (1968), using a school-based sample, found speech problems in approximately 20% of the cases. This inconsistency has been reported in the case study literature as well. It should be noted, however, that although children showing speech difficulties can manifest elective mutism, typically after they have been teased by playmates, this mutism tends to resolve when the stress is reduced (Gutzman, 1912). Intellectually, although most individuals with elective mutism fall within the average range (Kolvin & Fundudis, 1981; Wergeland, 1979), cases can be scattered across a wide range of functioning (Fundudis & Kolvin, 1981; Wright, 1968). Fundudis and Kolvin (1981) found that approximately 62% of their cases obtained a nonverbal IQ within one standard deviation of the mean. Outside of neurodevelopmental immaturity (Kolvin & Fundudis, 1981), few physical anomalies are reported in these children.

Family Variables

Perhaps the most dominant feature that has been associated with the diagnosis of elective mutism has been some form of family pathology (Brown, Fuller, & Gericke, 1963; Browne, Wilson, & Laybourne, 1963; Goll, 1979; Kolvin & Fundudis, 1981; Meyers, 1984; Pustrom & Speers, 1964; Rosenberg & Linblad, 1978; Wright, 1968). Over 30 years ago,

Parker, Olsen, and Throckmorton (1960) noted the association between elective mutism and specific familial factors, and more recent evidence continues to support these earlier contentions. Such factors include familial patterns of not speaking, parental shyness, impaired mother–child relationships, and, perhaps, socioeconomic status (Bradley & Sloman, 1975; Looff, 1971), although the importance of this latter factor has been contested (Kolvin & Fundudis, 1981). Rutter (1977) noted that these children often are overly dependent on their parents, typically with strong ties to their mothers. Furthermore, other investigators have suggested that this mother–child relationship is so interdependent that the normal process of separation-individuation is disrupted to a significant degree (Bradley & Sloman, 1975; Kaplan & Escoll, 1973). In addition, studies by Kolvin and Fundudis (1981) and Brown and Lloyd (1975) revealed a higher incidence of shyness or reserved personality traits in parents of children with elective mutism. Kolvin and Fundudis (1981) reported major personality problems, psychiatric concerns, marital discord, or a combination of these difficulties in about 58% of their cases. The issue of marital discord also has been raised by other investigators (e.g., Meijer, 1979; Subak, West, & Carlin, 1982). In fact, Meyers (1984) argued that the general relationship between family psychopathology and elective mutism should be included in the definition of this disorder.

The reported increased rates of psychopathology and, at least, increased shyness in families of children who are electively mute has led investigators to suggest that this disorder could be a learned phenomenon that is modeled by the family and, consequently, negatively reinforced by the parents/family by reducing elaborative speech demands (Cunningham et al., 1983; Halpern, Hammond, & Cohen, 1971; Kratochwill et al., 1979; Shaw, 1971; Sluckin, 1977). Interestingly, this also may help to explain the reported increased incidence of elective mutism in siblings of a child with this disorder.

Epidemiology

The DSM-III-R (American Psychiatric Association, 1987) noted that elective mutism is relatively rare in that it is found in less than 1% of clinic and school referrals. Earlier studies exploring the issue of prevalence have observed rates consistent with this assertion. For example, Salfield (1950) found that elective mutism was found in approximately 0.4% of child guidance clinic referrals. Using a similar population, Morris (1963) found a slightly higher rate of about 1%. Parker and associates (1960) found a 0.7% rate in their school-based sample. These findings are noteworthy in that a higher incidence rate would be expected in a clinic population. It is important to note, however, that these early studies were compromised by small sample sizes, poorly operationalized definitions, and the use of few formal assessment procedures.

Although large-scale epidemiological studies have been plagued by similar methodological issues, the prevalence of elective mutism in the general population appears to be quite low. Using a relatively stringent definition of elective mutism and individual clinical assessments, investigators in the Newcastle Epidemiological Study (Fundudis, Kolvin, & Garside, 1979) found elective mutism in only 2 out of 3,300 7-year-old children—a prevalence rate of approximately 0.61 per 1,000. Bradley and Sloman (1975), using a more liberal definition and a questionnaire technique for assessment, identified only 26 out of 6,865 nursery school children who had elective mutism—a prevalence rate of about 3.8 per 1,000. Employing similar assessment procedures and a liberal definition, Brown and Lloyd (1975) found that this disorder occurred in 42 out of 6,072 5-year-old children—a rate of approximately 6.9 per 1,000. Follow-up of these children approximately 1 year later revealed a prevalence rate of 0.66 per 1,000 for elective mutism, a rate similar to the Newcastle Epidemiological Study. Although somewhat variable, these findings tend to suggest that prevalence rates for this disorder likely are age-dependent, with the number of occurrences decreasing with advancing age. Hesselman (1983) noted in a comprehensive review of this topic, however, that there are likely to be many hidden (i.e., undiagnosed) cases.

In addition, there appears to be an increased incidence rate associated with demographic and socioeconomic variables. For example, elective mutism has been found to occur more frequently in immigrant families (Bradley & Sloman, 1975; Brown & Lloyd, 1975; Rosenberg & Lindblad, 1978) and in families from the Appalachian regions of the United States (Looff, 1971). A higher incidence rate also has been reported in non-first-born children of large families in which one parent was described as shy (Brown & Lloyd, 1975). Furthermore, slightly more females reportedly manifest elective mutism than their male counterparts, with rates varying from about 1.2:1 (Kolvin & Fundudis, 1981) to about 2.4:1 (Wilkins, 1985; Wright, 1968).

Lastly, elective mutism seems to occur largely during the preschool years, typically kindergarten (Meyers, 1984), although its clinical onset may vary widely. A review of the English literature on elective mutism by Wright and colleagues (1985) revealed that the age of onset was $\leq$ 6.0 years of age, with 4.9 years as the mean age of onset and 5.0 years the modal age. Similar findings were reported by Hayden (1980), who found about 79% of cases to have an onset in the preschool years or earlier, and by Wright (1968), who reported 3.6 years as the average age of onset. Despite the apparent existence of elective mutism prior to school entry, the age of referral tends to coincide with entry into formal schooling (Parker et al., 1960) or later (Kolvin & Fundudis, 1981; Wergeland, 1979). For example, Parker and associates (1960) found that approximately 70% of their children were referred during their kindergarten year (i.e., age 5.0 years). In general, although there appears to be a higher incidence of elective mutism during the preschool and early elementary school years, these cases tend to be most often reported between the ages of 5.0 and 7.0 years (Halpern et al., 1971; Sluckin, 1977), and the onset tends to be a slow, insidious development of shyness (Kolvin & Fundudis, 1981).

Etiology

Being relatively rare, it is no surprise that the etiological nature of this disorder has not been determined. Psychoanalytic reasons for this disorder have been proposed (Adams & Glasner, 1954; Browne et al., 1963; von Misch, 1952) along with behavioral (Kratochwill et al., 1979; Labbe & Williamson, 1984) and family-based rationales (Goll, 1979; Parker et al., 1960). Given the apparent heterogeneous nature of this disorder, it is likely that multiple etiological factors exist (Hesselman, 1983). For example, Wergeland (1979) speculated that etiological factors might include an inherited trait or a temperamental predisposition in combination with physical and/or emotional trauma at a sensitive developmental time period (e.g., periods of separation, formal school entry). Similarly, Kehrer and Tinkl-Damhorst (1974) proposed a list of conditions that they believed contributed to elective mutism. In addition to speech deficits, these investigators described a multitude of family system variables that also could be present. Although such multifactorial etiological explanations of elective mutism are intriguing, they remain largely speculative given the statistical difficulties presented by the rarity of this disorder.

To date, however, it would appear that family psychopathology is a common etiological factor (e.g., Kehrer & Tinkl-Damhorst, 1974; Subak et al., 1982). In nearly every case study presented in the recent literature, the issue of family psychopathology and/or family distress has been mentioned (Goll, 1979). This also is true for the literature in general (Hesselman, 1983). The exact nature of this etiological relationship has varied from mother's marital dissatisfaction (Pustrom & Speers, 1964), to a symbiotic relationship between mother and child (Bradley &

Sloman, 1975; Kaplan & Escoll, 1973), to parental modeling of the aberrant behaviors (Rosenberg & Linblad, 1978), to a combination of these variables. It is clear, however, that investigators from behavioral as well as psychodynamic persuasions have acknowledged the importance of family variables in the genesis of elective mutism. Even if family variables are discovered not to be major etiological agents, the importance of family psychopathology in perpetuating elective mutism likely will continue to be acknowledged. Despite the important influence of family factors on the development and/or perpetuation of elective mutism, these variables are curiously absent from descriptions of this disorder in the DSM-III-R.

Prognosis

Case study evidence suggests that symptoms can last from less than 1 year (Brown & Lloyd, 1975; Wright, 1968) to more than 12 years (Wergeland, 1979). For example, Wergeland (1979) found that the average duration of elective mutism in a small clinic sample was approximately 8 years. Furthermore, spontaneous remission rates of elective mutism have varied. Brown and Lloyd (1975) reported a significant drop in the incidence rate approximately 10 to 12 months after the beginning of school. In contrast, Hayden (1980) noted that spontaneous remission was quite low in elective mutism, and even when children would begin talking, they ultimately would stop again. Hayden also reported that treatment was unlikely to show immediate results in cases of greater than 12 years duration. Hayden concluded that elective mutism is a persistent disorder that can become more intractable over time. Similarly, Kolvin and Fundudis (1981) followed 24 elective mutes for 5 to 10 years and found that only 46% improved, typically by age 10, but the others remained electively mute. Moreover, some investigators have hypothesized that children with elective mutism actually may manifest a schizoid personality disorder at a later developmental period (Wolf & Barlow, 1979), although this has not received any empirical support (Kolvin & Fundudis, 1981). Elective mutism also has been hypothesized to be a possible antecedent of schizophrenia (Eldar, Bleich, Apter, & Tyano, 1985), although this requires further replication and substantiation.

Recent findings have suggested that the prognosis for elective mutism tends to be better for those children who have some type of early intervention (Wright et al., 1985) and perhaps for females (Kolvin & Fundudis, 1981), although this latter finding remains speculative at this time. Some investigators have reasoned that early intervention actually may serve to minimize the secondary difficulties that can be associated with this disorder (Nash, Thorpe, Andrews, & Davis, 1979). Relatedly, improvements also have been noted to coincide with a change in environments (Wergeland, 1979). In contrast, the prognosis tends to worsen for individuals who also evidence accompanying psychiatric problems, such as thought disorder or lower cognitive abilities (Wright, 1968). This is a particularly important finding given that elective mutism has been reported to be highly resistant to treatment (Elson, Pearson, Jones, & Schumacher, 1965; Kolvin & Fundudis, 1981; Kupietz & Schwartz, 1982; Lazarus, Gavilo, & Moore, 1983; Wergeland, 1979).

Response to Treatment

The treatment of elective mutism dominates the literature on this disorder, with case study methodology accounting for most of the work. Treatment methods have ranged from more psychodynamically based attempts to pure behavioral strategies designed to increase the child's verbal frequency in selected situations. A review of this literature is beyond the scope of this chapter, although recent and comprehensive literature reviews are available (American Psychiatric Association, 1989; Cunningham et al., 1983; Kratochwill et al., 1979; Labbe & Williamson, 1984), with the review conducted by Kratochwill and associates (1979) being particularly outstanding from a methodological perspective.

From a diagnostic perspective, however, children with elective mutism have shown a positive response to treatment. In fact, there appears to be emergent evidence for a differential response to various types of behavioral interventions depending on the exact behavioral manifestation of the disorder. For example, Piersel and Kratochwill (1981) noted that the intervention program used for a child with low speech frequency may be different than a program designed for a child who evidences no speech in selected situations (Labbe & Williamson, 1984). Recognition of the multidimensional nature of elective mutism, then, appears to have merit with respect to the response to selected treatment paradigms. Generally, a variety of behavioral therapy techniques, perhaps in combination with family interventions, appear to be most effective for this disorder at this time.

Summary

Definitional issues notwithstanding, the topography and associated features of elective mutism certainly seem to reflect the relatively unique nature of this disorder. In fact, some investigators have presented evidence along with conjecture that elective mutism actually may be a multidimensional disorder with different subgroups. The disorder is relatively rare, but it tends to be age-dependent, occurring more frequently during the preschool and early primary school years, although some investigators believe that elective mutism actually may be present for several years prior to referral. Although the findings are equivocal, there appears to be a slight trend in the literature for this disorder to be more prevalent in females than males, a reversal of the typical finding for many child psychiatric disorders. Etiology and prognostic issues continue to be elusive, although findings do implicate family psychopathology in each of these domains. Finally, the treatment of elective mutism reportedly is difficult, with low spontaneous remission rates. Some inroads have been made in this regard, however, particularly with respect to matching particular behavioral interventions to specific behavioral manifestations of the disorder.

DIAGNOSTIC ISSUES

Reliability

The data concerning the reliability of the criteria used for any diagnosis is crucial if there is to be confidence in that particular diagnosis (Quay & Werry, 1986). Unfortunately, there are no adequate data pertaining to the reliability of elective mutism and its inherent diagnostic criteria (Quay & Werry, 1986). This lack of information can be attributed, at least in part, to the fact that a large portion of the literature on this diagnosis is devoted to case studies, and this shortcoming impacts heavily on issues of reliability (Kratochwill et al., 1979). The idiosyncratic nature of the definitions used, the number and kind of subjects selected for presentation, and the assessment strategies employed ultimately have added little in the way of empirical findings with respect to the reliability of this diagnosis. Perhaps the primary question relating to the reliability of elective mutism is where do clinicians and researchers draw the line on the verbalization continuum (i.e., should it be zero speech)? Although some guidelines have been provided by the ICD-9 and the DSM-III-R, they lack depth and specific operational criteria. Consequently, at the present time, this distinction has been determined arbitrarily by investigators. Given that the literature appears to be dependent on case study methodology, even a case simulation addressing issues of diagnostic reliability would be a useful and welcome contribution.

Validity

Reliability sets the ceiling on validity, so the lack of information pertaining to the reliability of the diagnosis of elective mutism presents a critical stumbling block with respect to evolving this diagnosis further. Again, given the relative rarity of this disorder and the dependence on case study methodology for its description, this is not an oversight by the field but, rather, an issue of not having enough individuals to complete basic statistical analyses. Consequently, there appears to be little, if any, available information on the validity of this diagnosis.

Nonetheless, one of the major conceptual debates that surrounds elective mutism is whether it represents an extra dimension or "shading" of another disorder (Reed, 1963), as demonstrated by its inclusion as one of the disorders under sensitivity, shyness, and social withdrawal in ICD-9, or whether it represents a diagnostic entity or continuum of its own as demonstrated by DSM-III-R. To date, there have been two studies that have addressed this concern of discriminant validity (Kolvin & Fundudis, 1981; Wilkins, 1985).

Kolvin & Fundudis (1981) painstakingly collected 24 cases of children with elective mutism over a period of about 5 to 6 years. They attempted to use a strict definition of elective mutism (i.e., zero speech in certain situations) as compared to other studies with less stringent definitions of this disorder. These children were compared to a sample of children with speech retardation ($N = 84$) and a normal sample ($N = 102$) across a variety of variables that traversed biological and social-familial factors.

On the biological factors, Kolvin & Fundudis (1981) found that slightly more females than males (i.e., 54% vs. 46%) experienced elective mutism, as opposed to a clear trend in the opposite direction for the other disorder (i.e., 36% vs. 64%). This was consistent with the findings of Wright (1968), who noted a 2.4:1 female-to-male ratio. Although not directly consistent with the findings of Brown and Lloyd (1975), who found equal numbers of males and females, it is clear that this is one psychiatric diagnosis that does not show more affected males than females. In comparison to the normal and speech-impaired cohorts, the children with elective mutism also manifested a significantly later onset of speech (mean age = 27.3 months), even later than the children with speech disorders (mean age = 21.9 months). An increased incidence of enuresis (42%) and encopresis (17%) also was noted when compared to the other two groups. Although any measures of cognitive functioning undoubtedly would be confounded to some degree by the primary symptoms of the child with elective mutism, the IQ data that were available suggested that these children had significantly lower abilities (mean Wechsler Intelligence Scale for Children-Revised Performance IQ = 84.95) than either the normal (mean PIQ = 101.17) or speech-impaired (mean PIQ = 94.94) groups. This is relatively similar to the description of these children noted by Wright (1968).

On the social-familial factors, there did not appear to be any major differences between the groups in terms of socioeconomic status, with the elective mute sample representing a wide cross-section of backgrounds. However, there did appear to be a higher incidence of parental psychopathology in the sample of children with elective mutism. Specifically, 20% of mothers of the children with elective mutism had received some form of psychiatric assistance, as compared to only 8% of the mothers of the normal group. Similarly, 16% of the fathers of children with elective mutism had participated in psychiatric treatment, as compared to only 3% of the fathers of the normal group. There also seemed to be a tendency for children with elective mutism to be separated from their parents for at least 6 months during the first 5 years of life (25%), as compared to the normal group (14%), although this was not statistically significant.

More recently, Wilkins (1985) also compared a sample of 24 children with elective mutism to 24 matched controls with diagnosed emotional disorders. In contrast to most other studies, Wilkins used strict operational criteria for subject selection in this retrospective study. These criteria included: (a) mutism toward certain people or groups of people, or mutism in some definite setting, while the child was heard to speak fluently (with or without articulation difficulties) to other people or in other settings; (b) mutism present for at least 6 months; (c) an IQ on the WISC of 70 or more; (d) no symptoms of psychotic illness; and (e) both parents fluent English speakers so as to prevent linguistic factors complicating the study. Interestingly, Wilkins found three cases showing elective mutism exclusively in the home setting, a reversal of the pattern that is typically seen in these children. This sample was then matched to a heterogeneous group of children with emotional disorders by gender, chronological age, time seen, IQ, and area of residence. The diagnoses of this group included school refusal, phobic reactions, adjustment reactions, anxiety, depression, enuresis, and hysteria.

Similar to Kolvin and Fundudis (1981), Wilkins (1985) found that females with elective mutism outnumbered males by at least a 2:1 ratio. Also similar to the findings of Kolvin and Fundudis (1981), Wilkins found a greater likelihood of delayed speech and articulation difficulties in his sample of elective mutes. However, there was no difference between the groups on the incidence of enuresis. A comparison of cognitive abilities also revealed the children with elective mutism to be somewhat lower, falling within the low average to average range (mean

PIQ = 90.6), than the children with emotional problems (mean PIQ = 96.2).

When compared to the children with emotional disorders, Wilkins found that all of the children with elective mutism came from two-parent families as compared to 50% for the children with emotional disorders. However, this also accounted for the greater incidence of marital discord in the families of elective mutes. Furthermore, despite the preponderance of literature describing these children as shy, Wilkins also noted that these children were described as anxious, depressed, oppositional, and manipulative. Their mothers also were described as overprotective with a tendency toward spoiling the children.

In general, although not clearly definitive, these two studies do suggest that elective mutism is a disorder than can be distinguished from children with speech problems and from children manifesting a variety of psychiatric difficulties. These studies also stressed the higher female-to-male ratio and underscored the significance of family problems in this population. A variety of associated physical (e.g., enuresis, speech problems, speech delays) and psychological (e.g., anxiety, depression, oppositional) factors also were asserted by these studies. Lastly, these two studies do indicate the need for more frequent use of standardized criteria in diagnosing this disorder.

Proposed Changes in Diagnostic Criteria

Although hard scientific data pertaining to the diagnosis of elective mutism are lacking, largely due to the relative rarity of the disorder and to the preponderance of the case study methodology used for much of the research on this disorder, a number of conceptual issues should be addressed by future psychiatric nomenclatures in attempting to refine the diagnosis of elective mutism.

Generally, it would appear from the studies described earlier, in conjunction with the myriad of case studies, that elective mutism should be classified as a distinctive disorder as described in the DSM system. Moreover, given the relative rarity of this disorder, it would appear that a broader definition of elective mutism would serve to enhance the development and clinical utility of this diagnosis. This could be accomplished by merging the different perspectives espoused with respect to diagnosing this condition (e.g., zero speech vs. reluctant speech), perhaps placing it on a "continuum of silence." This continuum would include not only children who demonstrate the classic elective mutism (i.e., zero speech in selective situations), but also children with oddities in their verbal communication (e.g., low frequency, changed voices) in selected situations. Although the DSM-III-R does not state this position clearly, the concept of placing this disorder on a continuum would be consistent with the DSM-III-R definition (i.e., "The child with elective mutism may communicate . . . by monosyllabic or short, monotone utterances," American Psychiatric Association, 1987, p. 88). The data reviewed also support the issues of comorbidity addressed by the DSM-III-R, particularly family dysfunction, although care should be taken to rule out direct contributions of associated factors to the mutism (e.g., dysarthria). Broadening the definition of elective mutism in a systematic fashion would allow for more children to be identified under this diagnosis and, in turn, would permit more systematic, large-scale investigations of this disorder.

The placement of elective mutism on a continuum of silence not only would allow for more children to be identified as electively mute, but it also would serve to describe the possible multidimensional nature of this disorder more thoroughly. The case study data, although hampered by intrinsic methodological problems (e.g., lack of generalization), do suggest that multiple subtypes of elective mutism should be considered. This has been underscored particularly given the reported response to particular subtypes to certain behavioral interventions. The DSM-III-R already has begun to lay the foundation for this by describing associated features of this disorder but, from a treatment perspective, it may prove useful to subtype these cases further based on specific descriptions and models available in the literature. Again, this should allow for further exploration of this disorder with respect to response-to-treatment issues.

Finally, from a general perspective, it would seem important to place a time constraint on each case before an actual diagnosis is asserted. With nearly every other child psychiatric disorder there is a criterion addressing the amount of time that symptoms should be present before a specific diagnosis can be applied. However, given its reported resistance to treatment, it might be useful to invoke a shorter time frame rather than a longer one. Similarly, this would be supported, in part, by the finding that children who receive early intervention tend to have a better prognosis (Wright et al., 1985).

Given these general conceptualizations regarding the diagnosis of elective mutism, a number of specific proposed changes are offered (see Table 12.2). First, it is suggested that two forms of elective mutism be considered. The first form should be consistent with the classically described elective mute. This form should manifest zero speech in circumscribed situations (e.g., home, school, social), despite having relatively intact speech and language abilities. The second form should comprise children who manifest reluctant speech in selected situations, despite having relatively intact speech and language.

TABLE 12.2
Proposed Diagnostic Criteria for Elective Mutism

A. Persistent refusal or reluctance to talk in one or more major social situations. This may be manifested by zero speech in one or more situations, or by reluctant (i.e., low frequency) or odd speech (e.g., mumbling, odd voices) in one or more situations. The child may show this refusal or reluctance in his or her interactions with selected peers, adults (e.g., teachers), or even parents.
B. Although speech deficits or delays may be present, they do not significantly interfere with the individual's relative ability to speak or comprehend language.
C. The individual manifests distinctive behavioral features characterized by anxiety-depression, manipulative-oppositional, or mixed emotional features. Family psychopathology or marital discord also may be present, but it is not necessary for the diagnosis.
D. The individual is impaired in social, academic, or familial functioning.
E. The duration of the disturbance for at least 3 months.
F. The disturbance is not due primarily to mental retardation, pervasive developmental disorders, schizophrenia, specific expressive langauge disorder, or difficulties due to learning another language. Although other conditions can coexist with elective mutism, the key feature distinguishing elective mutism is the refusal or reluctance to speak in selected situations.

Types:

Elective Mutism, Zero Speech, Anxious-Depressed Type—This type of elective mutism is characterized by no speech in specific situations and personality features that are indicative of anxiety and/or depression. This type may represent the classic description of children with elective mutism.

Elective Mutism, Zero Speech, Manipulative-Oppositional Type—This type of elective mutism is characterized by no speech in specific situations and personality features that suggest manipulative and oppositional tendencies. These individuals may have frequent temper tantrums in the home setting, with the elective mutism being a form of oppositional behavior.

Elective Mutism, Zero Speech, Mixed Emotional Type—This type of elective mutism is characterized by no speech in specific situations and mixed personality features.

Elective Mutism, Reluctant Speech, Anxious-Depressed Type—This type of elective mutism is characterized by low frequency speech (i.e., one- to three-word utterances) in specific situations. This also can take the form of mumbling and/or the use of odd voices (e.g., radio announcer, Mickey Mouse) in their verbal communications. They rarely initiate conversations and will show personality features indicative of anxiety and/or depression.

Elective Mutism, Reluctant Speech, Manipulative-Oppositional Type—This type of elective mutism is characterized by low frequency speech (i.e., one- to three-word utterances) in specific situations. This also can take the form of mumbling and/or the use of odd voices (e.g., radio announcer, Mickey Mouse) in their verbal communications. They rarely initiate conversations and will show personality features indicative of manipulative and oppositional tendencies. These individuals may have frequent temper tantrums in the home setting, with the elective mutism being a form of oppositional behavior.

Elective Mutism, Reluctant Speech, Mixed Emotional Type—This type of elective mutism is characterized by reluctant speech in specific situations and mixed personality features.

Elective Mutism, Not Otherwise Specified—This should be reserved by unusual presentations of this disorder that cannot be classified into one of the types previously noted.

In addition, it will be important for specific personality characteristics to be associated with each form of elective mutism. Although different types of elective mutism have been offered based on primary personality features (e.g., Friedman & Karagan, 1973; Hayden, 1980; Heinze, 1932; Lesser-Katz, 1988; Reed, 1963; Waterink & Vedder, 1936), the general consensus from this literature seems to be that there are two major personality features that tend to dominate the majority of children manifesting elective mutism: anxious-depressed features and manipulative-oppositional features. These two types likely will not always be orthogonal to one another and, given the likelihood that other personality features might be involved, a third type with mixed emotional features should be considered. Given the success of the treatment literature in beginning to identify specific behavioral characteristics of elective mutes, and the effects noted with different behavioral features, this subdivision of elective mutism might prove clinically useful in establishing individual treatment strategies for selected individuals. Such a subdivision of this diagnostic category also may serve to facilitate research in this domain, particularly with respect to reliability and validity of the diagnosis.

Finally, it will be important for a specific length of time for symptoms to be present before the diagnosis of elective mutism can be applied. Although it seems that in a major portion of these cases the mutism appears to be transient, lasting about 5 months (Kolvin & Fundudis, 1981; Wright et al., 1985) to less than 1 year (Brown & Lloyd, 1975), the severity of the symptoms suggest that these children can be socially and academically compromised, particularly given that most of the cases appear to surface on formal school entry. In this regard, the criterion of a 6-month duration used by Wilkins (1985) in his definition of elective mutism seems to be a reasonable amount of time, and it would be consistent with the symptom duration prescribed for other childhood diagnoses (e.g., overanxious disorder, avoidant disorder of childhood and adolescents). However, given the severity of the symptoms, the likelihood of family psychopathology, the delicate age that these symptoms seem to emerge (i.e., preschool), and the relative rarity of this disorder, a 3-month duration might be more prudent and should be considered.

Summary

There is an abundance of diagnostic issues associated with elective mutism, with issues of reliability and validity leading the way. Despite these major empirical hurdles, it is clear from an examination of the available literature that clear guidelines for diagnosis of this disorder are long overdue, and would help to increase our understanding of this unique psychiatric disorder. The long history of case study literature and the recent comparative studies suggest that the diagnosis of elective mutism represents a distinctive diagnostic domain, and does not necessarily represent an extension of other forms of psychopathology. In order to increase research on children showing these symptoms, several suggestions have been offered in an effort to broaden the definition to some degree. This effort has attempted to preserve the position that the diagnosis of elective mutism should be reserved only for children showing zero speech in selective situations, but it also has attempted to extend the diagnosis along a continuum of silence to allow for comparative studies of children with unusual manifestations of this unique diagnosis. The application of specific personality features and a defined time of duration for symptoms to be present also should serve to improve the diagnostic clarity of elective mutism. Interestingly, these suggestions are not contrary to the position espoused in the DSM-III-R, but they are stated with more detail with respect to proposed criteria for elective mutism.

ASSESSMENT PROCEDURES

Given the basic behavioral feature of elective mutism (i.e., lack of speech in selective situations), it would appear that the diagnostic assessment of elective mutism would be a relatively simple task. It becomes evident, however, that this task has been extremely variable, poorly described and, in many instances, nonexistent. This section reviews methods and strategies that have been used in the diagnostic assessment of these children. Following this discussion, an assessment model designed to address the unique diagnostic issues presented by children with elective mutism is discussed. Finally, a brief discussion of selected measures that could be used with the proposed model is provided.

Current Assessment Procedures

A review of the case study literature, including the more recent literature available since 1980, would suggest that there has been as much variability in the diagnostic assessment of these children as there has been in the case descriptions. A cursory review of Table 12.1 reveals the wide variety of diagnostic tasks that investigators have used. In describing their case studies, some investigators have used vague descriptors (e.g., "a thorough evaluation involving all family members," Rosenberg & Lindblad, 1978; "diagnostic studies," Kass et al., 1967), whereas others described specific procedures and results (e.g., Kupietz & Schwartz, 1982). Furthermore, the amount and type of communication in specific settings are generally not measured but, instead, left to unsystematic anecdotal report.

Once a particular child was referred, the form and focus of the diagnostic assessment appeared to be dependent on the orientation of the professional who received the referral. For example, outside of a few investigators who have tended to focus on family functioning, an assessment of the home environment usually was not included. This is a major oversight in assessing a disorder that appears to be so closely tied to family dysfunction (Hesselman, 1983). By far the most frequent assessment strategies involved the use of observations, typically in one setting (e.g., the school), and a history of the presenting problem. Typically, this history taking of the presenting problem has included a cross-situational view of the child, an essential component to the diagnosis of elective mutism.

In addition, several investigators have attempted to assess other variables in order to describe associated features and/or to rule out other possible diagnoses (e.g., autism). Variables such as family functioning (Carr & Afnan, 1989), cognitive abilities (Louden, 1987), and neurological status (Kupietz & Schwartz, 1982) all have been used, but they have not typically been utilized in any systematic manner. For example, investigators have used nonverbal measures in an attempt to assess the cognitive abilities of these children. These measures tend to be those used in the assessment of hearing-impaired children and have included the Performance Scale of the Wechsler Intelligence Scales (Louden, 1987), Leiter International Performance Scale (Kupietz & Schwartz, 1982; Lazarus, Gavilo, & Moore, 1983), and the Peabody Picture Vocabulary Test (Lowenstein, 1979). However, few of these tests have been used in any systematic study of children with elective mutism.

Noteworthy among the case studies, however, is the work of Carr and Afnan (1989), who reported the case of a $6\frac{1}{2}$-year-old female who had a 4-year history of mutism. In an attempt to gain a more systematic appraisal of social-emotional functioning, Carr and Afnan used the Child Behavior Checklist (CBCL; Achenbach & Edelbrock, 1983) for both diagnostic assessment and evaluation of their intervention. Diagnostically, in addition to the elective mutism symptoms, these investigators noted that they were able to uncover a variety of conduct problems that were present simply by having both parents complete the

CBCL. Without these parental ratings of their child's behaviors, these behavioral difficulties may have been overlooked. Carr and Afnan reported that the CBCL also proved to be useful in measuring changes in the child's behavior following intervention.

In general, despite several noteworthy assessment strategies (e.g., Carr & Afnan, 1989), the literature would suggest that the diagnostic assessment of these children falls short of an adequate evaluation. Given the relative dearth of information pertaining to this diagnosis (e.g., reliability), a more systematic method for assessing and diagnosing these cases in a more comprehensive fashion appears warranted. This would allow for sufficient data to be collected so that clinicians and researchers can more adequately address the multiple questions that remain unanswered with respect to elective mutism.

Proposed Assessment Procedures

With the proposed expansion in the diagnostic criteria of elective mutism, the diagnostic assessment of children exhibiting symptoms of elective mutism will need to be more comprehensive and include a variety of functional domains. Although the electively nonverbal nature of these children always will pose difficulty for the clinicians and researchers who evaluate these children directly, it will be important for a broad-based assessment model to be used. Such a model, if sensitively constructed, would provide for assessment of the child across informants, settings, instruments, and time, and it also would help to improve the reliability of the diagnostic information obtained.

Multisetting, Multisource, Multi-Instrument Model

One model that attempts to account for the many variables present in personality appraisal is the multisetting, multisource, multi-instrument model (Martin, Hooper, & Snow, 1986). This is presented in Fig. 12.1. This assessment model is based on the *aggregation principle*, which asserts that data from any observation or measurement reflect two classes of phenomena: (a) the behavior the assessor intends to measure, and (b) the characteristics of the person, situation, time, instruments, or observer that the assessor did not intend to measure. To maximize the accuracy of the description or diagnosis, two or more observations or measurements of the same characteristic are added together, resulting in an aggregated measure that is more reliable than the individual component observations or measurements. Epstein (1983) and Eaton (1983) documented the place of aggregation in personality research and clinical diagnostic assessment. The multisetting, multisource, multi-instrument design (Martin et al., 1986) uses the aggrega-

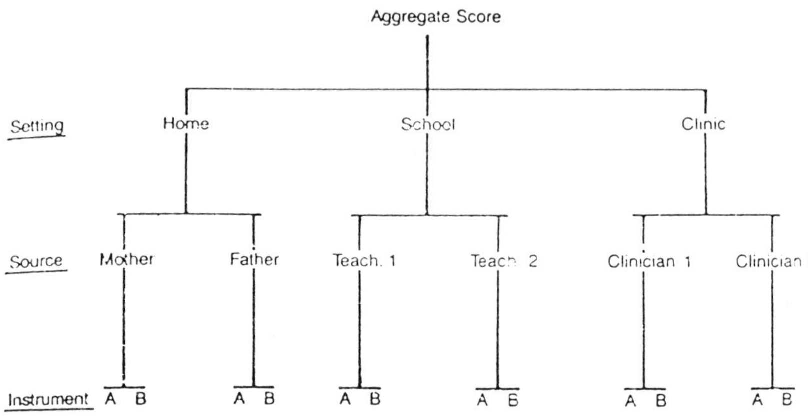

FIG. 12.1. The multisetting, multisource, multi-instrument model. From "Behavior Rating Scale Approaches to Personality Assessment in Children and Adolescents," by R. P. Martin, S. R. Hooper, and J. Snow, 1986, in H. M. Knoff (Ed.), *The psychological assessment of children and adolescents* (pp. 309–351), New York: Guilford Press.

tion principle in order to increase the reliability of a diagnosis, and it also allows for a broader coverage of primary and secondary diagnostic features of the child.

Most important, this design allows assessment to occur in multiple settings. For the majority of children this will involve the home, school, and perhaps the clinic. This is consistent with the position of Kratochwill and associates (1979), who noted that researchers should collect information on the frequency of verbal and nonverbal behaviors across a number of different settings. Generally, the chosen settings should include those of importance or relevance to the child, and those with characteristics that could differentially affect the child's behaviors (e.g., marital/family environment). Setting variance may be the single most crucial data point in the diagnosis of this disorder.

In addition, this assessment model uses multiple informants (i.e., at least two) from each setting. This allows for the reliability of the behavior to be checked within as well as between settings. Not only is this information important to asserting the diagnosis of elective mutism, but it also will serve to identify individuals with whom the child verbally interacts, and it aides in the establishment of specific targets for treatment. The use of multiple sources of information decreases the need to collect information solely from the child via direct interviews and observations by the clinician.

The third component of this model is more difficult to achieve and requires that two or more measurement devices be used to assess the same constructs for each information source in each setting. This component requires that the same or parallel measurement devices be used in each setting by each rater so as to facilitate direct comparisons. This is difficult to achieve, largely because of the relative dearth of instruments that have various forms of the same tool (e.g., parent, teacher, child, clinician versions). Consequently, although some instruments are available that permit this type of flexibility (e.g., CBCL), clinicians and researchers generally are left with attempting to approximate the spirit of this third component by using multiple assessment methods with each information source.

Diagnostic Instruments

In accordance with the proposed multisetting, multisource, multi-instrument assessment model for elective mutism, a variety of diagnostic instruments are available for use with these children. To date, however, it is clear from the case study literature that few, if any, standardized assessment procedures have been used with children with elective mutism (see Table 12.1). Consequently, the use of any type of formal assessment instrument to assist in the *diagnosis* of elective mutism, in conjunction with a thorough history of the behavioral symptoms, would be a major improvement over what has been employed thus far. Given the nonverbal nature of many of these children in the diagnostic situation, structured parent interviews, structured observations, and rating scales would appear to be the most viable diagnostic assessment strategies at this time. In addition, a variety of nonverbal measures designed to assess cognition and language would serve to assess the associated features that these children can manifest.

Although a variety of structured diagnostic interviews are available for use (e.g., Diagnostic Interview for Children and Adolescents, Schedule for Affective Disorders and Schizophrenia for School-Age Children), the Diagnostic Interview Schedule for Children-Parent Version (DISC-P; Costello, Edelbrock, Kalas, Dulcan, & Klaric, 1984) is one of the few structured interview techniques that is capable of obtaining a diagnosis of elective mutism according to DSM-III/DSM-III-R criteria. The DISC-P was designed to be administered to parents of children ages 6 to 18 years and follows a highly explicit format with clinical judgment kept to a minimum. Despite this structure, however, the questions of the DISC-P were organized in an attempt to follow a traditional clinical interview as much as possible. Reliability and validity of the DISC-P have been equivocal, with somewhat better findings noted for conduct problems as opposed to affective difficulties (Edelstein & Berler, 1987). One limitation of this scale for the diagnosis of elective mutism may be that, given the increased incidence of this disorder during the preschool years, it was not designed to be used with children under age 6.

Structured observations of children suspected of elective mutism also will be important. Not only should structured observations include observations of these children at home and school, but it should include observations in the social setting as well. Although these observations may be accomplished best by one observer, it may be helpful to have designated observers in each of these settings (e.g., parents, teachers). Specific information to be collected might include communicative intent, selected persons with whom the child chooses to speak, and samples of the child's school work. Perhaps one of the key behaviors to quantify is the child's speech. Speech samples would be crucial to the diagnosis of elective mutism, particularly with respect to determining setting variance, and they also would allow for the evaluation of the integrity of the child's speech. Tape recordings of the child's speech have been obtained without undue difficulties (Scott, 1977; Williamson et al., 1977).

Rating scales represent perhaps the most viable assessment strategies for children suspected of elective mutism. These scales could be helpful in formulating the diagnosis, determining the type of elective mutism present, and providing additional information pertaining to the child's social-emotional status. There are a variety of behavioral rating scales that could be useful in the diagnostic assessment of these children, such as the Personality Inventory for Children (Wirt, Lachar, Klinedinst, & Seat, 1977), the Revised Behavior Problem Checklist (Quay & Peterson, 1987), or the Louisville Behavior Checklist (Miller, 1981). However, one rating scale that seems to capture the spirit of the multisetting, multisource, multi-instrument design is the Child Behavior Checklist (CBCL; Achenbach & Edelbrock, 1983). The CBCL is a multi-instrument battery designed to obtain structured ratings regarding behavioral adjustment from the parent and teacher for children covering a wide age range. A Youth Self-Report for children ages 11 to 18 and a Direct Observational Form also are available.

The parent version of the CBCL extends downward to age 2 years and extends upward to age 16. The teacher version begins at age 6 years and is normed for adolescents through age 16. Both the parent and teacher versions of the CBCL produce general scores for adaptive functioning as well as for behavior problems (i.e., externalized, internalized, total), with the behavior problem areas being further subdivided into more refined factors tapping specific aspects of social and emotional functioning (e.g., social withdrawal, somatic complaints, etc.). Scores for the CBCL are analyzed separately for males and females. Psychometric findings suggest that this is a well-conceptualized behavioral rating system with an adequate normative base and satisfactory reliability and validity (Martin et al., 1986; McMahon, 1984). There is an advantage to this rating system in the diagnostic assessment of children suspected of having elective mutism, in that a variety of behaviors can be tapped across settings and raters without the clinician directly working with the child. These data should provide information related to the elective mutism as well as associated behavioral features that characterize these children.

More specific rating scales also should be used with these children and adolescents. Given the anxious features typically reported in these children, measures of anxiety would be useful in delineating the degree of anxiety present for an individual child. Child ratings such as the Revised Children's Manifest Anxiety Scale (Reynolds & Richmond, 1985), the Louisville Fear Survey for Children (Miller, Barrett, Hampe, & Noble, 1972), and the State-Trait Anxiety Inventory (Spielberger, 1983) could be helpful. Measures of depression also would seem pertinent and could include the Children's Depression Inventory (Kovacs & Beck, 1977), the Self-Rating Scale (Birleson, 1981), the Children's Depression Adjective Checklist (Sokoloff & Lubin, 1983), or the Perceived Competency Scale for Children (Harter, 1982). In addition, in conjunction with the belief that a subgroup of these children actually may be experiencing underlying feelings of anger, use of the State-Trait Anger Expression Inventory might prove fruitful (Spielberger, 1988).

Finally, despite the multitude of case studies on elective mutism that have been described, no specific checklist of symptoms has been devised that would directly assist investigators in their clinical and research endeavors with this disorder. Therefore, the Elective Mutism Rating Scale was developed by the authors from the case study literature on elective mutism. The rating scale was designed to be used primarily by clinicians in an effort to provide one method of systematic data collection for this population. Moreover, given the position that elective mutism should be viewed on a "continuum of silence," a three-point Likert format has been employed in developing this rating tool. To complete this rating scale, investigators need to indicate whether the specific behavior or characteristic is Not Similar (0), Somewhat Similar (1), or Very Similar (2) to the child or adolescent in question. The information necessary to complete this rating scale should be obtained from a variety of sources. No normative, reliability, or validity data have yet been generated with this rating scale, but it is hoped that its presentation will stimulate more detailed work with children and adolescents with elective mutism. In addition, once this instrument is further refined, perhaps parent, teacher, and child versions could be developed so as to preserve the multisetting and multisource components of the assessment. This proposed rating scale can be seen in Table 12.3.

There remains a multitude of assessment issues when working with

TABLE 12.3
Proposed Rating Scale for Elective Mutism

Directions: Please indicate whether these behaviors and characteristics are not similar (0), somewhat similar (1), or very similar (2) to your patient.

Behavior/Characteristic	*Not Similar*	*Somewhat Similar*	*Very Similar*
1. Marital discord in parents	0	1	2
2. Parental psychopathology	0	1	2
3. Sibling or other relative with reluctant or zero speech	0	1	2
4. Speech problems, but can communicate verbally	0	1	2
5. Shy and timid	0	1	2
6. Fears (e.g., strangers)	0	1	2
7. Oppositional	0	1	2
8. Passive-aggressive	0	1	2
9. Manipulative	0	1	2
10. Teased by siblings	0	1	2
11. Temper tantrums at home	0	1	2
12. Has been physically or sexually abused	0	1	2
13. Talks to a few selected friends but not to other children	0	1	2
14. Immature	0	1	2
15. Speech is normal at home, but softens/lessens as approaches school	0	1	2
16. Mother–child enmeshment	0	1	2
17. Learning a new language	0	1	2
18. Does not initiate conversations with children	0	1	2
19. Does not initiate conversations with teachers	0	1	2
20. Does not initiate conversations with parents	0	1	2
21. Does not initiate conversations with adults in social settings	0	1	2
22. Does not make requests (e.g., drink of water; bathroom)	0	1	2
23. Communicates via nonverbal gestures	0	1	2
24. Makes no spontaneous remarks, but may respond to questions with 1 to 3 word responses	0	1	2
25. Onset of mutism was gradual	0	1	2
26. Other psychiatric disorders	0	1	2
27. School performance is poor	0	1	2
28. Separation from parents for 6 months or more prior to age 6 years	0	1	2
29. Negativistic behavior at home	0	1	2
30. Will speak, but in a whisper, mumble, or odd voice	0	1	2
31. Delayed speech development	0	1	2
32. Immigrant family	0	1	2
33. Mutism symptoms present for more than 3 months. How long? ________	0	1	2
34. Nonverbally compliant	0	1	2

(continued)

TABLE 12.3
(Continued)

Behavior/Characteristic	*Not Similar*	*Somewhat Similar*	*Very Similar*
35. Family is socially isolated, with few friends or visitors	0	1	2
36. English is a second language	0	1	2
37. Refuses or reluctance to speak, but child can relate	0	1	2
38. Teased by peers	0	1	2
39. Wets bed	0	1	2
40. Wets self	0	1	2
41. Soils self	0	1	2
42. Close friend or family member was seriously ill or died at the onset of mutism	0	1	2
43. Maladaptive family functioning	0	1	2
44. Other developmental disorder(s)	0	1	2
45. Somatic complaints (e.g., stomach aches, headaches)	0	1	2

these children. In particular, the assessment of related characteristics and features of these children and their families continues to be important. The gathering of these data is important not only from a descriptive perspective, but also in terms of identifying potential treatment interventions. For example, it is important to assess the child's language abilities as comprehensively as possible so as to rule out a primary language disturbance as one of the contributors to this disorder. Nonverbal receptive language measures, such as the Peabody Picture Vocabulary Test-Revised (Dunn & Dunn, 1981), may be helpful in this regard. Similarly, there is an issue with respect to the intellectual and academic functioning of these children, with some investigators suggesting that this label should be used only for children with "normal" cognitive abilities (Hesselman, 1983). The Performance Scale of the Wechsler scales, the Test of Nonverbal Intelligence, and the Kaufman Assessment Battery for Children (Kaufman & Kaufman, 1983) all would be useful in attempting to gain cognitive estimates for these children. In the academic achievement domain, the Peabody Individual Achievement Test-Revised (Markwardt, 1989) provides a nonverbal measure of academic skills.

Finally, given the association of family dysfunction to the diagnosis of elective mutism, it will be important for more thorough assessments of family functioning to be obtained. This could include the Parenting Stress Index (Abidin, 1983) and the McMaster Family Assessment (Miller, Epstein, Bishop, & Keitner, 1985), which attempt to tap selected aspects of family functioning and stress; the Locke–Wallace Marital Adjustment Test (Locke & Wallace, 1959), which was designed to measure marital satisfaction; the O'Leary–Porter Scale (Porter & O'Leary, 1980), which was designed to assess the frequency of overt parental conflict that occurs in front of the child; and other instruments designed to assess parental psychological adjustment, such as the Beck Depression Inventory (Beck, Rush, Shaw, & Emery, 1979) and the Revised Minnesota Multiphasic Personality Inventory (Hathaway & McKinley, 1989).

Summary

The diagnostic assessment of elective mutism has depended largely on clinical observations, generally in one setting, and perhaps a history of the presenting problem. This is amply illustrated in the case study literature. To improve the psychometric underpinnings of this diagnosis, a number of suggestions have been offered with respect to the diagnostic assessment of elective mutism. In particular, it will be important for the assessment strategies to attempt to follow a multisetting, multisource, multi-instrument design in order to encompass all of the primary diagnostic features of this diagnosis. This broad-based assessment model also will serve to describe primary and secondary features of elective mutism more clearly and to improve the reliability and validity of this diagnosis.

Furthermore, the use of selected rating scales directly related to the diagnosis of elective mutism should be employed. Such assessment techniques will contribute to placing children on a continuum of silence and would be consistent with proposed changes in the diagnostic criteria. In this regard, a specific rating scale for elective mutism was proposed based on the literature, although its reliability, validity, and clinical utility remain to be determined. Taken together, this information will not only provide a more firm foundation with respect to the reliability and validity of the diagnosis of elective mutism, but it also will help to differentiate it from other primary psychiatric disorders to a greater degree.

SUMMARY AND CONCLUSIONS

This chapter has presented a review of information related to the diagnosis of elective mutism. Definitional issues were discussed and a detailed description of this diagnostic entity was provided, largely from the case study literature, across a variety of parameters (e.g., etiology, prognosis, response to treatment). In particular, the heterogeneous presentation of children manifesting this disorder was highlighted, with an emphasis placed on the multiple subtypes that might comprise this disorder. The obvious lack of reliability and validity information pertaining to this unique diagnosis was illuminated, although studies have come to the forefront over the past several years that have directly addressed issues of discriminant validity.

Based on this literature, a number of specific suggestions regarding this diagnosis were offered, although it should be stressed that the current DSM-III-R criteria do seem to address many of these suggestions indirectly. Generally, these suggestions call for the diagnosis of elective mutism to remain an independent diagnostic entity at this time. The comparative studies that are available seem to suggest that these children are distinct from children manifesting other forms of psychopathology. Moreover, the literature suggests that the diagnosis should not be treated as an "all or none" type of phenomenon but, rather, conceptualized on a "continuum of silence." This would allow for both the pure definition of elective mutism to be preserved (i.e., zero speech in selected situation) and for other possible variants of this disorder to be reported and studied (i.e., low frequency speech). In addition, the literature reported a preponderance of cases manifesting selected personality characteristics (i.e., anxious-depressed, manipulative-oppositional), and these characteristics should be considered in the multidimensionality of this disorder as well, particularly with respect to treatment.

Assessment strategies for diagnosing this disorder also were discussed although, at present, there are no guidelines for the assessment of children suspected of being electively mute. The multisetting, multisource, multi-instrument model was offered in an effort to encourage clinicians and researchers to expand their assessment of these children, and to increase diagnostic reliability via use of the aggregate principle. A variety of specific assessment techniques were discussed to operationalize this model, with a particular emphasis on rating scale technology.

Reports of elective mutism have existed for well over 100 years but, given its general rarity, it is no accident that it has not been studied more intensively. Consequently, critical questions remain with respect to this diagnostic entity, and it will be important for these concerns to be addressed so as to evolve the clinical utility of this diagnosis further. It is hoped that the issues and suggestions presented in this chapter have begun to address these concerns, and that they set the stage for future work with this disorder.

REFERENCES

Abidin, R. (1983). *Parenting Stress Index.* Charlottesville, VA: Pediatric Psychology Press.

Achenbach, T. M., & Edelbrock, C. (1983). *Manual for the Child Behavior Checklist and Revised Child Behavior Profile.* Burlington, VT: University of Vermont, Department of Psychiatry.

Adams, M. H., & Glasner, P. J. (1954). Emotional involvements in some forms of mutism. *Journal of Speech and Hearing Disorders, 19,* 59–69.

American Psychiatric Association. (1952). *Diagnostic and statistical manual of mental disorders.* Washington, DC: Author.

American Psychiatric Association. (1968). *Diagnostic and statistical manual of mental disorders* (2nd ed.). Washington, DC: Author.

American Psychiatric Association. (1980). *Diagnostic and statistical manual of mental disorders* (3rd ed.). Washington, DC: Author.

American Psychiatric Association. (1987). *Diagnostic and statistical manual of mental disorders* (3rd ed., rev.). Washington, DC: Author.

Amman, H. (1958). Schweigende kinder [silent children]. *Heilpaedagogische Werkblaetter, 27,* 209–216.

Barlow, K., Strother, J. A., & Landreth, G. (1986). Sibling group play therapy: An effective alternative with an elective mute child. *School Counselor, 34,* 44–50.

Beck, J. R., & Hubbard, M. G. (1987). Elective Mutism in a missionary family: A case study. *Journal of Psychology and Theology, 15,* 291–299.

Beck, A. T., Rush, A. J., Shaw, B. F., & Emery, G. (1979). *Cognitive therapy for depression.* New York: Guilford Press.

Birleson, P. (1981). Validity of depressive disorder in childhood and the development of a self-rating scale: A research report. *Journal of Child Psychology, Psychiatry and Allied Disciplines, 22,* 73–88.

Blake, P., & Moss, T. (1967). The development of socialization skills in an electively mute child. *Behavior Research and Therapy, 5,* 349–356.

Bozigar, J. A., & Hansen, R. A. (1984). Group treatment for elective mute children. *Social Work, 29,* 478–480.

Bradley, S., & Sloman, L. (1975). Elective mutism in immigrant families. *Journal of American Academy of Child Psychiatry, 7,* 510–514.

Brown, B. J., Fuller, J., & Gericke, C. (1975). Elective mutism: A review and a report of an unsuccessfully treated case. *Journal of the Association of Workers for Maladjusted Children, 3,* 27–37.

Brown, B. J., & Lloyd, H. A. (1975). Controlled study of children not speaking at school. *Journal of the Association of Workers for Maladjusted Children, 3,* 49–63.

Browne, E., Wilson, V., & Laybourne, P. C. (1963). Diagnosis and treatment of elective mutism in children. *Journal of the American Academy of Child Psychiatry, 2,* 605–617.

Carr, A., & Afnan, S. (1989). Concurrent individual and family therapy in a case of elective mutism. *Journal of Family Therapy, 11,* 29–44.

Commission on Professional and Hospital Activities. (1978). *International classification of diseases-(9th rev.)-Clinical modification.* Ann Arbor, MI: Author.

Costello, A. J., Edelbrock, C., Kalas, R., Dulcan, M. K., & Klaric, S. J. (1984). *Development and testing of the NIMH Diagnostic Interview Schedule for Children in a clinical population. Final report to the Center for Epidemiologic Studies.* Rockville, MD: National Institute for Mental Health.

Croghan, L. M., & Craven, R. (1982). Elective mutism. Learning from the analysis of a successful case history. *Journal of Pediatric Psychology, 7,* 85–93.

Cunningham, C. E., Cataldo, M. F., Mallion, C., & Keyes, J. B. (1983). A review and controlled single case evaluation of behavioral approaches to the management of elective mutism. *Child and Family Behavior Therapy, 5,* 25–49.

Dunn, L. M., & Dunn, L. M. (1981). *Peabody Picture Vocabulary Test-Revised.* Circle Pines, MN: American Guidance Service.

Eaton, W. O. (1983). Measuring activity level with actometers: Reliability, validity, and arm length. *Child Development, 54,* 720–726.

Epstein, S. (1980). The stability of behavior: II. Implications for psychological research. *American Psychologist, 35,* 790–806.

Edelstein, B. A., & Berler, E. S. (1987). Interviewing and report writing. In C. L. Frame & J. L. Matson (Eds.), *Handbook of assessment in childhood psychopathology, Applied issues in differential diagnosis and treatment evaluation* (pp. 163–184). New York: Plenum.

Eldar, S., Bleich, A., Apter, A., & Tyano, S. (1985). Elective mutism: An atypical antecedent of schizophrenia. *Journal of Adolescence, 8,* 289–292.

Elson, A., Pearson, G., Jones, C. D., & Schumacher, E. (1965). Follow-up study of childhood elective mutism. *Archives of General Psychiatry, 13,* 182–187.

Friedman, R., & Karagan, N. (1973). Characteristics and management of elective mutism in children. *Psychiatry in the Schools, 10,* 249–252.

Fundudis, T., Kolvin, I., & Garside, R. (1979). *Speech retarded and deaf children. Their psychological development.* London: Academic Press.

Goll, K. (1979). Role structure and subculture in families of elective mutists. *Family Process, 18,* 55–68.

Gutzman, H. (1912). *Vorlesungen ueber sprachheilkunde* [Lectures on speech medicine]. Berlin: Fischer.

Halpern, W. I., Hammond, J., & Cohen, R. A. (1971). Therapeutic approach to speech phobia: Elective mutism reexamined. *Journal of American Academy of Child Psychiatry, 10,* 94–107.

Harter, S. (1982). The Perceived Competency Scale for Children. *Child Development, 53,* 87–97.

Hathaway, S. R., & McKinley, J. C. (1989). *Minnesota Multiphasic Personality Inventory-2.* Minneapolis, MN: National Computer Systems.

Hayden, T. L. (1980). The classification of elective mutism. *Journal of the American Academy of Child Psychiatry, 19,* 118–133.

Heimlich, E. P. (1981). Patient as assistant therapist in paraverbal therapy with children. *American Journal of Psychotherapy, 35,* 262–267.

Heinze, H. (1932). Freiwillig schweigende kinder [Voluntarily silent children]. *Z. Kinderforsch, 40,* 235–256.

Hesse, P. P. (1981). Colour, form, and silence (A formal analysis of drawings of a child who did not speak). *Arts in Psychotherapy, 8,* 175–184.

Hesselman, S. (1983). Elective mutism in children 1877–1981: A literary summary. *Acta-Paedo-Psychiatricia, 49,* 297–310.

Hill, L., & Scull, J. (1985). Elective mutism associated with selective inactivity. *Journal of Communication Disorders, 18,* 161–167.

Hoffman, S., & Laub, B. (1986). Paradoxical intervention using a polarization model of co-therapy in the treatment of elective mutism: A case study. *Contemporary Family Therapy: An International Journal, 8,* 136–143.

Kaplan, S. I., & Escoll, P. (1973). Treatment of two silent adolescent girls. *Journal of American Academy of Child Psychiatry, 12,* 59–72.

Kass, W., Gillman, A. E., Mattis, S., Klugman, E., & Jacobson, B. J. (1967). Treatment of selective mutism in a blind child: School and clinic collaboration. *American Journal of Orthopsychiatry, 37,* 215–216.

Kaufman, A. S., & Kaufman, N. L. (1983). *Kaufman Assessment Battery for Children (K-ABC) administration and scoring manual.* Circle Pines, MN: American Guidance Service.

Kehrer, H. E., & Tinkl-Damhorst, N. (1974). Verhaltenstherapic bei elektivem mutismus [Behavioral therapy with elective mutism]. *Acta paedo-psychiatry, 41,* 34–44.

Kolvin, I., & Fundudis, T. (1981). Elective mute children: Psychological development and background factors. *Journal of Child Psychology and Psychiatry, 22,* 2219–232.

Kovacs, M., & Beck, A. (1977). An empirical-clinical approach toward a definition of childhood depression. In J. Schulterbrandt & A. Raskin (Eds.), *Depression in childhood: Diagnosis, treatment, and conceptual methods* (pp. 1–26). New York: Raven Press.

Kratochwill, T. R. (1981). *Selective mutism: Implications for research and treatment.* Hillsdale, NJ: Lawrence Erlbaum Associates.

Kratochwill, T. R., Brody, G. G., & Piersel, W. C. (1979). Elective mutism in children. In B. B. Lahey & A. E. Kazdin (Eds.), *Advances in clinical child psychology* (Vol. 2, pp. 193–233). New York: Plenum.

Kupietz, S. S., & Schwartz, I. L. (1982). Elective mutism: Evaluation and behavioral treatment of three cases. *New York State Journal of Medicine, 7,* 1073–1076.

Kussmaul, A. (1877). *Die Storungen der Sprache* [Language disorders] (Band 12. Anhang, in: Handbuch d. spec. Pathol. Ther.). Lipzig: F. C. W. Vogel.

Labbe, E. E., & Williamson, D. A. (1984). Behavioral treatment of elective mutism: A review of the literature. *Clinical Psychology Review, 4,* 273–293.

Lachenmeyer, J. R., & Gibbs, M. S. (1985). The social-psychological functions of reward in the treatment of a case of elective mutism. *Journal of Social and Clinical Psychology, 3,* 466–473.

Laybourne, P. C. (1979). Elective mutism. In J. D. Noshpitz (Ed.), *Basic handbook of child psychiatry* (Vol. 2, pp. 475–481). New York: Basic Books.

Lazarus, P. J., Gavilo, H. M., & Moore, J. W. (1983). The treatment of EM in children within the school setting. Two case studies. *School Psychology Review, 12,* 467–472.

Lerea, L., & Ward, B. (1965). Speech avoidance among children with oral-communication defects. *Journal of Psychology, 60,* 265–270.

Lesser-Katz, M. (1986). Stranger reaction and elective mutism in young children. *American Journal of Orthopsychiatry, 56,* 458–469.

Lesser-Katz, M. (1988). The treatment of elective mutism as stranger reaction. *Psychotherapy, 25,* 305–313.

Lipton, H. (1980). Rapid reinstatement of speech using stimulus fading with a selectively mute child. *Journal of Behavior Therapy and Experimental Psychiatry, 11,* 147–149.

Locke, H. J., & Wallace, K. M. (1959). Short marital adjustment and prediction tests: Their reliability and validity. *Marriage and Family Living, 21,* 251–255.

Looff, D. H. (1971). *Appalachia's children: The challenge of mental health.* Lexington, Kentucky: University Press of Kentucky.

Louden, D. M. (1987). Elective mutism: A case study of a disorder of childhood. *Journal of the National Medical Association, 79,* 1043–1048.

Lowenstein, L. F. (1979). The result of 21 elective mute cases. *Acta Paedopsychiatrica, 45,* 17–23.

Markwardt, F. C., Jr. (1989). *Peabody Individual Achievement Test-Revised.* Circle Pines, MN: American Guidance Service.

Martin, R. P., Hooper, S., & Snow, J. (1986). Behavior rating scale approaches to personality assessment in children and adolescents. In H. M. Knoff (Ed.), *The psychological assessment of children and adolescents* (pp. 309–351). New York: Guilford Press.

McMahon, R. J. (1984). Behavioral checklists and rating forms. In T. H. Ollendick & M. Hersen (Eds.), *Child behavioral assessment: Principles and procedures* (pp. 80–105). New York: Pergamon Press.

Meijer, A. (1979). Elective mutism in children. *Israeli Annals of Psychiatry and Related Disciplines, 17,* 93–100.

Meyers, S. V. (1984). Elective mutism in children: A family systems approach. *American Journal of Family Therapy, 12,* 39–45.

Miller, I., Epstein, N., Bishop, D., & Keitner, G. (1985). The McMaster family assessment device: Reliability and validity. *Journal of Marital and Family Therapy, 11,* 345–356.

Miller, L. C. (1981). *Louisville Behavior Checklist Manual-Revised.* Los Angeles: Western Psychological Services.

Miller, L. C., Barrett, C. L., Hampe, E., & Noble, H. (1972). Revised anxiety scales for the Louisville Behavior Checklist. *Psychological Reports, 29,* 503–511.

Mora, G., De Vault, S., & Schopler, E. (1962). Dynamics and psychotherapy of identical twins with elective mutism. *Journal of Child Psychology and Psychiatry, 3,* 41–52.

Morin, C., Ladouceur, R., & Cloutier, R. (1982). Reinforcement procedure in the treatment of reluctant speech. *Journal of Behavior Therapy and Experimental Psychiatry, 13,* 145–147.

Morris, J. V. (1953). Cases of elective mutism. *American Journal of Mental Deficiency, 57,* 661–668.

Nash, R. T., Thorpe, H. W., Andrews, M. M., & Davis, K. (1979). A management program for elective mutism. *Psychology in the Schools, 16,* 246–256.

Nadoleczny, M. (1926). *Die sprachstöerungen im Kindesalter* [Language disturbances in childhood]. Leipzig: Vogel.

Paniagua, F. A., & Saeed, M. A. (1988). A procedural distinction between elective and progressive mutism. *Journal of Behavioral Therapy and Experimental Psychiatry, 19,* 207–210.

Parker, E. B., Olsen, T. F., & Throckmorton, M. C. (1960). Social case work with elementary school children who do not talk in school. *Social Work, 5,* 64–70.

Piersel, W. C., & Kratochwill, T. R. (1981). A teacher implemented contingency management package to assess and treat selective mutism. *Behavioral Assessment, 3,* 371–382.

Pigott, H. E., & Gonzales, F. P. (1987). Efficacy of videotape self-modeling in treating an electively mute child. *Journal of Clinical Child Psychology, 16,* 106–110.

Porter, B., & O'Leary, K. D. (1980). Marital discord and childhood behavior problems. *Journal of Abnormal Child Psychology, 8,* 287–295.

Pustrom, E., & Spears, R. W. (1964). Elective mutism in children. *Journal of the American Academy of Child Psychiatry, 3,* 287–297.

Quay, H. C., & Peterson, D. R. (1987). *Manual for the Revised Behavior Problem Checklist.* Coral Gables, FL: Authors.

Quay, H. C., & Werry, J. S. (Eds.). (1986). *Psychological disorders of childhood* (3rd ed.). New York: Wiley.

Reed, G. F. (1963). A re-appraisal. *Journal of Child Psychology and Psychiatry and Allied Disciplines, 4,* 99–107.

Reynolds, C. R., & Richmond, B. O. (1985). *Revised Children's Manifest Anxiety Scale (RCMAS).* Los Angeles, CA: Western Psychological Services.

Rosenberg, J. B., & Lindblad, M. B. (1978). Behavior therapy in family context: Treating elective mutism. *Family Process, 17,* 77–82.

Rothe, C. (1928). Sprachscheue kinder [Speech-shy children]. *Zeitschrift fur Ohrenheilkunde, 62,* 904–909.

Rutter, M. (1977). Speech delay. In M. Rutter & L. Hersov (Eds.), *Child psychiatry: Modern approaches* (pp. 698–716). Oxford: Blackwell Scientific Publications.

Salfield, D. J. (1950). Observations on elective mutism children. *Journal of Mental Science, 96,* 1024–1032.

Scott, E. A. (1977). A desensitization program for the treatment of mutism in a 7 year-old girl: A case report. *Journal of Child Psychiatry, 18,* 263–270.

Shaw, W. H. (1971). Aversive control in the treatment of elective mutism. *Journal of American Academy of Child Psychiatry, 10,* 572–581.

Sluckin, A. (1977). Children who do not talk at school. *Child Care, Health and Development, 3,* 69–79.

Sluzki, C. E. (1983). The sounds of silence: Two cases of elective mutism in bilingual families. *Family Therapy Collections, 6,* 68–77.

Sokoloff, R., & Lubin, B. (1983). Depressive mood in adolescent, emotionally disturbed females: Reliability and validity of an adjective checklist (C-DACL). *Journal of Abnormal Child Psychology, 11,* 531–536.

Spielberger, C. D. (1983). *Manual for the State-Trait Anxiety Inventory.* Palo Alto, CA: Consulting Psychologists Press.

Spielberger, C. D. (1988). *State-Trait Anger Expression Inventory (STAI).* Odessa, FL: Psychological Assessment Resources, Inc.

Spieler, J. (1944). *Schweigende und sprachscheue kinder* [Silent and speech-shy children]. Olten: Verlag Otto Walter.

Subak, M. E., West, M., & Carlin, M. (1982). Elective Mutism: An expression of family psychopathology. *International Journal of Family Psychiatry, 3,* 335–344.

Tramer, M. (1934). Elective mutismus bei kindern [Elective mutism in children]. *Z. Kinderpsychiat, 1,* 30–35.

Trüper, J. (1897). Ein knabe mit sprechhemmungen auf psycho-pathischer grundlage [A boy with speech inhibitions based on psychopathy]. *Zeitschrift fur Kinderfehler, 5,* 138–143.

Von Mish, A. (1952). Elekitiver mutsimus in kindesalter [Elective mutism in childhood]. *Zsitachriftfuer Kinderpsychiatrie, 19,* 49–87.

Waterink, J., & Vedder, R. (1936). Quelques cas de mutisme thymogenique chez des enfants tres jeunes et leur traitement [Several cases of thymogenic mutism in very young children and their treatment]. *Z. Kinderpsychiatrica, 3,* 101–112.

Weber, A. (1950). Zum eclektiven mutismus der kinder [An elective mutism in childhood]. *Z. Kinderpsychiatrica, 17,* 1–15.

Wergeland, H. (1979). Elective mutism. *Acta psychiatrica Scandinavia, 59,* 218–228.

Wilkins, R. (1985). A comparison of elective mutism and emotional disorders in children. *British Journal of Psychiatry, 1,* 198–203.

Williamson, D. A., Sanders, S. H., Sewell, W. R., Haney, J. N., & White, D. (1977). The behavioral treatment of elective mutism: Two case studies. *Journal of Behavior Therapy and Experimental Psychiatry, 8,* 143–149.

Wirt, R., Lachar, D., Klinedinst, J., & Seat, P. (1977). *Multidimensional description of child personality: A manual for the Personality Inventory for Children.* Los Angeles: Western Psychological Services.

Wolf, S., & Barlow, A. (1979). Schizoid personality in childhood. *Journal of Child Psychology and Psychiatry, 20,* 29–46.

World Health Organization. (1965). *International classification of diseases* (8th ed.). Geneva: Author.

World Health Organization. (1978). *International classification of diseases* (9th ed.). Geneva: Author.

Wright, H. H., Miller, M. D., Cook, M. A., & Littmann, J. R. (1985). Early identification and intervention with children who refuse to speak. *Journal of the American Academy of Child Psychiatry, 24*, 739–746.

Wright, H. L. (1968). A clinical study of children who refuse to talk in school. *Journal of the American Academy of Child Psychiatry, 7*, 603–617.

Epilogue: Child Psychopathology

Stephen R. Hooper
University of North Carolina School of Medicine

The chapters in this volume have covered the major psychiatric disorders that typically appear during childhood and adolescence as identified in the DSM-III-R. When the modern history of childhood psychiatric diagnosis and classification is traced (Mattison & Hooper, chapter 1), it is clear that there has been enormous growth over the past 20 to 30 years. This is amply illustrated by the fact that in 1952 the DSM-I did not contain any psychiatric disorders that were specific to the child and adolescent populations, and a text such as the present one may not even have been conceivable at that time. Currently, it is clear from the chapters contained within this volume that there is great enthusiasm and interest in childhood and adolescent psychiatric disorders and, from this, greater clarity and refinement of their classification will continue to evolve.

As mentioned at the beginning of this volume, with this increased interest in child and adolescent psychiatric disorders comes the potential for confusion among practicing clinicians and researchers. To recapitulate, this confusion is created by issues related to (a) how to diagnose psychopathology, (b) what correspondence exists between currently employed criteria and research findings with children and adolescents, (c) how the criteria were developed, and (d) what particular assessment strategies or models would be most useful in arriving at a specific diagnosis. The current volume and its companion (*Developmental Disorders*) were designed to address these diagnostic and classification issues of childhood and adolescent psychiatric disorders. The major goal for each chapter in this volume was to provide diagnostic and assessment guidelines for the clinician and researcher that were based on the scientific literature for specific psychiatric disorders. As such, it is hoped that the data-based nature of many of these chapters has provided further guidance for the continued evolution of psychiatric classification for children and adolescents (i.e., DSM-IV). Although a wealth of information was provided by the contributors for each of the psychiatric disorders discussed, there were a variety of general themes that emerged across the chapters, and these deserve mention.

First, the current DSM system (i.e., DSM-III-R) and other types of psychiatric nosologies are dynamic in nature, and this feature is a testament to the ongoing evolution of our understanding of childhood and adolescent disorders. It is quite appropriate that the developers of the DSM-III and DSM-III-R viewed these versions as "only one still frame in the ongoing process of attempting to better understand mental disorders" (American Psychiatric Association, 1980, p. 12). Each of the chapters in this volume traces the historical evolution and progression of a respective psychiatric disorder, with each disorder having its own unique developmental history. For example, at one point in time autism was viewed as intimately related to schizophrenia. However, more recent work has viewed these disorders as separate and distinct, with current efforts suggesting that there may be a closer alignment between schizoid personality disorder and childhood schizophrenia (Russell, chapter 2). Some diagnostic entities have had a long-standing history, such as attention deficit-hyperactivity disorder, and have continued to undergo change and be the subject of much debate (Guevremont & Barkley, chapter 5). Others, such as gender identity disorder of childhood (Zucker, chapter 9), tic disorders (Towbin, Riddle, Leckman, & Cohen, chapter 10), elimination disorders (MacLean & Brayden, chapter 11), and elective mutism (Hooper & Linz, chapter 12), have only recently been included formally in childhood psychiatric nosologies.

Furthermore, given the evolution of our understanding of selected diagnoses of childhood and adolescence, there has been some debate as to whether they should remain within a psychiatric nosology. This applies especially to tic disorders and elimination disorders. Specifically, Towbin, Riddle, Leckman, and Cohen have made a convincing argument for keeping tic disorders within a psychiatric classification system, despite mounting evidence that they are neurologically based, noting that one deciding factor should be where individuals seek treatment (i.e., individuals with tic disorders traditionally have sought treatment in mental health settings). A similar argument could be made for other disorders as well (e.g., should ADHD be considered a psychiatric disorder or a developmental disorder?).

MacLean and Brayden noted a parallel set of circumstances for the elimination disorders; however, these investigators provided creative solutions to this dilemma based on the available scientific literature and sound clinical rationale. Specifically, MacLean and Brayden suggested that *primary* manifestations of these disorders should be considered developmental disorders and, consequently, coded on Axis II. When these behaviors are manifested as *secondary* symptoms, then they should be considered more psychiatric in nature because the normal developmental progression has been disrupted. This conceptualization represents a significant departure from the category Special Symptoms Not Elsewhere Classified, which is where these disorders were relegated in DSM-II.

Second, this dynamic, everchanging nature of psychiatric classification systems has contributed to further refinement in how child and adolescent disorders are defined. Although there is little argument that the DSM system could benefit from greater clarity of the definitions for many of the disorders, the DSM-III and DSM-III-R ushered in a new era in terms of how psychiatric disorders should be defined. The DSM system has attempted to be more descriptive, with specific criteria being presented for each disorder and a multiaxial system for conceptualizing diagnoses. This has led investigators to direct more attention to specific operational criteria for respective diagnoses.

In this volume, suggestions for improvement are offered for most diagnoses. The criteria associated with conduct disorders (Routh & Daugherty, chapter 4) and anxiety disorders (Mattison, chapter 6) are the only ones that remain unchanged, although for different reasons. For conduct disorders, the investigators noted that the field seemed to be in general consensus about the criteria, whereas for anxiety disorders no changes were proposed given the relative lack of literature available for children and adolescents at this time. Mattison did note, however, that these data are undoubtedly on the horizon, and recent work with children on panic disorder (Black & Robbins, 1990; Vitiello, Behar, Wolfson, & McLeer, 1990), obsessive-compulsive disorder (Riddle et al., 1990), and overanxious disorder (Bowen, Offord, & Boyle, 1990) supports that notion.

Most of the contributors made modest suggestions in the diagnostic criteria, such as in schizophrenia (Russell), major depressive disorder (Newman & Garfinkel, chapter 3), tic disorders (Towbin, Riddle, Leckman, & Cohen, chapter 10), attention deficit-hyperactivity disorder (Guevremont & Barkley), and anorexia/bulimia (Garner, Shafer, & Rosen, chapter 8), whereas others asserted more radical changes in the development of specific diagnostic criteria. For example, major changes were asserted for the criteria for eating disorders of infancy and early childhood (Mayes, chapter 7), in what may be one of the more extensive reviews available on this topic, and for elimination disorders (MacLean & Brayden). Major changes also were suggested for elective mutism (Hooper & Linz), although these changes are based largely on case study methodology and will require further substantiation. In addition, many of the chapters highlight the importance of a developmental perspective in childhood psychopathology (e.g., Guevremont & Barkley; MacLean & Brayden), the need for well-defined behavioral criteria (e.g., Guevremont & Barkley; Zucker), and issues of severity (Garner, Shafer, & Rosen).

Third, given refinement in the diagnostic criteria, there has been an increased appreciation of the complexities involved in childhood and adolescent psychiatric disorders. Nearly all of the chapters directly or indirectly address the heterogeneity of specific psychiatric disorders. This is illustrated by discussions on the diagnostic components of specific disorders (e.g., Guevremont & Barkley; Hooper & Linz; Zucker) as well as more specific subtypes of a given disorder (e.g., Hooper & Linz; MacLean & Brayden; Towbin, Riddle, Leckman, & Cohen). Specific subtypes also are suggested for particular diagnostic entities that were based on age parameters, such as eating disorders (Garner, Shafer, & Rosen; Mayes). This multidimensional conceptualization also contributed to numerous discussions of etiology, with many of the discussions incorporating a biological perspective (Mattison; Newman & Garfinkel). Regardless of one's perspective, the literature presented in these chapters strongly implicates the heterogeneity within, as well as between, the disorders of childhood and adolescence.

The increased refinement in diagnostic criteria also has increased the number of questions surrounding comorbidity. Although the DSM and ICD systems approach the issue of comorbidity from different vantage points (Rutter & Gould, 1985), with the DSM system being the more liberal of the two, it is clear that this issue pervades childhood psychopathology and subsequent research-related endeavors (e.g., is any given subject depressed, anxious, or both?). One reason for this is the dependence of both classification systems on categorical data. Although most of the chapters do not directly challenge the categorical nature of the DSM system, the possibility of conceptualizing psychiatric disorders on a continuous or dimensional basis as opposed to a categorical basis is raised, with support being offered for a continuous conceptualization of conduct disorders (Routh & Daugherty). Nearly all of the chapters address the issue of comorbidity, with noteworthy discussions occurring for schizophrenia (Russell), major depressive disorder (Newman & Garfinkel), attention deficit-hyperactivity disorder (Guevremont & Barkley), tic disorders (Towbin, Riddle, Leckman, & Cohen), and anxiety disorders (Mattison). It is hoped that the refinement noted in many of the diagnostic criteria contained within these chapters will contribute to the clarification of some of the issues related to comorbidity for selected diagnoses. Relatedly, few if any of the chapters address issues of resiliency (e.g., why are some children more resilient to psychiatric disorders than others?). Along with comorbidity concerns, issues of psychiatric vulnerability and resiliency undoubtedly will become the focus of future clinical and research energies (e.g., Fergusson, Horwood, & Lawton, 1990).

Fourth, in contrast to the assessment of developmental disorders, the assessment of childhood and adolescent psychiatric disorders has lagged behind the development of their classification. In general, the evolution of diagnostic criteria and differential diagnosis for selected disorders has forged ahead without the benefit of standardized assessment tools. Typically, the most frequently employed procedure has been the traditional clinical interview. More recently, however, there has been an increased interest and utilization of standardized techniques and tools. Specifically, nearly all of the chapters discuss the use of semistructured or structured diagnostic interviews. These interviews tend to be general in their application (e.g., K-SADS), but more specific structured interviews have been developed for specific populations, such as gender identity disorders (Zucker) and eating disorders (Garner, Shafer, & Rosen).

Rating scales also have begun to be used regularly in clinical and research endeavors. As with the structured and semistructured interviews, rating scales have been developed for general (e.g., CBCL) as well as more specific (e.g., depression, attention deficits, tics) concerns. In fact, some investigators have called for their use to be mandatory for selected disorders, such as attention deficit-hyperactivity disorder (e.g., Guevremont & Barkley). Recent work also has shown their utility in determining internal consistency estimates for a variety of child diagnoses in the DSM-III (Hodges, Saunders, Kashani, Hamlett, & Thompson, 1990).

The assessment of child and adolescent psychopathology also has progressed as a result of the introduction of a variety of assessment methodologies. In the search for the "gold standard" assessment model, a variety of clinical and actuarial models have been described (Routh & Daugherty). In addition, the multisetting, multisource, multi-instrument assessment model described by Hooper and Linz for elective mutism should also be applicable to a variety of other disorders. It is noteworthy that none of the chapters advocate for a single test approach (i.e., one test, one unstandardized clinical interview) in the assessment and diagnosis of childhood psychopathology. It is also noteworthy that assessment strategies have moved from projective to objective techniques. Although this should not be interpreted as the death knell for projective testing, it does highlight the need for more reliable, valid, and data-based assessment of child psychological functioning.

Although relatively recent, the use of more standardized and objective assessment methods and models will contribute to increased estimates of reliability and validity for individual diagnoses. Some information exists for selected diagnoses, such as anxiety disorders (Mattison), but it is woefully lacking for others. In fact, for some of the diagnoses this information is nonexistent (e.g., elective mutism). The data provided by the field studies on selected diagnoses for DSM-III (APA, 1980) and the large-scale studies of the ICD-9 (Gould, Shaffer, Rutter, & Sturge, 1988; Remschmidt, 1988) provided a significant beginning, but it is clear that more extensive studies concerning the reliability and validity of diagnoses for children and adolescents are needed. In this regard, Rutter and Tuma (1988) noted that there are far too many diagnostic categories than can be justified by the available reliability and validity information, and perhaps this should be heeded in future research endeavors and psychiatric classification efforts. Generally, very few of the diagnostic categories can demonstrate utility with respect to etiology, prognosis, or response to treatment.

There remain a plethora of issues that confront clinicians and researchers in the field of child psychopathology, although it is fair to say that much progress has been registered to date. It is hoped that this volume has contributed to clarifying some issues and raising others. It also is hoped that the chapters contained in this volume have contributed, in some fashion, to the ongoing evolution and refinement of an accurate and clinically useful psychiatric classification system for children and adolescents. Given the amount of information presented in each of these chapters, there is no doubt that the future for the diagnosis and assessment of childhood and adolescent psychiatric disorders will continue to show dynamic changes with respect to our understanding of developmental psychopathology and its appraisal.

REFERENCES

American Psychiatric Association. (1952). *Diagnostic and statistical manual of mental disorders*. Washington, DC: Author.

American Psychiatric Association. (1980). *Diagnostic and statistical manual of mental disorders* (3rd ed.). Washington, DC: Author.

Black, B., & Robbins, D. R. (1990). Case study: Panic disorder in children and adolescents. *Journal of the American Academy of Child and Adolescent Psychiatry, 29,* 36–44.

Bowen, R. C., Offord, D. R., & Boyle, M. H. (1990). The prevalence of overanxious disorder and separation anxiety: Results from the Ontario Child Health Study. *Journal of the American Academy of Child and Adolescent Psychiatry, 29,* 753–758.

Fergusson, D. M., Horwood, L. J., & Lawton, J. M. (1990). Vulnerability to childhood problems and family social background. *Journal of Child Psychology, Psychiatry, and Allied Disciplines, 31,* 1145–1160.

Gould, M. S., Shaffer, D., Rutter, M., & Sturge, C. (1988). UK/WHO Study of ICD-9. In M. Rutter, A. H. Tuma, & I. S. Lann (Eds.), *Assessment and diagnosis in child psychopathology* (pp. 37–65). New York: Guilford Press.

Hodges, K., Saunders, W. B., Kashani, J., Hamlett, K., & Thompson, R. J. (1990). Internal consistency of DSM-III diagnoses using the Symptom Scales of the Child Assessment Schedule. *Journal of the American Academy of Child and Adolescent Psychiatry, 29,* 635–641.

Remschmidt, H. (1988). German Study of ICD-9. In M. Rutter, A. H. Tuma, & I. S. Lann (Eds.), *Assessment and diagnosis in child psychopathology* (pp. 66–83). New York: Guilford Press.

Riddle, M. A., Scahill, L., King, R., Hardin, M. T., Towbin, K. E., Ort, S. I., Leckman, J. F., & Cohen, D. J. (1990). Obsessive compulsive disorder in children and adolescents: Phenomenology and family history. *Journal of the American Academy of Child and Adolescent Psychiatry, 29,* 766–772.

Rutter, M., & Gould, M. (1985). Classification. In M. Rutter & L. Hersov (Eds.), *Child and adolescent psychiatry: Modern approaches* (2nd ed., pp. 304–321). Oxford: Blackwell.

Rutter, M., & Tuma, A. H. (1988). Diagnostic classification: Some outstanding issues. In M. Rutter, A. H. Tuma, & I. S. Lann (Eds.), *Assessment and diagnosis in child psychopathology* (pp. 437–452). New York: Guilford Press.

Vitiello, B., Behar, D., Wolfson, S., & McLeer, S. V. (1990). Case study: Diagnosis of panic disorder in prepubertal children. *Journal of the American Academy of Child and Adolescent Psychiatry, 29,* 782–788.

Author Index

D

E

I

L

M

S

Y

Z

Subject Index